The Biology of Musical Performance and Performance-Related Injury

Alan H. D. Watson

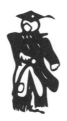

THE SCARECROW PRESS, INC.
Lanham, Maryland • Toronto • Plymouth, UK
2009

SCARECROW PRESS, INC.

Published in the United States of America
by Scarecrow Press, Inc.
A wholly owned subsidary of
The Rowman & Littlefield Publishing Group, Inc.
4501 Forbes Boulevard, Suite 200, Lanham, Maryland 20706
www.scarecrowpress.com

Estover Road
Plymouth PL6 7PY
United Kingdom

British Library Cataloguing in Publication Information Available

Library of Congress Cataloging-in-Publication Data

Watson, Alan H. D., 1953–
    The biology of musical performance and performance-related injury / Alan H. D. Watson.
        p. cm.
    Includes bibliographical references and index.
    ISBN-13: 978-0-8108-6358-3 (cloth : alk. paper)
    ISBN-10: 0-8108-6358-8 (cloth : alk. paper)
    ISBN-13: 978-0-8108-6359-0 (pbk. : alk. paper)
    ISBN-10: 0-8108-6359-6 (pbk. : alk. paper)
    [etc.]
    1. Music—Performance—Physiological aspects. 2. Music—Performance—Psychological
aspects. I. Title.
ML3820.W27 2009
612.002'478—dc22   2008034025

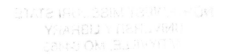

To Doris Watson, who taught me what it means
to communicate through music.

Contents

CD Contents: Teaching Materials   vii

Preface   xi

Acknowledgments   xvii

Reference Abbreviations   xix

1 Introduction to the Tissues of the Body   1

2 Posture and the Back in Musical Performance   17

3 The Shoulder, Arm, and Hand: Structure and Problems   42

4 Breathing in Singing and Wind Playing   101

5 The Voice: Management and Problems   139

6 The Embouchure and Wind Playing   193

7 The Structure and Organization of the Brain   213

8 How the Performance of Music Affects the Brain   232

9 Hearing and the Processing of Musical Sound by the Brain   276

10 Performance-Related Stress and Its Management   332

Index   353

About the Author   369

CD Contents

Teaching Materials

FIGURES

Copies of color versions of all of the figures in jpeg format.

VIDEO FILES

Video files are in Windows Media file (.wmv) format, which can be played on Windows Media Player. Apple users can play them on QuickTime by downloading Flip4Mac Windows Media Components freeware from the QuickTime download center. This program or Windows Media Player for Mac can also be obtained from the Microsoft Windows download center.

video 3-1 Tendon Linkages.wmv: "Tendon linkages in the hand" (a demonstration of Lindburg-Comstock syndrome)

video 4-1 plethysmograph sing.wmv: "Recording chest and abdominal movements during singing" (demonstrates the use of inductive plethysmography to record respiratory movements in singers)

video 4-2 plethysmograph wind.wmv: "Recording chest and abdominal movements during wind playing" (demonstrates the use of inductive plethysmography to record respiratory movements in wind players)

video 4-3 Konno Mead sing.wmv: "Using Konno-Mead diagrams to understand breathing movements during singing"

video 4-3 Konno Mead wind.wmv: "Using Konno-Mead diagrams to understand breathing movements during wind playing"

video 5-1 normal larynx.wmv: "Movements of the vocal folds" (as seen using stroboscopic video laryngoscopy). Images and video clips from the Voice Clinic of the University of Iowa Department of Otolaryngology–Head and Neck Surgery, Iowa City; used with permission.

video 5-2 singers formant.wmv: "Voice projection; the singers' formant" (demonstration of the enhancement of vocal projection through formant manipulation, in the mezzo-soprano voice)

video 5-3 edema nodules.wmv: "Problems with the vocal folds; Reinke's edema and vocal nodules." Images and video clips from the Voice Clinic of the University of Iowa Department of Otolaryngology–Head and Neck Surgery, Iowa City, and Clark Rosen, M.D., University of Pittsburgh Voice Center; used with permission.

ANIMATIONS (POWERPOINT)

animation 2-1 stand-sit.ppt: "Lumbar lordosis and posture" (the effect of standing and sitting postures on lumbar curvatures)

animation 2-2 violin posture.ppt: "The case of the twisted violinist" (postural problems arising from holding the violin between the shoulder and cheek)

animation 2-3 piano posture.ppt: "Piano posture" (the effect of seat position and height on posture at the piano)

animation 3-1 shoulder.ppt: "Moving the shoulder joint" (the shoulder joint and its stabilization by rotator cuff muscles)

animation 3-2 shoulder problems.ppt: "Problems with the shoulder" (bursitis and rotator cuff syndrome)

animation 3-3 lumbricals.ppt: "Control of finger movement" (the role of the extensor and flexor muscles that lie in the forearm, and of the lumbrical muscles of the hand)

animation 3-4 retinacula of the wrist.ppt: "Wrist position during instrumental performance (1)" (the role of the retinacula in containing tendon movement at the wrist)

animation 3-5 wrist position.ppt: "Wrist position during instrumental performance (2)" (the effect of radial and ulnar deviation on tendons and nerves at the wrist)

animation 3-6 ulnar nerve.ppt: "Ulnar nerve entrapment at the elbow" (problems affecting the ulnar nerve)

animation 4-1 breathing.ppt: "Breathing movements" (the role of the diaphragm and abdominal wall muscles in breathing)

animation 4-2 breathing (continuous).ppt: (the action from the previous animation running as a continuous loop)

animation 5-1 larynx-height.ppt: "Laryngeal movements in swallowing and yawning" (the actions of muscles that raise and lower the larynx)

animation 5-2 larynx-breathing.ppt: "The vocal folds and breathing" (actions of the principal muscles that open and close the glottis during breathing)

animation 5-3 larynx-voice quality.ppt: "Voice quality" (muscles controlling the larynx in whispering, breathy phonation, flow phonation, and pressed phonation)

animation 5-4 larynx-pitch.ppt: "Control of vocal pitch" (muscles and laryngeal movements involved in changing vocal pitch)

animation 5-5 vocal fold cycle.ppt: "Movements of the vocal folds during phonation" (views of vocal fold movements and the flow glottogram over the vocal fold cycle) animation 5-6 vocal fold cycle (continuous).ppt: (as above but running as a continuous loop)

animation 5-7 voice timbre.ppt: "Vocal timbre" (schematic view of the principles behind changes in voice timbre with changing register)

SOUND PRESENTATIONS (POWERPOINT)

SP 9-1 sound identification.ppt: "Identifying the sounds of instruments" (harmonic structure of complex sound and the role of timbre in sound identification)

SP 9-2 Tartini tones.ppt: "Tartini tones" (demonstration of the appearance of a third pitch in the Tartini tone illusion)

SP 9-3A, B, C Missing fundamental illusions (demonstration of the properties of the missing fundamental illusion in which virtual pitch is generated by an incomplete harmonic series):

SP9-3A.ppt: "The missing fundamental illusion 1"

SP9-3B.ppt: "The missing fundamental illusion 2: The illusion fails at high frequencies"

SP9-3C.ppt: "Pitch perception using 'best fit' "

MUSIC EXTRACT

Smetana quartet Mavron.wma: An extract from Smetana's quartet "Ma Vlast," last movement, Vivace, which contains a musical representation of tinnitus. Played by the Mavron Quartet (Christiana Mavron, Katy Rowe, Rebekah Brown, and Abigail Blackman). See the acknowledgments.

Preface

The performance of music at the highest level requires a degree of skill that certainly matches and arguably exceeds that of most other physical activities, yet while the training of musicians deals extensively with the structure of music, its history, and its interpretation, it has until recently almost entirely neglected the physical demands that it makes on the body. The teaching of instrumental and singing technique has traditionally and indeed necessarily been based on the subjective experience of individual teachers, sometimes resting on erroneous notions of the way in which the body works. One of the reasons for this is that our conscious sensations do not always provide a reliable guide to what our body is doing. As a result, it is often necessary to fall back on metaphor or vague subjective descriptions to try to convey what is being demanded of the pupil. This is a major barrier to passing on the knowledge gained through a lifetime of performance, as the pupil is often left confused about how an important aspect of technique is achieved. While it must be acknowledged that objective information of the many physical processes crucial to performance remains far from complete, there nevertheless exists a considerable body of knowledge that would be very useful to practicing musicians if only they could access it. Unfortunately, this is scattered through the science literature, frequently in publications that are hard to obtain for those outside a large academic institution. Furthermore, it is generally couched in the arcane language of science, which will be opaque to most musicians unless they are provided with an introduction to the world and vocabulary of biology. The object of this book is to help performers overcome this barrier by presenting them with accurate information on the biological principles that underlie their craft. From this beginning they can move forward to develop a rational approach to the development of technique. It should also allow those who would like to delve deeper into the science to access and interpret original sources and perhaps ultimately to become involved in studies that will extend our understanding of performance biology.

Although the physical challenges faced by musicians might be similar to those of athletes, they differ in one crucial respect: while the combination of declining physical powers and accumulated injury leads most athletes to retire in their thirties, musicians are expected to maintain elite levels of performance throughout a career that typically spans many decades. It is therefore not enough for musicians to reach a high level of proficiency by the time they leave a music college or conservatoire. They must be equipped with a technique that is sustainable in the long term and capable of supporting the intense levels of playing demanded of the contemporary performer. If you speak to any professional musician, he or she will tell you either from personal experience or from that of close colleagues that the profession carries a considerable risk of a career-threatening injury. Until recently, however, health problems were rarely discussed openly among players and managers. One reason for this was the not unjustified feeling that any admission of weakness might cost the sufferer his or her hard-won position in the highly competitive world of professional music. This is slowly beginning to change, in no small measure through the efforts of a group of musicians who, having suffered playing-related problems, have been moved to write about their experiences, the lessons they have learned from them, and the strategies they have developed both to overcome them and to avoid further difficulties. Large employers of musicians such as orchestras and opera companies are increasingly expected to look after the health of their players. Within the UK, this has been formalized by new endeavors such as the Healthy Orchestra Charter and the Sound Ear Initiative. Of course as with all forms of occupational health, prevention is the most effective form of treatment, but this requires that good practice be instilled in players from the very earliest stages of their training. Even a cursory examination of the postures adopted by many professional musicians on stage amply demonstrates that such an approach is long overdue. For schemes aimed at reducing the risk of injury to performers to be viable, however, information on which these can be based must be widely available, and this is one of the objectives of this book.

Over the last two decades, arts medicine has emerged as a distinct discipline and a considerable number of treatment centers for it have sprung up, particularly in the United States and in some European countries such as Germany, the Scandinavian countries, and more recently Spain and the UK. This has arisen from the realization that not only do the intense physical demands made on professional musicians make them at least as vulnerable to injury as professional athletes, but that their satisfactory treatment also requires a similarly specialized approach. The growth of this discipline has undoubtedly been aided by the fact that many clinicians have an interest in music. Finding practitioners with the necessary skills and insights to provide rapid and accurate diagnosis and treatment, however, still remains something of a lottery. It is difficult for health professionals such as doctors or physiotherapists to develop expertise in the treatment of a particular type of patient if they see only one or two a year. Many of the problems suffered by musicians are well known to medicine, but for effective treatment it is vital that these are viewed in their vocational context. From this perspective many aspects that might initially appear perplexing quickly become clear and we can progress from treating the symptoms to tackling the root cause. It is also important to realize that the level of function that must be restored in an injured musician to allow a return to even a basic level of professional performance is much greater than that which would be acceptable for most other patients presenting with similar problems. Furthermore, the treatment may have to be modified in light of the particular instrument played, similar to how athletes are rehabilitated differently based on their sports.

The information presented in this book may therefore be of value to health professionals who find themselves treating injured musicians for the first time.

Fortunately, in some countries there now exist national organizations that actively foster links between medicine and the arts, for example, Médecine des Arts (France), the Deutsche Gesellschaft für Musikphysiologie und Musikermedezin (Germany), and the Performing Arts Medicine Association (PAMA) in the U.S. These each take their own approach, but in the UK the British Association of Performing Arts Medicine (BAPAM—BAPAM.org.uk) has set up regional clinics for the initial diagnosis of performance-related health problems (in dancers and actors as well as musicians), from which performers can be referred to doctors and other health professionals who are specialists in their treatment and rehabilitation. Together with the Musicians Benevolent Fund, BAPAM is also increasingly involved in health promotion and injury prevention.

An area of research that has emerged even more recently than arts medicine is that of performance biology—the objective study of the physical and mental processes that underlie singing, instrumental performance, and dance. This field has the ultimate aim of putting musical performance training on a rational basis so that not only are the most effective strategies used, but the chance of developing an injury is minimized. Early investigations in the field were often not rigorous enough and suffered from small numbers of study subjects, but this is slowly beginning to change. Notable centers for the study of music biology, psychology, and medicine are now found in such places as the Institute for Music Physiology and Musicians' Medicine in Hannover, Germany, the University of Montreal, Harvard Medical School, and the Royal College of Music in London. In addition, many researchers have made contributions to music biology as a sideline from their main research. The field is currently in the state that sports biology reached several decades ago, but some music teachers are already trying to apply the available information to the teaching and treatment of musicians. Many institutions have set up courses covering at least some areas of performance biology and medicine; however, the lack of a suitable textbook is a major impediment to the wider development of such courses, which should form part of the core curriculum of all music schools. This book is intended to remedy this situation by providing a broad introduction to the major areas of human biology of relevance to performers.

One often feels, when reading the literature of music biology, that although musicians are interesting subjects for anatomists, physiologists, and neuroscientists, they are by and large passive participants in many studies and don't always receive the return they deserve for their participation. The science of performance has a great deal to offer performers and it has been my experience in Cardiff that if they are interested in these matters, musicians can quickly assimilate sufficient knowledge to take an active part in and ultimately direct such studies for their own ends. Another object of the book is therefore to help facilitate this transition. It is not simply an account of human anatomy or physiology to which have been added a few examples of medical problems found in musicians. Each chapter is written specifically from the viewpoint of musical performance and makes heavy use of relatively unknown literature sources on music biology, which provide important information that is not to be found in standard biology or medical textbooks. For example, you will not find a discussion of the limitations to individual finger movement even in the definitive text of *Gray's Anatomy*, and no medical textbook provides an account of current research into respiratory strategies of relevance to singers or discusses theories of the control of register or voice projection. With this book I have endeavored, wherever possible, to address questions that musicians need answers to and to point out some of the limitations of current knowledge. I have also sought to assess the validity of some key notions that are commonly held by musicians, although I will not pretend that I can provide the last word on any of these issues. Rather, the position presented here is a starting point from which I hope musicians themselves will carry the baton onward.

This book originated from a series of lectures given at Cardiff University and the Royal Welsh College of Music and Drama. Preparing these lectures brought home to me the difficulty for musicians (and indeed biologists) of finding accessible sources of information on music biology. For musicians this is exacerbated by having to deal with the language of biology, and the book tries to assume no prior knowledge of this. Even for biologists, some of the most active areas, such as the study of what goes on in the brain when we listen to music, can be quite impenetrable. This is not only because of the terminology used, but also because of the difficulty of trying to untangle different methods and approaches, which can generate results that may at first appear conflicting or confusing. Here then is a starting point, but keep in mind that this field is still in its infancy; it will be clear to those who read the book that many concepts of central importance are in urgent need of comprehensive reevaluation and study. The ease with which physiological data can now be collected, digitized, and analyzed with modest computing resources means that a great deal can be achieved with relatively inexpensive equipment if directed at a well-defined and manageable objective. However, it is all too easy to collect large amounts of data from which it is difficult to extract vocationally meaningful conclusions. It is therefore essential that experienced professional musicians, as well as those with a background in science or medicine, be involved at all stages of such studies, from setting the initial objectives, through experimental design and execution, to analysis and interpretation. If this book encourages just a few performers in taking on such a role, it will have made an important contribution to ensuring that musicians will in the future have a solid body of information on which to build their technique.

HOW TO USE THIS BOOK

For some readers, it will be sufficient that the book serves as a source of reference or of background information on the biology of technique. For others it will form a bridge that will provide access to the original literature on music biology as it currently stands and as it evolves. Each chapter therefore ends with a list of references of the main sources of information on which it is based. The chapters' differing lengths reflect to some extent the depth of our understanding in each area. In the hope that the book will encourage the development of courses in music biology in music colleges and conservatoires, I have produced a set of teaching aids, which can be found on the accompanying CD. One element is a set of simple illustrations that are intended to present key anatomical information in a clear and approachable way. You will find them printed in black and white in the text, but on the disc most are produced in color, which will make them more engaging and perhaps easier to interpret. Written descriptions of movements and postures can sometimes be difficult to understand, though they are easily appreciated when seen. The disc therefore includes a set of animations that illustrate some key concepts of posture, movement, and laryngeal function. These are in the form of PowerPoint presentations but can be run even if you do not have the program by clicking on pptview.exe in the appropriate directory. You can then select the animation you require, whereupon it will open fullscreen and run automatically with preset timings. Alternatively, if you have PowerPoint, you can open them with the program and manipulate or disable the timings. One of the disappointing aspects of reading accounts of auditory illusions—important for our appreciation of music—is that they can't be heard unless you have access to facilities for generating or manipulating sound waveforms. The CD therefore also contains a number of PowerPoint files (labeled Sound Presentations) that reproduce the auditory effects discussed in chapter 9. Once the files are opened fullscreen, some will run automatically while others will produce the sounds only when the loudspeaker symbols are clicked. For some, you will also need to use the Page Down key to go to the next screen. If you are using them in a lecture hall, the clarity of the illusions will depend on the quality of the sound system, though for private listening even an inexpensive set of headphones is adequate. The disc also contains an excerpt from Smetana's Quartet "Ma Vlast" (From My Life), which gives a musical rendition of a hearing problem known as tinnitus. This is played by the Mavron Quartet (see the acknowledgments). Finally, I have created a number of short videos, mainly dealing with breathing for singers and wind players and with aspects of laryngeal function.

Acknowledgments

I am most grateful for the generosity of Roger Chaffin, Robert Harrison, Michael Karnell, Clark Rosen, Johan Sundberg, and Ingo Titze for giving me permission to reproduce images from their work; to Buddug Verona James for discussions on singing technique and for her involvement in the respiratory recordings shown in the book and heard on the disc; to Robert Santer, who was involved in creating the video of tendon anomalies; and to the Mavron Quartet (Christiana Mavron and Katy Rowe [violins], Rebekah Brown [viola], and Abigail Blackman [cello], www.mavronquartet.co.uk) for making the recording of the Smetana Quartet that appears on the CD. Louise Atkins of the Royal Welsh College of Music and Drama (RWCMD) played a major role in collecting and analyzing the respiratory data from wind players that form the basis of some of the figures and videos. This is part of a project to raise awareness in musicians of the physical aspects of performance and has been supported by a grant for public engagement in science from the Wellcome Trust, held by Kevin Price and me. I would also like to acknowledge Zoe Smith, who has encouraged the integration of the material that forms this book into the music curriculum of the RWCMD, and Sanchita Farruque of the British Association of Performing Arts Medicine, who was brave enough to try some of the support materials on a variety of audiences. Finally, I am greatly indebted to Kevin Price (head of brass teaching at RWCMD) for acting as a sounding board for many of the ideas presented here, for liaising with performers who have contributed to the production of some of the illustrative material, and for helping to ensure that the treatment of the material is vocationally relevant to working musicians. The fact that this project has come to fruition owes a great deal to his support and enthusiasm.

Reference Abbreviations

Below is a list of abbreviations used in the references at the end of each chapter and the corresponding full name for each publication.

Acta Anat Basel (Basel)	*Acta Anatomica* (Basel)
Acta Otolaryngol	*Acta Otolaryngologica*
Adv Cog Psychol	*Advances in Cognitive Psychology*
Adv Neurol	*Advances in Neurology*
Am J Med	*American Journal of Medicine*
Am J Orthod	*American Journal of Orthdontics*
Am J Otol	*American Journal of Otolaryngology*
Am J Physiol	*American Journal of Physiology*
Am J Psychiatry	*American Journal of Psychiatry*
Am J Psychol	*American Journal of Psychology*
Anat Rec	*Anatomical Record*
Anat Rec A Discov Mol Cell Evol Biol	*Anatomical Record A: Discoveries in Molecular, Cellular, and Evolutionary Biology*
Angle Orthod	*Angle Orthodontist*
Ann Allergy	*Annals of Allergy*
Ann NY Acad Sci	*Annals of the New York Academy of Sciences*
Ann Otol Rhinol Laryngol	*Annals of Otology, Rhinology and Laryngology*
Annu Rev Psychol	*Annual Review of Psychology*
Arch Environ Health	*Archives of Environmental Health*
Arch Med Res	*Archives of Medical Research*
Arch Néerl Phon Expér	*Archives Néerlandaises de Phonétique Expérimentale*
Arch Otorhinolaryngol	*Archives of Otorhinolaryngology*
Arch Phys Med Rehabil	*Archives of Physical Medicine and Rehabilitation*
Aust Dent J	*Australian Dental Journal*
Behav Brain Res	*Behavioral Brain Research*
Behav Res Ther	*Behaviour Research and Therapy*
Biofeedback Self Regul	*Biofeedback and Self Regulation*

Biol Psychol	*Biological Psychology*
BMC Dermatol	*Biomed Central Dermatology*
BMC Neurosci	*Biomed Central Neuroscience*
Brain Cogn	*Brain and Cognition*
Brain Res Brain Res Rev	*Brain Research: Brain Research Reviews*
Brain Res Cogn Brain Res	*Brain Research: Cognitive Brain Research*
Brit J Psychol	*British Journal of Psychology*
Br Dent J	*British Dental Journal*
Cereb Cortex	*Cerebral Cortex*
Clev Clin Q	*Cleveland Clinic Quarterly*
Clin Anat	*Clinical Anatomy*
Clin Biomech (Bristol, Avon)	*Clinical Biomechanics* (Bristol, Avon)
Clin Neurphysiol	*Clinical Neurophysiology*
Clin Sci (Lond)	*Clinical Science (London)*
CMAJ	*Canadian Medical Association Journal*
Cogn Brain Res	*Cognitive Brain Research*
Curr Opin Neurobiol	*Current Opinion in Neurobiology*
Ear Hear	*Ear and Hearing*
Epilepsy Behav	*Epilepsy and Behavior*
Eur J Anat	*European Journal of Anatomy*
Eur J Neurosci	*European Journal of Neuroscience*
Eur J phys	*European Journal of Physiology*
Eur Respir J	*European Respiratory Journal*
Exp Brain Res	*Experimental Brain Research*
Folia Phoniatr (Basel)	*Folia Phoniatrica* (Basel)
Forsch Komplementarmed Klass Naturheilkd	*Forschende Komplementärmedizin und Klassiche Naturheilkunde*
Hand Clin	*Hand Clinics*
Hum Brain Mapp	*Human Brain Mapping*
Hum Mov Sci	*Human Movement Science*
Int J Dermatol	*International Journal of Dermatology*
Int J Pediatr Otorhinolaryngol	*International Journal of Pediatric Otorhinolaryngology*
Int J Ther Rehab	*International Journal of Therapy and Rehabilitation*
J Acoust Soc Am	*Journal of the Acoustical Society of America*
JAMA	*Journal of the American Medical Association*
J Am Dent Assoc	*Journal of the American Dental Association*
J Anat	*Journal of Anatomy*
J Appl Physiol	*Journal of Applied Physiology*
J Asthma	*Journal of Asthma*
J Biomech	*Journal of Biomechanics*
J Bone Joint Surg Am	*Journal of Bone and Joint Surgery (American volume)*
J Clin Neurosci	*Journal of Clinical Neuroscience*

J Cogn Neurosci	*Journal of Cognitive Neuroscience*
J Consult Clin Psychol	*Journal of Consulting and Clinical Psychology*
J Hand Surg (Am)	*Journal of Hand Surgery* (American volume)
J Hand Surg (Br)	*Journal of Hand Surgery* (British volume)
J Hand Ther	*Journal of Hand Therapy*
J Int Double Reed Soc	*Journal of the International Double Reed Society*
J Manipulative Physiol Ther	*Journal of Manipulative and Physiological Therapeutics*
J Music Theory	*Journal of Music Theory*
J Neurol Sci	*Journal of Neurological Science*
J Neurophysiol	*Journal of Neurophysiology*
J Neuroradiol	*Journal of Neuradiology*
J Neurosci	*Journal of Neuroscience*
J Res Music Educ	*Journal of Research in Music Education*
J R Soc Med	*Journal of the Royal Society of Medicine*
J Speech Hear Res	*Journal of Speech and Hearing Research*
J Voice	*Journal of Voice*
Learn Mem	*Learning and Memory*
Logoped Phoniatr Vocol	*Logopedics, Phoniatrics, Vocology*
Md Med J	*Maryland Medical Journal*
Med Hypotheses	*Medical Hypotheses*
Med J Aust	*Medical Journal of Australia*
Med Prob Perform Artists	*Medical Problems in Performing Artists*
Mem Cognit	*Memory and Cognition*
Mov Disord	*Movement Disorders*
Muscle Nerve	*Muscle and Nerve*
Nat Neurosci	*Nature Neuroscience*
Nat Rev Neurosci	*Nature Reviews Neuroscience*
Neuroendocrinol Lett	*Neuroendocrinology Letters*
Neuroreport	*Neuroreport*
Neurosci Lett	*Neuroscience Letters*
Neurosci Res	*Neuroscience Research*
Obstet Gynecol	*Obstetrics and Gynecology*
Occup Med (Lond)	*Occupational Medicine* (London)
Otolaryngol Clin North Am	*Otolaryngologic Clinics of North America*
Otolaryngol Head Neck Surg	*Otolaryngology: Head and Neck Surgery*
Plast Reconst Surg	*Plastic and Reconstructive Surgery*
Proc Natl Acad Sci USA	*Proceedings of the National Academy of Sciences* (U.S.)
Psychol Music	*Psychology of Music*
Psychol Sci	*Psychological Science*
Respir Physiol	*Respiratory Physiology*
Sci Am	*Scientific American*
Semin Neurol	*Seminars in Neurology*

Speech Hear Res	*Speech and Hearing Research*
Trans Med Soc Lond	*Transactions of the Medical Society of London*
Trends Cogn Sci	*Trends in Cognitive Sciences*
Trends Neurosci	*Trends in Neuroscience*

Chapter One

Introduction to the Tissues of the Body

Before we examine the biological principles that underlie the performance of music, it is first necessary to know something about the structure of the basic tissues that make up the body. The objective of this chapter is therefore to provide a brief introduction to this topic; taking the time to go through it carefully will make it easier to understand the following chapters. It is important to recognize, however, that this is not intended to provide a comprehensive overview of human body structure, but is highly focused on subjects that are central to the rest of the book. It does not, for example, deal with the circulatory system or with the major organ systems of the body. Even the subjects that are covered are dealt with on a need-to-know basis, in order to get readers who are musicians into the sections of the text that concern them as quickly as possible. If they find the biology interesting, some may wish to delve more deeply into conventional textbooks at a later date, and this will undoubtedly add to their appreciation of the issues presented here. However, such books generally have little to say on the specific aspects of biology that are central to musical performance.

This chapter deals with the basic elements of the body excluding the organs, that is, bone, cartilage, and joints; muscles and tendons; the skin; and the organization of the spinal cord. It deals with sensation and in particular with the nature of pain. The section on skin will also address some matters of particular relevance to musicians in the form of a discussion of contact dermatitis. The succeeding chapters will build on what is presented here and provide additional basic information as necessary for the understanding of performance-related function and injury. Information is introduced where its relevance for performers is best appreciated, so it should not be necessary to keep flipping from one chapter to another to get the complete picture. For example, the section on tendon sheaths will be found close to where the problems associated with tendons are discussed. An account of the respiratory system is left entirely to the chapter on breathing strategies, and an overview of the organization of the brain is presented in the chapter that immediately precedes those dealing with music and the brain, the auditory system, and stress, all of which are dependent on the foundation this chapter provides.

BONE, CARTILAGE, AND JOINTS

When you think of bone, what probably comes to mind is the dry skeleton and with it the idea that bone is an inert and unchanging structural material like concrete, but this is far from the truth. Both the calcium and the phosphates that make up the hard material in bone are important chemicals used by all cells in the body for a variety of purposes. While a major function of bone is to provide structural support for the body, it also acts as a reserve supply of these materials. Bone also responds to the demands that are made upon it and will slowly increase in mass if great forces are applied to it. Historically this is seen, for example, in English longbowmen, whose bows required a force of up to 65 kilograms to draw. Examination of skeletons of archers recovered from the Tudor warship the *Mary Rose* reveals that the bones of the load-bearing left arm show significantly greater development than those of the drawing arm. A similar phenomenon is seen today in tennis players, in whom the mineral content of the bones of the racket arm may be up to 20 percent greater than in the other.

On the other hand, bone mass can also be lost. This is known as osteoporosis and is common in elderly people of both sexes, but particularly in women, in whom it is a consequence of the hormonal changes that take place at menopause. This reduction in bone mass makes one more vulnerable to hip fractures and spinal deformity. In life, bone is therefore an active tissue. Far from being dry, it not only contains cells that regulate its structure but also a good blood and nerve supply to maintain them. As a result, breaking a bone is a very painful experience. The structure of large bones is designed to provide maximum strength with a minimum of weight. The central section of the long bones of the arms and legs is made up of a cylinder of dense bone surrounding a hollow core. The core contains marrow, a tissue that is responsible for the production of red blood cells, the carriers of oxygen, and white blood cells, which fight disease. Toward the ends of the long bones, the marrow is replaced by spongy bone, which, though light, is capable of supporting considerable force.

During embryological and early postnatal development, bone develops from a more flexible material called cartilage, which provides a matrix for the deposition of calcium and phosphate. There are many other forms of cartilage in the body, however. Cartilage forms the ligaments that hold bones in position and the tendons that transmit the forces generated by muscles to the bones. Cartilage also contributes to several important components that in turn contribute to the structure of joints. We will see in a later chapter that the skeleton of the larynx is constructed entirely from cartilage, though bone may be deposited there later in life. Cartilage is created by cells that secrete a variety of structural fibers with differing properties. Some of these are elastic, while others such as collagen are thicker and less extensible. These fibers give the cartilage its tensile strength. The gaps between the fibers are filled with space-filling molecules, many of which help the tissue to retain water. Together these create a gel in which the fibers are embedded. This gives the cartilage great stiffness and a resistance to compression. The structural advantages of materials that combine a meshwork of fibers within an incompressible matrix are reflected in their widespread use in engineering, from prestressed concrete and fiberglass to the carbon fiber and other composites used by the aeronautics industry.

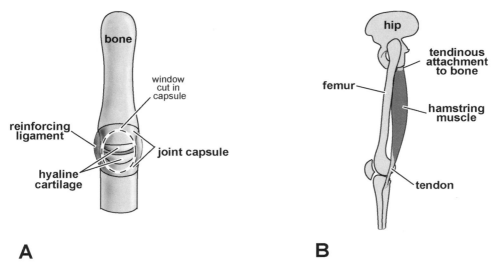

Figure 1-1. A. The structure of a synovial joint. The surfaces of the bone that make contact in the joint are covered with smooth, hard-wearing hyaline cartilage. The joint is enclosed in a capsule, which is usually reinforced by ligaments and contains lubricating synovial fluid. B. The relationship between muscle and tendon is shown in this diagram of a hamstring muscle, which runs from the pelvis to the bones of the lower part of the leg. A thin strip of tendinous tissue (cartilage) attaches the muscle to the hip (its origin). At the other end, a long, thin tendon (the "hamstring") emerges from the muscle and runs down the side of the knee to its attachment site on the side of the lower leg (its insertion).

Where bones come together, they are connected by joints. Some of these allow little to no movement, such as the ones between the bones of the skull, but most are present to permit some degree of movement, that is, they allow the bones to articulate with one another. The joints that are most important for the purposes of this book are what are called synovial joints, and we will here concern ourselves exclusively with these (fig. 1-1A). The surface of normal bone is covered with a fine membrane called the periosteum, which is not sufficiently robust to resist the friction and wear at the contact surfaces of a moving joint. These surfaces are instead covered with a special form of cartilage called articular or hyaline cartilage. This provides a smooth, glassy surface that is resistant to wear and is self-repairing, which is important as these moving joints must remain intact for a lifetime. If the bony surface of the joint is shallow (e.g., the shoulder joint), a rim made up of a different type of cartilage must be laid down to give it added depth. In order to reduce the friction between the moving surfaces, they are lubricated with a watery fluid (synovial fluid) produced by membranes (synovial membranes) that lie within the joint. To stop the fluid from draining into the surrounding tissues, each joint is enclosed in a sac called the joint capsule. The joint is usually reinforced with ligaments that run between the bones to keep the two sides in close proximity and to limit the degree of movement in certain planes. The ligaments, which are also made of cartilage, are often fused with the capsule. In some cases (such as the jaw joint), a disk of cartilage is also interposed between the two joint surfaces.

The possible range of movement at a joint depends on the shape or the articular surfaces. The elbow joint and the last two joints in the fingers are known as hinge joints because they allow movement in only one plane. Joints such as those at the wrist and at the base of the finger and thumb allow limited movement in two planes, while the shoulder and hip joints are ball-and-socket joints that allow a much greater range of movement.

MUSCLES AND TENDONS

The joints between the bones are moved by what is known as skeletal muscle. Such muscle is composed of hundreds of thousands of long muscle fibers, each of which is capable of contracting under the control of the nervous system. The fibers are rather strange cells as each is formed from the fusion of many smaller cells. Most cells have only a single nucleus, which contains the genetic blueprint of the whole animal, but from which is translated the parts required by the particular cell type. Because of how they are formed, muscle fibers each contain many nuclei. Muscle fibers, even within the same muscle, may have different properties. Some are known as fast-twitch fibers because they contract rapidly, but these are easily fatigued. Slow muscle fibers by contrast not only do not contract so quickly, but can remain contracted for longer periods without becoming exhausted. The balance between slow and fast muscle fibers depends on what the muscle is used for, how it has been trained, and the genetic makeup of the individual. Muscles have a variety of forms depending on their role in the body. Some, such as those in the abdominal wall, are flat sheets, while others such as the biceps are more rounded in cross-section. We generally think of muscles as being anchored to a fixed bone at one end and a moving one at the other. Under these circumstances, the fixed end of the muscle is described as its origin and the moving end its insertion. It is not unusual, however, to find that the bone at either end may be moved depending on the posture adopted. For example, a muscle on the front of the thigh may raise the leg when we walk but pull the trunk forward at the waist when we sit up from a recumbent position. Similarly, a muscle at the back of the thigh may bend the knee if the weight of the body is supported by the other leg or rotate the pelvis backward if the foot is planted firmly on the ground (fig. 1-1B). Although many muscles are attached to bone at both ends, others insert into sheets of fibrous connective tissue (e.g., abdominal muscles) or even the skin or other muscles (e.g., the muscles of the face and embouchure). Where the attachments are made to bone, some tendinous tissue forms the connection. This may be difficult to see at the origin, where the muscle often appears to spring directly from the bone. The tendon at the other end is usually elongated into a strap or sheetlike structure (fig. 1-1B). Long tendons can be used to improve the mechanical advantage of the muscle, but they also allow the muscle to lie some distance away from the joint from which it acts. In the case of the hand, the major power muscles that flex and extend the fingers lie in the forearm. They can therefore be much larger and stronger than would be possible if they all lay within the hand itself, which contains much smaller muscles that provide the fine control necessary for dextrous finger movements.

There are two other major classes of muscle. One of these is exclusive to the heart. Cardiac muscle requires quite different properties from skeletal muscle. First, as the heart beats throughout life it must be very resistant to fatigue. It must also provide a conductive path for waves of electrical excitation to spread across the heart. Many cardiac muscle fibers will contract rhythmically even in the absence of signals from the nervous system. The other major type of muscle is smooth muscle. This is found mainly in the hollow organs such as the gut and bladder, and lining the airways of the lungs. It is also present in the walls of the arteries. This smooth muscle directs blood to different places as the need arises by regulating the width of different arteries. For example, when we run, the muscular walls of the arteries supplying the muscles relax to increase their access to oxygen and nutrients. More blood is also directed through the arteries running in the skin to dissipate the heat that the muscles produce. By contrast, when we eat a heavy meal, the smooth muscle in the arteries in the muscles and skin contracts to make them narrower, while the arteries supplying the gut and the liver increase in diameter to support digestion.

SKIN AND EPITHELIA

Epithelia are sheets of cells that cover the external and internal surfaces of the body, forming a barrier between the tissues of the body and the external environment or the contents of organs such as the gut or bladder, but they may also be modified for other roles such as secretion of fluids, mucus, or other compounds. For the purposes of this book we need consider only two types of epithelia. The first covers the outer surface of the body and we call this the skin (fig. 1-2). The second, which we will see in chapter 5, lines the back of the nose, the throat, and the larynx.

The skin has several major functions. One is to provide a covering for the body that is both resistant to abrasion and a barrier to the uncontrolled loss of water. The epithelium, which forms the outer region or epidermis or outer layer of the skin, is composed of many layers of flattened cells, which are constantly lost from the surface and replaced from below (fig. 1-2A). It is a somewhat nauseating truth that the material that collects on the air filters of the London Underground is mostly composed of skin cells! Only the cells in the inner layers are alive, but these are tightly bound together to prevent water in the underlying tissues from escaping to the surface. The cells on the outer layers are dead, but they provide a tough surface that is resistant to damage due to rubbing or scraping. The cells are modified to resist abrasion by being desiccated and by containing granules of keratin, a tough protein that also makes up fingernails and hair.

The epidermis does not have a blood supply, but the dermis (the layer of the skin that lies directly beneath it) is well supplied by blood vessels. When the body becomes overheated, the blood vessels expand so that heat can be more efficiently lost by radiation from the skin surface. Heat is also lost by the evaporation of sweat, which is released from sweat glands that are found in the dermis but which send ducts all the way up to the skin surface. Most of the body is covered with hair growing from hair follicles that are modifications of the epidermis that push down to its border with the

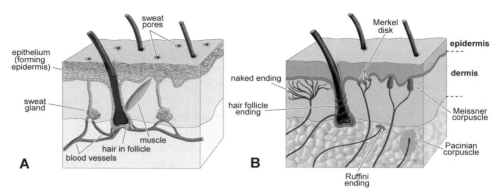

Figure 1-2. A. The structure of the skin. The outer layer of the skin (epidermis) is formed by a multilayered epithelium of flattened cells. The outer cells are dead and are gradually sloughed off to be replaced by those beneath, which are continually being produced by the innermost layer. Beneath the epidermis lies the dermis, which contains the sweat glands and hair follicles. Small muscles attach to the walls of the hair follicle; these raise the hair if we are cold or frightened. B. Sensory nerve endings in the skin. The sensory nerves that supply the skin carry a variety of types of sensation, such as pain. Some are known as naked endings in which the branches at the end of the axons are not structurally modified. Other endings are associated with cellular structures that have an effect on their sensitivity to different types of stimuli. Some endings lie below the dermis, while others lie more superficially at the boundary between the dermis and epidermis. The more superficial endings are responsible for the finest forms of tactile discrimination.

dermis, where the cells that produce the hair get their blood supply. Sebaceous glands also empty their contents into the hair follicles, producing a thin grease that flows onto the hair and the skin surface, which helps to make the skin more water resistant and so prevents it from drying excessively, which could cause it to crack. Each hair follicle is attached to a small muscle that can pull the hair erect (fig. 1-2A). This originally evolved as a mechanism to conserve heat; though the hair on our skin is generally too fine and sparse for this to have much effect, the response still occurs, creating what we call "goose bumps." Each of these represents the effects of a muscle attached to a single hair follicle. The hairs also stand up when we are frightened or excited, causing sensations that we may experience as "creeping," "hair rising on the back of the neck," or "shivers down the spine," depending on the context. This sometimes happens when we have a strong emotional reaction to a piece of music.

Like many other body tissues, the properties of the skin change depending on how it is used. Where it experiences great friction or pressure it becomes thicker and may form calluses. This is important for guitarists and players of bowed string instruments, as the calluses that build up on the pads of the fingers allow high pressures to be exerted to keep the string in contact with the fret or fingerboard without causing pain or blister formation. Playing an instrument can cause the skin to become modified or damaged in less helpful ways, however. In violin and viola players, pressure and abrasion can lead to changes in the texture and color of the skin on the side of the neck where it makes contact with the instrument. Particularly when combined with poor hygiene, this may also lead to acne or infection. The altered skin is commonly known as "fiddler's neck" and ranges from a mild thickening or discoloration to dry, itchy, or infected skin (Blum and Ritter 1990; Onder et al. 1999; Harvell and Maibach 1992). Occasionally, swelling that initially appears to be due to skin thickening is the result of cysts in the salivary glands, which lie beneath the jawline or on the cheek, where they can be compressed by the instrument. Allergic or toxic reactions to compounds associated with the instrument can also contribute to the symptoms of fiddler's neck (Gambichler, Boms, and Freitag 2004). Some string players develop allergies to rosin (colophony), a compound derived from the sap of pine and spruce trees, or components of instrument varnish such as propolis. Propolis, also known as bee glue, is a resin collected from the buds and bark of trees such as the poplar and used to seal gaps in the hive. In some individuals, contact with these materials produces dermatitis (a general term indicating a swelling of the tissues in the skin) or an eczema-like reaction. Many exotic hardwoods such as rosewoods, cocobolo, and ebony, which are used in recorders and in high-quality clarinets and oboes, can also induce allergic skin responses. Some chin rests may also be carved from rosewoods. Allergic reactions are not only seen in players, but can also pose a significant problem for instrument makers, as the dust from these woods quite often triggers asthmalike symptoms. The chemicals in the wood that are responsible are not unique to a single species of tree, so some experimentation may be required to find a suitable alternative for an offending chin rest or woodwind instrument. Boxwood is generally a safe replacement as it does not contain significant quantities of known allergens. Problems can also arise from stains that have been used on wood. For example, paraphenylenediamine, a stain used to give the appearance of ebony to paler and more common woods, is a well-known allergen. As a result, chin rests and fingerboards that appear to be ebony but are not can be a source of contact dermatitis on the neck or fingers.

If the symptoms of fiddler's neck are caused mainly by the pressure of the instrument on the skin, a number of approaches may be used to reduce them (Harvell and Maibach 1992; Blum and Ritter 1990). Attention to hygiene and ensuring that any cloths used over the chin rest are always clean are obvious measures. Men may find it beneficial to grow a beard, though occasionally this causes its own problems if the hair is curly and becomes ingrown. Changing the setup to increase the load-bearing area of the skin surface may also offer some benefit. It has been suggested that one way of achieving this is to move the chin rest toward the midline of the instrument (Blum and Ritter 1990); however, one objective study of different chin rests found that higher pressures were exerted with this type of rest than with two others whose contact surfaces were positioned more to one side (Okner, Kernozek, and Wade 1997).

Contact with certain metals can also cause skin problems. Nickel is particularly well known for this, though other metals such as chromium have also been implicated to a lesser extent. Nickel is a component of alloys used in the manufacture of many brass instruments and their mouthpieces, inexpensive flutes, and the fittings of other woodwinds. It is frequently employed in the form of nickel silver, which is actually an alloy of copper, zinc, and nickel. However, the situation is complicated by the fact that the alloy that forms the bulk of the instrument may be covered by a plating of another metal. Heat, abrasion, and interactions with sweat or saliva all conspire to increase the risk of contact dermatitis with metals. Indeed, the flaking of skin around the mouth (cheilitis) in brass players or flutists is sometimes due solely to physical abrasion of the thin, wet skin around the lip (Thomas, Rueff, and Przybilla 2000). Where a reaction to metal is the cause, a thin coating of a more inert metal such as silver or gold may provide a solution. Alternatively, a mouthpiece with a plastic rim or one made entirely of plastic can be used. Nickel is sometimes present in the metal elements of violin and viola chin and shoulder rests and so can contribute to the development of fiddler's neck. It is used as a coating for steel guitar strings and in the overwound strings of many instruments. If this irritates the skin of the fingers, an alternative choice of string is generally available; for example, bronze or aluminum is often used in overwindings. In electric guitars, however, almost all available strings have a major nickel component.

THE CENTRAL AND PERIPHERAL NERVOUS SYSTEM

For the purposes of description, the nervous system is usually divided into the central nervous system, which is made up of the brain and spinal cord, and the peripheral nervous system, which comprises the nerves that supply the skin, muscles, joints, and organs. The structure of the brain and its role in musical performance are dealt with in chapters 7 and 8. Here we will confine our considerations to the spinal cord and the peripheral nervous system.

The Spinal Cord

The vertebrae that form the skeleton of the spine each incorporate a hollow space for the spinal cord. The cord is therefore surrounded by bone, so each vertebra must have a pair of openings through which nerves pass to reach the rest of the body (see chapter 2). These nerves are called the segmental nerves and they supply the muscles, the skin, and the organs. The region of skin innervated by each segmental nerve is called a dermatome, and in the thorax (chest region), these can be viewed as horizontal strips on the surface of the skin. The pattern is more complicated in the cervical (neck) region and in the lumbosacral (lower back) region, where the segmental nerves must supply the limbs as well as the trunk. In these regions the nerves from several spinal segments fuse together and then branch again in complex patterns to form a network or plexus. In the case of the arm this is called the brachial plexus and for the leg, the lumbosacral plexus (see chapters 2 and 3). We will see later that compression of the branches of the brachial plexus can cause problems in musicians, for example, where they emerge from the vertebral column, or where they pass between the muscles of the neck or through a narrow space between the collarbone and the rib cage.

If we were to peer into the narrow tunnel that runs down the center of the vertebral column, we would see that each segmental nerve is formed by the fusion of many small rootlets that arise as a continuous series from both the dorsal and ventral surfaces of the spinal cord (fig. 1-3A). At each spinal level, the dorsal bundles fuse to form a single dorsal root and the ventral bundles, a ventral root. The dorsal and ventral roots then join to create the segmental nerve. The section of cord giving rise to each segmental nerve is regarded as a functional unit and is named after the vertebrae

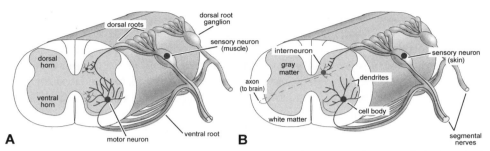

Figure 1-3. The organization of the spinal cord. There are three types of nerve cells in the spinal cord: sensory neurons, motor neurons, which supply the muscles, and interneurons, which make connections between other neurons. Each neuron has a cell body, which contains the nucleus, and an axon that connects it to other neurons. Motor neurons and interneurons also have many dendrites that sprout from the cell body and lie within the gray matter, while the surrounding white matter carries axons up and down the cord. The gray matter is divided into the dorsal horn, which is mainly concerned with processing sensory information, and the ventral horn, which contains the motor neurons. A. A sensory neuron that carries information from a muscle runs into the ventral horn to contact motor neurons, though it also interacts with interneurons in the dorsal horn. B. A sensory neuron comes from the skin and ends in the dorsal horn on an interneuron that carries sensory information up the cord to the brain.

through which the nerve passes. However, the spinal cord is much shorter than the vertebral column. It terminates in the midlumbar region (in the small of the back), and the segmental nerves of the lower segments of the cord must run for some distance down the central tunnel within the spine so that they can emerge at the appropriate vertebral level. These abundant downward running roots are called the cauda equina because of their superficial resemblance to a horse's tail.

Seen in cross-section, the spinal cord is round or oval, but it has a central butterfly-shaped area which, because of its color, is called the gray matter (fig. 1-3B). This is surrounded by a border of paler tissue known as white matter. Regions of gray and white matter are found throughout the central nervous system; in order to understand their significance we need to consider the nature and diversity of nerve cells (more details of this can be found in chapter 8). Figure 1-3 shows the structure of several types of nerve cells (or neurons). Each has a central spherical region called the cell body from which arise a number of short branches and one long branch. The cell body contains the nucleus where the genetic material of the cells is packaged into chromosomes, which contain the blueprints for all of the proteins that make up the cell. These proteins are manufactured outside the nucleus but within the cell body and have many different roles. They may be used to build structures within the cell, be involved in communication between or within cells, or control the manufacture of other molecules required by the cell. The short branches that emerge from the cell body are called dendrites and the single long process, the axon (fig. 1-3B). The axon carries information in the form of pulses of electricity to other nerve cells, either nearby or at distant sites within the nervous system or outside of it. Usually the axons from nerve cells in the same region run together in bundles, and these form the white matter. This can therefore be considered the cabling of the nervous system. The axons finally end in a series of fine branches, which contact the dendrites and cell bodies of other neurons. Information is passed from the axon to the dendrite by the release of chemicals called neurotransmitters. Generally these will either excite or inhibit the follower cell. The dendrites therefore represent the input end of the neuron, and the axon, the output end. The contacts between neurons are found in the gray matter and consequently, this is where the nervous system carries out all of its complex functions. In the spinal cord, the gray matter makes up the central core while the white matter runs along the periphery; however, in many regions of the brain it is the other way around.

Nerve Cells in the Spinal Cord

Nerve cells can be divided into three broad categories: motor neurons, sensory neurons, and interneurons. We will examine each of these in turn.

Motor neurons. These have their cell bodies in the ventral region (ventral horn) of the gray matter within the spinal cord, which faces the front when we are standing upright. The axons of the motor neurons leave the spinal cord through the ventral roots and pass into the segmental nerves, which convey them to the muscles. The axons of motor neurons can be very long. A motor neuron supplying a muscle in the hand will have its cell body in the cervical (neck) region of the spinal cord, so its axon will be more than a meter long. As all of the proteins needed by the cell are manufactured in the cell body, they must be transported along the entire length of the axon if they are required at its terminal end. The cell must therefore not only construct and maintain the axon but also maintain an active transport system, which requires energy to run it. To put this task into perspective, if we imagine the motor neuron cell body to be the size of a tennis ball, the axon running to a muscle in the hand would at this scale be about two kilometers long!

Many motor neurons are needed to control each muscle and together these are known as its motor pool. Every motor neuron contacts many muscle fibers. The group of fibers driven by one motor neuron is called a motor unit (fig. 1-4); however, these are nonoverlapping as each muscle fiber is driven by only a single motor neuron. The motor neurons within the motor pool are not equivalent. Some control large motor units composed of thousands of fibers, and others much smaller ones. When fine movements requiring little strength are needed, the small motor units are activated first. The strength of contraction can be gradually increased by recruiting additional small units. As the contraction increases further, the increments of force gradually get bigger because the newly recruited motor units become increasingly large. This is called the size principle of motor recruitment and makes the most efficient use of the motor neurons in the pool, as the greatest degree of control is needed when the forces generated by the muscle are small. In a strongly contracted muscle, adding a small motor unit would have little effect and so it is most appropriate to recruit large motor units under these circumstances. The number of motor neurons needed in the motor pool of a particular muscle depends on what it is used for, not simply on its absolute size. For example, a small lumbrical muscle in the hand that contributes to its dexterity and needs fine control has about a hundred motor neurons, whereas a muscle in the shin, though two hundred times as powerful, has only seven times as many (Hamilton, Jones, and Wolpert 2004). A single one of the six muscles that move the eye, which

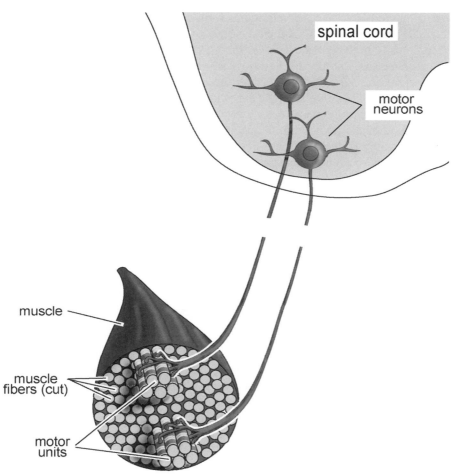

Figure 1-4. The control of muscles by motor neurons. Muscles are composed of large numbers of long, thin muscle fibers that contract when they are stimulated by motor neurons. Each muscle is supplied by tens of thousands of motor neurons that constitute its motor pool. Each motor neuron contacts a small number of muscle fibers that make up what is called a motor unit. Because every muscle fiber is supplied by only one motor neuron, the motor units are controlled entirely independently.

must be controlled very precisely, has nearly three thousand motor neurons (Feinstein et al. 1955). The size principle has considerable significance for instrumentalists because it means that the greatest control over movement is achieved only when the forces used are at a minimum. This is just one of several reasons why a conscious effort should be made to relax the fingers as much as possible during playing in order to eliminate excessive or inappropriate muscle contraction.

Sensory neurons. The second class of nerve cell that we need to consider is the sensory neuron. These neurons carry information from the skin, muscles, joints, and organs to the central nervous system. They have an unusual structure, however, as the cell body does not lie at the end of the axon, but on a side branch part of the way along its length (fig. 1-3). The cell bodies form a cluster known as the dorsal root or segmental ganglion. The axons then continue on their way to the spinal cord, where they end mostly in the dorsal region of the gray matter (the dorsal horn).

There are several categories of sensory neurons, each of which carries a particular type of sensation. We will first consider the nerve cells that supply the skin and are concerned with temperature and pain and with different types of tactile sensation. The information they carry is described as exteroceptive because in the main it concerns the interaction of the body with the external world. Figure 1-2B is a diagram of the skin showing the peripheral endings of the main classes of exteroceptive sensory neurons. Some of these axons have unadorned, naked endings and others are encapsulated by other types of cells that modify their response properties. Some naked endings respond to painful stimuli or to temperature, while others wrap around hair follicles and are activated by hair movement. In the superficial layers of the skin, two types of encapsulated endings are found, Meissner's corpuscles and Merkel cell endings. The sensory nerve cells associated with Meissner's corpuscles respond transiently to indentation of the skin and so can detect brief, rapidly changing contact. Merkel cell endings have a more prolonged response to contact. Because the endings of these nerve cells are clustered close together in the most sensitive regions of the body, such as the fingertips and the lips, they provide detailed information of the shape or texture of the surface that is making contact with the skin. They would therefore allow the precise position of a string or a key under the pad of the finger to be monitored. In the deeper layers of the skin there are two additional categories of encapsulated sensory endings, the Pacinian and Ruffini corpuscles. Pacinian corpuscle endings are sensitive to vibration such as that from a string or from the surface of the instrument. Ruffini endings respond to shear stresses generated when the outer layers of the skin are being dragged parallel to the surface, creating tension with the deeper layers. This might occur when our grip is slipping or in string playing, when the finger is rocked to create vibrato. The relevance of these different exteroceptive sensations for musicians is therefore obvious.

Not all sensory nerve cells respond to exteroceptive information. An important component of sensation originates from the body itself. This is known as proprioception. Proprioceptors (fig. 1-3A) provide information about the degree of muscle contraction and the level of tension in tendons (for example, as a consequence of the weight being supported) and the angle at which a joint is being held. We do not need to look at our arms or fingers to have an awareness of their position. Proprioception plays a major role in such basic activities as the maintenance of balance as well as in the control of highly skilled movements. Proprioceptive feedback is particularly important when we are learning a new activity such as playing an instrument. For many instruments, one of the crucial early skills that must be acquired is the ability to position the hands and fingers accurately without looking at them, and this depends on proprioception. It is also important when learning the fingering of a new piece of music. After the brain has sent the signal to activate the muscles, their performance is monitored by proprioception. Through repetition, the movements are refined by comparing what is actually happening with what was intended. Though part of this monitoring process comes from what we hear, a significant part also comes from how the movement feels. An internal image of technique (motor memory) is thus gradually built up until the movements become accurate and automatic. This is particularly crucial for violinists, cellists, and viola players, who must devote a significant proportion of practice time to establishing the precise positioning of the fingers on which accurate intonation depends.

Interneurons. The sensory neurons and motor neurons carry information to and from the spinal cord, respectively, but by far the most abundant nerve cells within the nervous system are those that connect neurons. These are called interneurons (fig. 1-3). Within the spinal cord they are necessary for many simple activities such as reflexes. They also carry information from the cord to the brain and vice versa. Though we will not consider the details of how they operate, they are responsible for all the complex functions that are carried out by the central nervous system, some of which are discussed in chapters 8 and 9.

The Peripheral Nervous System

The peripheral nervous system is composed of the nerves that run from the spinal cord to supply the rest of the body. These nerves therefore carry the axons of sensory and motor neurons, but in addition they contain axons belonging to what is known as the autonomic nervous system. This component of the nervous system will be dealt with in chapter 10 as it plays an important role in the response of the body to stress. The neurons of the autonomic nervous system control the smooth muscle of the organs and arteries. They also supply the sweat glands of the skin, the secretory tissue that keeps the lining of the nose and throat moist, the salivary glands, and glands in the stomach and intestine that secrete digestive enzymes.

Bundles of axons are easily damaged and so nerves are structured to give them protection. Where they pass in narrow channels close to the bone or between muscles, they may be compressed or trapped when the muscles contract, and where they cross joints they may rub against the bone or be stretched significantly as the joint is flexed or extended. The major nerves therefore have a tough outer sheath that helps to limit the degree of stretching, while within they are reinforced by fibers such as collagen. To prevent the axon bundles from being crushed, the spaces between them are packed with fatty tissue that plays a similar role to bubble wrap. Small nerves, such as those running along the sides of the fingers, are less well protected and are sometimes pinched against the bone when a string is plucked or by the pressure needed to support an instrument. Unless severed completely, nerves that are damaged will often regrow, but this is a slow process as it runs at a rate of about one millimeter per day.

THE NATURE OF PAIN AND ITS TREATMENT

Because pain is a major symptom of many performance-related physical problems, it is important to understand the nature and properties of its various manifestations. Sensations that we interpret as pain are carried by a particular class of sensory nerve endings that require very strong stimuli to activate them, that is, they have a high threshold. Biologists and clinicians make a clear distinction between nociception, which is the perception of intense sensory stimulation indicative of tissue damage, and pain itself, which is the unpleasant subjective sensation that this creates in our minds. Whether we perceive a noxious stimulus as pain depends on our mental state. A serious wound incurred in battle or when fleeing from danger may not feel painful until much later, when the immediate threat has diminished. On the other hand, quite innocuous physical stimulation of the skin may under some circumstances feel exceedingly painful. In the context of performance-related injury, pain may be made worse by anxiety or by changes that occur in the central nervous system when a noxious signal lasts for a prolonged period of time.

The electrical pulses that run along all sensory nerves are identical, regardless of whether the sensation that gives rise to them is perceived as pleasant, unpleasant, or neutral. If we use the analogy of a telephone network, each type of sensation (modality) has its own line carrying similar electrical signals that represent words, regardless of their import. However, though the line that carries nociceptive information is similar to the rest, it is given a priority because it runs to the "red emergency telephone." This is the one we cannot afford to ignore. It always gets our attention and triggers an alarm that the brain labels as pain. The sensation of pain therefore originates there and not in the peripheral nervous system or spinal cord.

There are two phases to nociception. When we suffer an injury such as a cut or a blow, there is an initial sharp, well-localized pain that comes from rapidly transmitting sensory nerve fibers (Aδ fibers). This is followed by a duller and more diffuse pain, carried by slower conducting sensory fibers (C fibers), that lasts for a longer period of time. The C fibers also respond to noxious heat but can be stimulated by the active chemical ingredient in chili powder (capsaicin), which interacts with the same proteins in the nerve ending that are influenced by heat. In other words, to the nervous system, real heat and the effect of capsaicin are identical. Capsaicin can be used to deactivate these sensory fibers and this is why people who eat a lot of spicy food cease to be strongly affected by it. In some situations capsaicin is used therapeutically to reduce the sensitivity to pain.

Pain is essential to normal life, as it often prevents severe injury by alerting us to dangerous situations; for example, it stops us from drinking very hot liquids, from maintaining skin contact with sharp or hot objects, or from putting weight on injured joints and ligaments. Low levels of pain or discomfort encourage us to change position regularly, whether awake or asleep, thus preventing skin pressure sores or the maintenance of stressful postures.

Nerve cells communicate with each other using chemicals called neurotransmitters. In the case of sensory nerve cells, this is the amino acid glutamate. However, the sensory neurons of the pain system also contain small proteins (peptides) such as substance P or CGRP, which are released within the gray matter of the spinal cord by the axons of sensory neurons, together with glutamate. Indeed, the sensation of moderate to severe pain is dependent on this release of substance P. The peptides are also released from the other end of the sensory neurons, at the endings that lie within the skin, muscles, and joints. Here, substance P induces the release of other chemicals (e.g., histamine) from cells within the damaged tissue, and together these not only promote inflammation but also increase the sensitivity of nociceptive sensory endings to further stimulation. This is known as hyperalgesia. Some nociceptive nerve endings are completely unresponsive to mechanical stimulation until they have been sensitized in this way. In addition, other compounds promoting inflammation and hyperalgesia are formed from the breakdown of damaged cells at the site of injury. Among these are the prostaglandins. Painkillers such as aspirin and ibuprofen block the production of prostaglandins and so not only reduce pain, but also limit inflammation. For this reason they are often described as nonsteroidal anti-inflammatories (NSAIDs) to distinguish them from the steroid compounds that are used to reduce inflammation alone.

The effect of prolonged stimulation of nociceptive sensory nerve cells is to cause a buildup of substance P within the spinal cord. This leads to a progressive increase (windup) in the activity of the pain pathways, which increases the sensitivity to pain (secondary hyperalgesia). In addition, sensory endings from the undamaged area around the wound, endings that normally carry innocuous sensations perceived as touch, may start to generate the sensation of pain. This is known as allodynia and is the result of changes in the circuitry within the spinal cord that handles sensation. Normally this quickly returns to normal as the peripheral swelling resolves and the injury heals; however, in long-term (chronic) pain states it can become very difficult for the spinal circuits to switch back to more normal states of sensation.

Though, as described above, different types of sensation run to a large extent in distinct channels, there is nevertheless a degree of interaction between them. This is central to the well-known "gate theory" of pain processing. This proposes a mechanism by which the access of the nociceptive sensory signals to the pain pathways that ascend from the spinal cord up into the brain can be blocked under certain circumstances. One way in which this can be achieved is by the simultaneous intervention of a mild sensory stimulus. We are all familiar with this process. When we collide with some hard object, we rub the affected area to close the "gate" and hence lessen the pain. The gate can also be closed by the action of drugs such as opium and its derivatives (e.g., laudanum, morphine), which have been used for centuries to control severe pain. How this is achieved has only quite recently been discovered. It transpires that the nervous system contains its own opium-like chemicals called endorphins and enkephalins. These are neurotransmitters used by nerve cells that block pain by preventing the transfer of information from the nociceptors to the spinal pain pathways. Morphinelike drugs mimic this action but in a more powerful way. The ability of our mental state to influence pain perception comes about partly via pathways that descend from the brain to stimulate the endorphin- and enkephalin-containing nerve cells. Descending pathways also use other means to close the pain gate, such as reducing the buildup of substance P in the spinal cord. However, the brain can not only reduce our sensitivity to pain, it can also enhance it. If you are apprehensive about receiving an injection, it will be a more painful experience than if you are unconcerned, or if the nurse skillfully distracts your attention at the moment the needle goes in. Pain perception is not only influenced by expectation but also by mood. For example, anxiety and depression both enhance pain perception, as does a negative outlook and tendency to expect the worst (sometimes known as catastrophization). People with a more positive outlook, and greater ability to cope with life's problems, are more likely to have higher thresholds to pain.

This may be linked to a feeling of having a degree of control over the situation that leads to the pain. For this reason, psychological as well as pharmacological strategies have an important role in the treatment of chronic pain states.

A comprehensive account of the current understanding of the phenomenon of pain can be found in the definitive book on the subject by Melzac and Wall (Wall, McMahon, and Koltzenburg 2006). Though this weighty tome contains a great deal of information about the origin and treatment of different types of pain, it also makes clear just how much we do not yet understand about pain states and how to manipulate them.

REFERENCES

Blum, J., and G. Ritter. 1990. Violinists and violists with masses under the left side of the angle of the jaw known as "fiddler's neck." *Med Prob Perform Artists* 5 (4):155–60.

Feinstein, B., B. Lindegard, E. Nyman, and G. Wohlfart. 1955. Morphologic studies of motor units in normal human muscles. *Acta Anat (Basel)* 23 (2):127–42.

Gambichler, T., S. Boms, and M. Freitag. 2004. Contact dermatitis and other skin conditions in instrumental musicians. *BMC Dermatol* 4 (1):3.

Hamilton, A. F., K. E. Jones, and D. M. Wolpert. 2004. The scaling of motor noise with muscle strength and motor unit number in humans. *Exp Brain Res* 157 (4):417–30.

Harvell, J., and H. I. Maibach. 1992. Skin diseases among musicians. *Med Prob Perform Artists* 7:114–20.

Okner, M. A. O., T. Kernozek, and M. G. Wade. 1997. Chin rest pressure in violin players: Musical repertoire, chin rests and shoulder pads as possible mediators. *Med Prob Perform Artists* 12:112–21.

Onder, M., A. B. Aksakal, M. O. Oztas, and M. A. Gurer. 1999. Skin problems of musicians. *Int J Dermatol* 38 (3):192–95.

Thomas, P., F. Rueff, and B. Przybilla. 2000. Cheilitis due to nickel contact allergy in a trumpet player. *Contact Dermatitis* 42 (6):351–52.

Wall, P. D., S. B. McMahon, and M. Koltzenburg. 2006. *Wall and Melzack's textbook of pain.* 5th ed. Philadelphia: Elsevier/Churchill Livingstone.

Chapter Two

Posture and the Back in Musical Performance

Even in players with good posture, many instruments impose asymmetrical stresses on the muscles of the back, and at professional as well as amateur levels, many performers make life difficult for themselves by assuming unnecessarily tortuous positions while playing. If you watch the posture of musicians when they return to the stage to acknowledge the applause, you will often see that they still stand asymmetrically when not playing (or even carrying) their instruments. In order to avoid playing-related injury it is therefore important not only to minimize the stresses on the body while performing, but also to reduce or eliminate the spillover of playing posture into everyday life. It can become a rather tedious habit to find yourself being distracted from the music by analyzing the postures of performers on stage, particularly if you insist on sharing your observations with your companions; however, it is very instructive. Large ensembles such as orchestras are the most interesting in this regard, as they allow a direct comparison between players of the same instruments. It will soon become obvious that postures vary widely and some are inherently more risky than others in terms of potential injury. When you have read the material in this chapter and the next, much of this will become clear to you, as the principles behind correct posture are quite straightforward. Promoting safe and sustainable posture is also fundamental to optimizing musical performance and should be a component in instrumental teaching from the earliest stages. This is much easier to instill right from the beginning than to correct later. In this chapter we shall start by exploring the anatomy of the back. We will then look in some detail at the origins of back pain, how this is related to the playing posture of different instruments, and how it can best be avoided. Finally, we shall examine the vexing question of seating, a subject that is only just beginning to get the attention it deserves.

STRUCTURE OF THE VERTEBRAL COLUMN (SPINE)

The spine or vertebral column is composed of a series of thirty-three bones (vertebrae) that run from the base of the skull to the pelvis (fig. 2-1A). These are divided into five

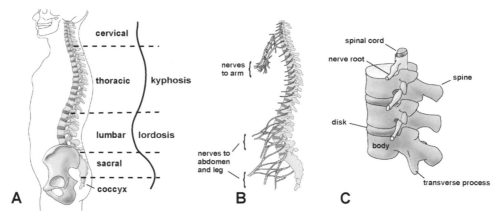

Figure 2-1. The vertebral column and pelvis as seen from the side. **A.** There are seven cervical vertebrae in the neck, twelve thoracic vertebrae each supporting a pair of ribs, five lumbar vertebrae, five sacral vertebrae that are fused to the pelvis, and four coccygeal vertebrae that form a single bony mass. Each section of the vertebral column is curved in a characteristic fashion when the body is held erect. **B.** The root of a large segmental nerve emerges from between each pair of vertebrae. Many of the cervical roots merge and branch in a complex fashion to supply the arm; an equally complex system of lumbar and sacral roots supplies the leg. **C.** A more detailed view of the origin of the segmental nerves as they emerge from the central space within the vertebral column, which carries the spinal cord.

groups. The neck is supported by the upper seven or cervical vertebrae; the twelve thoracic vertebrae are each attached to a pair of ribs; five lumbar vertebrae support the abdomen; the five sacral vertebrae are immobile, being rigidly fixed to the pelvis; and the final four vertebrae are fused together to form the coccyx, a rudimentary tail-like structure. Figures 2-1C and 2-2A, B, show some of the typical features of the vertebrae. The central element is a short column of spongy bone called the vertebral body, which carries the weight of the trunk. The area of the vertebral body increases progressively from the first cervical to the last lumbar vertebra as the length of the column and the weight that it must bear increases. Behind the vertebral body is a channel that contains the spinal cord and this is protected by an arch of bone (the neural arch). A pair of segmental nerves arise from the spinal cord at the level of each vertebra and emerge through openings on each side of the neural arch (figs. 2-1B, C). A number of bony projections arise from the arch. These provide attachment sites for ligaments and muscles that support the spine. They also carry the smooth articular surfaces of some of the joints that link adjacent vertebrae or support the ribs. Usually there is one dorsal process called a spine, which sticks out from the apex of the arch (and therefore points toward the skin surface), and one transverse process emerging from each side.

The flat upper and lower surfaces of the bodies of adjacent vertebrae do not make direct contact with one another. Instead they are separated by the cushionlike intervertebral disks, which act as shock absorbers (fig. 2-2). These have a tough, fibrous, ring-like outer wall (the annulus fibrosus) composed of several layers of cartilage whose fibers run in different directions like the reinforcement of a cross-ply tire. The annulus fibrosus is firmly attached to the vertebral bodies above and below. At the center of

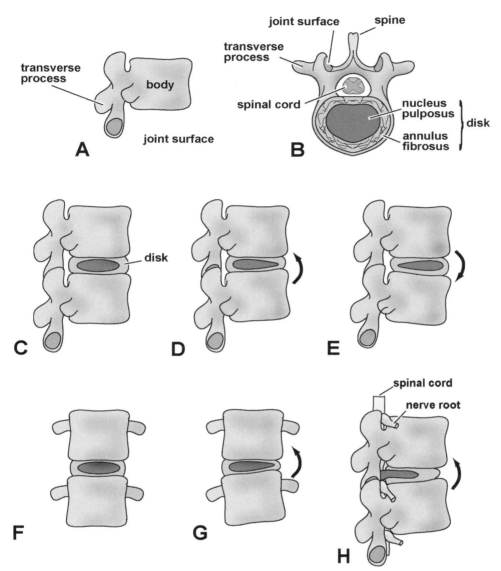

Figure 2-2. The lumbar vertebrae and their disks. A, B. One of the lumbar vertebrae viewed (A) from the side and (B) from above. The main load-bearing parts of the vertebrae are the vertebral bodies. These sit one above the other, separated by the intervertebral disks. The disks have a distortable, gelatinous core (nucleus pulposus) contained by a fibrous wall (annulus fibrosus) that acts rather like the wall of a tire. Behind this lies the channel containing the spinal cord. The spine and transverse processes provide attachment sites for the muscles and ligaments of the back. Adjacent vertebrae are linked by several small joints that help maintain alignment when the vertebral column is flexed, extended, or rotated. C–G. Views of the upper lumbar vertebrae as seen from the side (C–E) and directly in front (F–G) showing how the nucleus pulposus of an intervertebral disk is distorted as the vertebrae move relative to one another. H. If the annulus ruptures, the nucleus pulposus may be extruded so that it compresses either the spinal cord or the nerve roots emerging from it. This is known as a prolapsed or "slipped" disk.

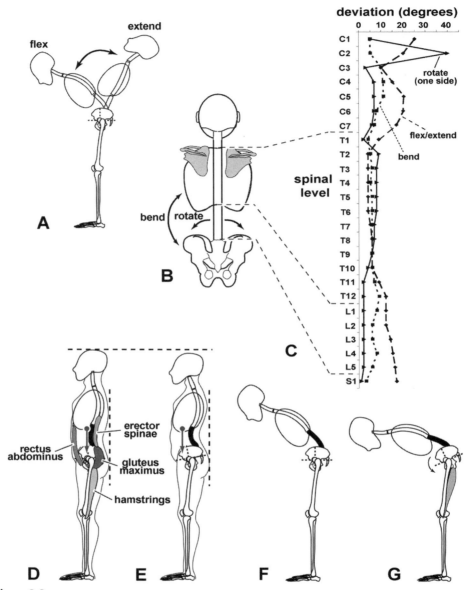

Figure 2-3

the disk is a deformable gel-filled core called the nucleus pulposus. In a young adult, the nucleus pulposus is 90 percent water with the remaining 10 percent being made up of water-absorbing proteins. Water is incompressible, and so provides a good buffer between the bony surfaces of the vertebral bodies, but the wall of the nucleus pulposus is flexible and can be distorted as the angle between the vertebrae changes when the spine is tilted forward or back, or from side to side. The degree of distortion that is possible in the nucleus pulposus is limited by the annulus fibrosus. In effect,

Figure 2-3. A–C. Ranges of spinal movement. The movements of the vertebral column can be described as flexion, extension, rotation, and lateral bending (A, B). The total range of movement is the sum of the movement possible at the joints between adjacent vertebrae, shown graphically in C. The joints of the thoracic vertebrae (T1–T12) allow the least movement, partly because of the rigidity of the rib cage, while those of the neck (C1–C7) have the most freedom. The joint between the first two neck vertebrae (C1–C2) allows the greatest degree of rotation (about 40° to either side). The lumbar vertebrae bear the weight of the trunk but are supported only by muscles, and so although considerable flexion and extension and a smaller amount of lateral bending are possible, rotation is severely limited by the shape of the small joints between them, thus imparting some degree of stability. D–G. Standing posture. In the diagrams shown here and in figure 2-5, the dashed reference lines centered on the hip joint indicate the degree of pelvic rotation in various postures relative to the joint's position in an erect stance. D. When standing fully erect, maximum height is attained. The center of gravity of the trunk lies in front of the vertebral column and so the trunk must be held erect by the active involvement of muscles of the back, abdomen, and legs (arrows). If the muscles are allowed to relax, the abdominal wall becomes more prominent and the pelvis rotates forward. This increases the curvature of the lumbar spine (increased lordosis) and the shoulders move forward, resulting in a reduction of height. F. When the trunk bends forward during standing, the first 60° of the movement is brought about by flexion of the lumbar spine, which reverses its curvature (i.e., it becomes kyphotic). G. In normal individuals, a further 25° of flexion can be achieved by allowing the pelvis to rotate forward. This rotation is limited by the length of the hamstring muscles, which run from the back of the pelvis to below the knee. Further rotation requires flexing of the knee to give the muscle more play.

the vertebrae roll over the nucleus pulposus as if it were a rubber ball sitting at the center of the disk, giving the spine its flexibility. The compression acting on the disk when we are upright forces some of the water out, and though the nucleus can counter this to some degree by absorbing salts to draw water in again by osmosis, the spine typically shortens by a couple of centimeters in the course of a normal day. When we lie down at night, the pressure on the disk is relieved and the water content increases again. As we get older the proportion of water in the nucleus pulposus is reduced by approximately one-third and this, together with the fact that older people tend to stand less erect, is one of the main reasons height declines with age.

If the vertebrae were only linked via the intervertebral disks, the spine would be very unstable, and constant and considerable muscular effort would be required to hold it erect. In practice, the degree to which adjacent vertebrae can move relative to one another is restricted by the presence of smaller accessory joints (zygapophysial joints) that link vertical flanges that rise from the neural arches of adjacent vertebrae. These joints are stabilized by short ligaments that limit their range of movement and further reduce the amount of muscular work needed to maintain an erect posture.

The degree of movement that is possible between adjacent vertebrae varies considerably in different regions of the spine. Bowing forward is described as flexing the spine, while bending backward is known as extension (fig. 2-3A). The first cervical vertebra (the atlas) lacks a vertebral body, but the shape of the load-bearing joints that support the skull allows significant flexion and extension movements (as in nodding) but virtually no rotation of the head on the neck (turning the head from side to side). In contrast, the joint between the atlas and second cervical vertebra (the axis) is the one at which the most rotation can take place. This allows the head to turn through an angle of about 40° to each side (fig. 2-3C). The thoracic vertebrae carry the ribs; at the front of the chest these are linked either to each other or to a flat plate of bone called the sternum (breastbone) (fig. 2-4A). The linkages between the ribs and the sternum are made of flexible cartilage, but the box formed by the chest wall is quite rigid. This considerably restricts the range of movement possible between the thoracic vertebrae (fig. 2-3C). It might be expected that the lumbar vertebrae would have a much greater freedom of movement, and this is certainly true for flexion and extension; however, the amount of side-to-side bending and the degree of rotation possible at each joint are actually rather small. This is a consequence of the position and orientation of the facets of the accessory joints between the vertebrae. If the degree of movement between the lumbar vertebrae were greater, it would put intolerable demands on the muscles of the back that maintain lumbar stability. The total flexibility of the spine in any one direction is of course the sum of the movement possible at each joint, so even though the relative motion between pairs of adjacent vertebrae is small, when this is summed over the twenty-five movable joints that lie between them, the total angle through which the spine can be bent is considerable. The head can be flexed and extended on the cervical vertebrae through a total angle of 100°, while for the entire vertebral column this angle can be as much as 250° (Kapandji 2000), though we generally see such extreme bending only in gymnasts.

Even in a person with normal posture who is standing or sitting erect, the spine is far from straight. If the body is held in what is known as vertical alignment (with the shoulder joint lying on a vertical line above the hip and ankle joints), the spine exhibits several pronounced curvatures. These are described by the terms *kyphosis* and *lordosis*. If we think of the curves as being shaped like the letter "C," kyphosis refers to the situation where the opening of the C faces the front of the body, while in lordosis the opening faces the back (fig. 2-1A). When we stand erect, the cervical spine has a slight lordosis, the thoracic spine has a clear kyphosis, the lumbar spine exhibits a marked lordosis, and the fused sacral and coccygeal vertebrae are together kyphotic. This can change when other postures are adopted. When we sit in a chair and slump forward, the lumbar spine straightens and ultimately becomes kyphotic. Somewhat confusingly, while many writers apply the terms *kyphosis* and *lordosis* to the normal curvatures of the erect spine as I have done here, others use them only to describe curvatures that deviate from the norm. When seen from directly behind, the spine should appear straight. A strong lateral curvature of the spine (scoliosis) is usually symptomatic of disease, though small lateral deviations can develop as a result of everyday activities such as habitually carrying a heavy bag by a strap over one shoulder. If this posture is maintained, it can lead to discomfort or pain. We will return to this topic later when discussing the playing postures of instrumentalists.

The vertebrae are held in position by a series of ligaments that help to limit the potential displacement between them. Some of these run along the walls of the central space that carries the spinal cord. One such ligament (the ligamentum flavum) runs down the roof of the neural arches beneath the spines of the vertebrae. Unlike most of the other ligaments, which are relatively inextensible, the ligamentum flavum is elastic and thus holds the spine under tension when it is in the erect position. A long, broad external ligament links the front of the bodies of the vertebrae for the entire length of the vertebral column, while a narrower one links the back of the vertebral bodies. Short external ligaments run between adjacent spines and transverse processes. The cervical vertebrae receive additional support from a large sail-like ligament (the nuchal ligament) that passes downward from the back of the skull. This not only braces the vertebrae of the neck, but also provides an attachment site for several muscles.

We have already seen that the annulus fibrosus of the intervertebral disks links the bodies of vertebrae. The smaller joints that link the vertebrae to each other and to their ribs are held together by sheets of tissue that form a joint capsule (see chapter 1). These capsules not only limit the vertebrae's range of movement but also serve to contain the synovial fluid, which lubricates the joint. Though the spinal ligaments are important in keeping the vertebrae in alignment, they do not impart much strength to the vertebral column which, being composed of a series of blocks stacked one above the other, remains quite unstable. The load that would collapse the unsupported spine is several hundred times less than the weight it must support as we carry out our normal daily activities; it is only through the action of muscles that the necessary stability can be achieved. In addition, even when we stand erect, the center of gravity of the trunk lies in front of the vertebral column, which must be actively braced by muscles against a force that is trying to flex it forward.

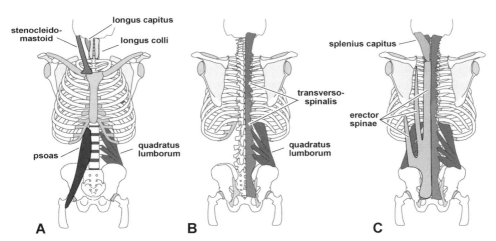

Figure 2-4. **The basic organization of the postural muscles of the back. A. The vertebral column seen from the front showing some of the major muscles acting on the head and neck. The longus capitus muscles act on the head, pulling it downward, while the longus colli flex the neck forward. The sternocleidomastoid, which rotates the head to the opposite side and upward, runs from the skull, just behind the ear, to the collarbone and sternum. The psoas muscle runs from the side of the lumbar vertebral bodies to the femur and can act to increase lumbar lordosis. The quadratus lumborum runs from the transverse processes of the lumbar vertebrae to the edge of the pelvis and can flex the trunk to the side. B. The vertebral column from the back. The deep muscles of the vertebral column are collectively called transversospinalis. They stabilize the individual vertebrae and contribute to their ability to move relative to one another. C. The superficial muscles that act directly on the vertebral column are collectively known as the erector spinae. These, and the splenius capitus muscle, are the major muscles responsible for extending the spine when active on both sides and for rotating the spine when acting on one side only.**

MUSCLES ACTING ON THE SPINE

The basic layout of the major muscles acting on the vertebral column is shown in figure 2-4.

The Neck

We will first consider the muscles of the neck, which can be divided into three groups: 1) those that link the vertebrae to each other, 2) those that run between the vertebral column and the base of the skull, and 3) those that are not attached to the vertebrae but act on the neck indirectly.

Attached to the front of the neck vertebrae are the prevertebral muscles (fig. 2-4A), which flex the neck (i.e., pull the head forward and down). The longus colli series (literally, the long muscles of the neck) run between the cervical and upper thoracic vertebrae and therefore act only on the neck, while the longus capitus muscles (the long muscles of the head) are attached at one end to the cervical vertebrae and at the other to the base of the skull and therefore act mainly to tilt the head forward. In addition, two small rectus (straight) muscles run between the skull and the first of the cervical vertebrae to stabilize the head. The head and neck are also moved by two large muscles that run like guy ropes from behind the ear to the collarbone and the sternum. These are the sternocleidomastoid muscles, which can often be seen forming a V-shaped ridge in people with thin necks. Because their attachment to the skull lies behind the axis of rotation and the point of balance of the head on the neck, they turn the face upward when they contract together. If only one is active, the face is also turned to the opposite side. Because of their attachment to the sternum, the sternocleidomastoids can also be considered accessory muscles of respiration (see chapter 4).

The organization of the muscles at the back of the neck, which extend it (tilting the head upward), is rather more complicated. One set of muscles (e.g., the upper muscles of the transversospinalis and erector spinae groups) runs from the cervical to the upper thoracic vertebrae and act only on the neck, while another set (e.g., splenius capitus) runs from the vertebrae to the back of the skull and tilts the head backward (fig. 2-4B, C). In addition, there are two sets of small rectus and oblique muscles that run from the upper two cervical vertebrae to the back of the skull to stabilize the head. A number of muscles also connect the vertebral column to the back of the skull and the shoulder blade (scapula). The shoulder blade is not directly attached to the trunk but is suspended from it by several sets of muscles and is therefore highly mobile (see chapter 3). The position of the shoulder blade has considerable significance for the playing posture adopted by violin and viola players, and so some of the muscles attached to it will be considered here (see fig. 3-3). Of particular significance in this context are those that raise the left shoulder and pull it inward when the instrument is held under the chin. The shoulder blade is shaped like an inverted triangle, with a prominent ridge or spine running approximately horizontally across the back. Sets of small muscles, the levator scapulae, run down from the upper cervical vertebrae to the inner corner of the triangle and pull it upward. Below these are two broad rhomboid muscles that pull the inner edge of the shoulder blade toward the spine. Over the surface of these lies a triangular sheet of muscle called the trapezius, the upper part of which runs from the back of the skull and the nuchal ligament to the spine of the scapula and is active when the shoulders are shrugged. As these shoulder muscles are attached at each end to a movable structure (the scapula or the vertebral column), their effect depends on which end is held in a fixed position. Therefore, although they are usually described in terms of their effect on the scapula, if this is held fixed by the action of other muscles, it is the head or neck that is moved. This is an important general principle of muscle action that is sometimes not made clear in standard descriptions of their actions, and we will encounter it again later. In fact, in many actions, there is a degree of movement of the bones at both ends of such muscles, within the tolerances set by the actions of other muscles, ligaments, and joints. From the foregoing account it will be appreciated that there are many superimposed layers of muscles in the neck and shoulders. These are often chronically and unnecessarily held in tension as a result of emotional stress, and many tension-relieving strategies (e.g., massage) pay particular attention to this area.

The Thoracic and Lumbar Spine

There are no muscles equivalent to longus colli running on the front surface of the vertebral bodies of the lower thoracic or lumbar vertebrae. This region of the vertebral column is flexed mainly by the muscle that forms the front wall of the abdomen, the rectus abdominus (popularly known as the "six pack"), which runs between the lower ribs and the midregion of the pelvis (figs. 2-3D, 4-3). In this it is aided by the action of the psoas muscle (fig. 2-4A), which runs from the lateral surfaces of the bodies of the lumbar vertebrae to the top of the femur (thighbone). The psoas can also move the thigh, but when the femur is carrying the weight of the body, its position is fixed, so the action of the psoas is to flex the lumbar spine. On either side of the rectus abdominus, the muscular wall of the abdomen is formed by three sheets of oblique and transverse muscle fibers (fig. 4-3). The abdomen is a sealed chamber, so if all of the muscles in its walls contract at the same time, the pressure within it rises, and as its circumference is reduced, the visceral organs are pushed up toward the chest cavity. If the breath is held at the same time, keeping the volume of the chest constant, the trunk becomes rigid, like an inflated ball, and can provide support to resist forward flexion of the spine. This is a common strategy we use when trying to lift a heavy weight from the floor and is seen in its most extreme form in weightlifters.

The arrangement of the muscles on the dorsal surface of the back is quite complicated; however, they are usually divided into a deep group and a superficial group (fig. 2-4B, C). The muscles of the deep layer run between the transverse process of one vertebra and the spinous or transverse process of a vertebra several segments above. These muscles stabilize and extend the vertebral column when active on both sides at the same time and cause rotation when active on one side only. The more superficial muscles, collectively called the erector spinae, run between the spinal processes of the vertebrae, or between the bases of the ribs. When the erector spinae on both sides are active simultaneously, they cause extension of the vertebral column, and when active on one side only, lateral bending. When the actively extended back is viewed from behind, two muscular columns are visible beneath the skin on either side of a central groove. The groove represents the position of the spinous processes of the vertebrae and the columns, the collective bulk of the deep and superficial muscle masses. In addition to these muscles, a broad sheet (the quadratus lumborum) runs from the back of the pelvis to the transverse processes of the lumbar vertebrae and the base of the lowest rib, forming part of the muscular wall at the back of the abdomen. Its action contributes to the lateral bending of the lumbar spine.

If we bend forward from the waist, starting from the fully erect standing position with the knees straight, the movement through the first 60° is that allowed by the joints between the vertebrae. The weight of the trunk is supported by progressively increasing activity in the erector spinae and deep muscles of the back. The pelvis is held fixed by the action of the large muscles of the buttocks (the gluteus maximus) and the hamstring muscles at the back of the thighs (fig. 2-3D–G). The gluteus maximus runs from the back of the pelvis to the femur while the hamstrings run from the back of the pelvis to the lower leg, just below the knee. We normally think of these muscles in terms of their ability to move the femur or flex the knee joint; however, when the leg is fixed and the knee locked to carry our weight, these muscles instead rotate the pelvis backward. When we need to bend the trunk forward beyond 60°, the gluteus maximus and hamstring muscles relax, allowing the pelvis to rotate forward relative to the femur by about 25°, the weight being borne by the elasticity of the muscles and their tendons. The length of the hamstrings determines the maximum possible angle of forward pelvic rotation. If the knees are bent, this slackens the hamstrings, allowing the pelvis to be rotated much further. For the same reason, the angle of the knees is one factor that determines the pelvic rotation possible when we are sitting.

Because the center of gravity of the trunk lies in front of the vertebral column, there is a tendency for it to flex forward during standing (fig. 2-3E). If this is allowed to happen, the shoulders slump, causing the curvature of the thoracic spine to increase (kyphosis). The pelvis rotates forward, increasing the lumbar curvature of the spine (lordosis), and as a result, the abdomen bulges outward. When we stand fully erect (fig. 2-3D), our height increases because the tendency to flex forward is resisted by the muscles of the back. The rectus abdominus muscle helps to rotate the pelvis upward under these circumstances, reducing lordosis. In young people, who generally have good muscle tone, these corrective actions are easily maintained, but in older people the loss of muscle strength makes this more difficult, particularly if the mass of the abdomen is increased by obesity. The slumped posture may, as a result, become permanent, or at least habitual. This can be exacerbated by conditions such as osteoporosis, which involves a general loss of bone mass throughout the skeleton and is particularly significant for posture through its effects on the vertebrae. Osteoporosis is common in older women, in whom it is often a consequence of the reduction of circulating steroid hormones after menopause.

The majority of musicians do much of their professional playing while seated. The posture of the spine in sitting is quite different from that in standing. This can be seen in animation 2-1. An excellent review of the effect of sitting on the spine and its consequences for seat design can be found in Harrison et al. (1999). Sitting in any posture puts greater pressure on the intervertebral disks than does standing. This leads to a greater loss of fluid from the nucleus pulposus. The main structures through which the weight of the body is transmitted to the seat of the chair are the lowest points on the pelvis. These are called the ischial tuberosities. The forces acting on these points while we are seated erect on a hard chair rotate the pelvis backward, which reduces lumbar lordosis (fig. 2-5A, animation 2-1). The use of seats with a lumbar support limits this, reducing disk pressure and consequently the severity of the symptoms of low back pain. If the body is allowed to recline farther backward from the erect position, the lumbar spine will reverse its curvature to become kyphotic (fig. 2-5C, animation 2-1). As a result, lumbar support becomes even more important for comfortable sitting. The angle between the trunk and the thighs also has an effect on lumbar curvature through the action of the postural muscles acting on the legs. It has been suggested that when sitting erect, an angle of about 135° between the thighs and the trunk minimizes the tension on the lumbar spine because it allows a reduction in the activity of the thigh muscles, which act on the pelvis and spine (Keegan 1953), and increases lordosis. This is possible because such a posture brings the center of gravity of the upper body directly over the ischial tuberosities, minimizing the tendency of the weight of the trunk to rotate the pelvis (fig. 2-5B, animation 2-1). Under these circumstances, the degree of lumbar curvature lies between that of standing or sitting and approximates to the degree of lordosis seen in the unloaded spine—the so-called neutral position (Adams et al. 2002). To achieve such a posture, either the seat of the chair needs to slope downward at an angle of 45° from horizontal, which would be rather impractical, or, alternatively, the sitter needs to move to its front edge to allow the thighs to slope downward. Office chairs that allow the seat to be tilted typically have a range of adjustment of 7°–15°.

BACK PAIN

About three-quarters of us experience back pain (particularly low back pain) at some stage in our lives. This may reflect an obvious physical injury such as a muscle strain or damaged disk, but often it is impossible to determine the precise source of the pain. In some cases, what have been termed *psychosocial factors* appear to play a significant role in back pain. For example, individuals who find themselves in unrewarding situations (such as unstimulating jobs with poor working conditions) or have illnesses such as depression are more likely to complain of physical problems, as the lack of other compensations makes them more aware of their discomfort. In addition, one symptom of stress is a general increase of muscle tension, particularly in the back, neck, face, and jaw. Directly or indirectly, this may lead to postural problems and back pain.

At one time it was widely accepted that an exaggerated lordosis would inevitably lead to back pain, but objective studies have found little evidence for this (White and Panjabi 1990). Apart from people employed in heavy manual labor, one of the groups in whom back pain is most common is pregnant women. Here the pain derives from the strain of supporting the weight of the growing fetus, which causes the center of gravity of the abdomen to move farther forward from the vertebral axis. This may be exacerbated by the softening of ligaments, including those of the spine, that occurs during pregnancy. In young musicians, occupation-related back pain is most likely to be due to muscle or ligament strains related to maintaining playing postures for long periods of time. In the majority of cases, low back pain is self-limiting, that is, with rest from the stressful position it resolves itself over a period of time. Apart from pain relief, the most suitable treatment is exercise aimed at strengthening the postural muscles that support the back, with the aim of improving the alignment of the vertebral column and reducing the pressure on the disks (Horvath 2002; Paull and Harrison 1997; Richardson and Jull 1995). Bed rest, which was once a commonly prescribed treatment, is now regarded as quite unhelpful as it causes rapid weakening of precisely the sets of muscles that support the spine. Of course, rather than waiting for problems to develop, it is better to adopt a posture that minimizes the risk of developing back pain and to keep the postural muscles in good condition (see below).

Another type of soft-tissue injury that results in back pain is what is commonly known as a "slipped" disk. This is an inappropriate term as the disk does not slip out of position; instead, weakness or damage to the annulus fibrosus allows the nucleus pulposus to push outward through it (fig. 2-2H). This most commonly occurs on straightening the spine following a prolonged period of forward bending (flexion). The disks that are most vulnerable are those of the lower cervical or lower lumbar vertebrae. It is not unusual for more than one disk to be affected; the persistence of pain following treatment is sometimes due to the fact that this has not been recognized. The extruded nucleus pulposus almost always emerges from the back of the disk, and the pain is the result of the pressure this exerts either on the spinal cord or on the nerve roots that emerge from it. The nerve supply to the disks themselves is confined to the outer part of the annulus fibrosus so that we normally have no sensation of pressure in the core. However if the disk degenerates, the sensory nerve endings may invade the nucleus pulposus, causing chronic pain (Freemont et al. 1997)

AVOIDING OCCUPATIONAL BACK PAIN

Lifting and Carrying

One of the reasons the muscles and ligaments of the back are vulnerable to injury is that they run very close to the central axis of the vertebral column, which means that they have a very poor mechanical advantage (i.e., they have a small lever arm) when they act to resist flexion of the spine. As a result, the stresses they are subjected to if the back is bent forward during lifting are extremely large. The farther away from the body the weight being lifted is held, the greater the effective lever arm the weight exerts on the spine and the greater the force that must be resisted by these muscles and ligaments and the disks of the vertebrae. Vertical lifting should therefore be carried out with a straight back using the large muscles of the thighs to provide the power for the lift (fig. 2-5D). The weight should be held as close to the body as possible to reduce its leverage. If instead it is lifted with straight legs and a bent back, it must be supported almost entirely by the erector spinae muscles (fig. 2-5E). In this posture, the downward force on the spine acts across the face of the intervertebral joints, something they are not well designed to cope with. Lifting with the body twisted to the side should also be avoided, as the stresses on the back under these circumstances are about three times as great as if the body is held straight (Hall 2003). Many musical instruments are either in themselves heavy or require robust protection for transport, which adds significantly to their weight. Their awkward shapes may also tempt the owners to adopt risky lifting postures when moving them in confined spaces. The difficulties cannot be eliminated completely if the player is alone, but simple strategies such as adding wheels to cases, or carrying cases on the back using straps over both shoulders so that the weight is supported symmetrically, will greatly reduce the risk of injury. When moving pianos on their wheels, the main impetus should come from pushing rather than pulling. When pushing against the piano, the force exerted on the vertebral column acts to extend the spine. This is counteracted by the rectus abdominus muscle, which is both large and has a high mechanical advantage for flexing the spine (fig. 2-5F). When pulling, the force exerted on the body flexes the spine and this must be resisted by the erector spinae muscles, whose mechanical advantage, as we have seen, is poor.

Playing

Many instruments can be played either standing up or sitting down. As we have seen, the pressure on the disks is lower during standing, so where possible this posture should be adopted for playing. While this is not always possible, for example, when playing in an orchestra or other ensemble, it can at least be used during practice, which often represents a period of several hours a day. Of course even when standing care must be taken to adopt good posture. For example, there is often a tendency to lean forward unnecessarily, which puts extra strain on the back and should be avoided. This may be exacerbated by having the music stand set too low, or may reflect eyesight problems that make reading music from a distance difficult. If the forward leaning is related to the weight of the instrument, frequent short rests should be inserted into practice sessions, and a conscious effort should be made to gradually build up the strength of the erector spinae muscles in order to be able to maintain good posture for the duration of the bouts of playing needed in performance. Tenseness in the muscles of the back, shoulders, neck, and arms due to performance anxiety, worries about making mistakes, or concern that the instrument may slip increase fatigue and have a negative influence on posture. As we are often unaware of such chronic tension, it is necessary to make a conscious effort to take a subjective inventory of tension at regular intervals during playing. An optimum posture is one in which your grip on the instrument is sufficiently firm but flexible, while the playing fingers are relaxed. The back should be supported but not rigid, and the shoulders and neck relaxed. Great players make playing look easy because they have found ways to make playing easy on themselves. Optimizing their posture and eliminating unnecessary tension allows them to play close to the physical limits of the body when necessary, and well within these limits at other times.

The postures adopted by performers on different instruments can be divided into two broad categories: those that at least appear symmetrical and those that are clearly

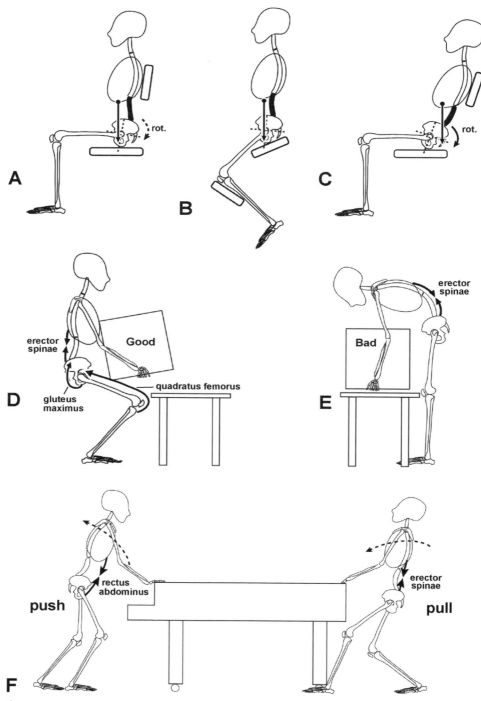

A

rot.

B

C

rot.

D

erector
spinae

Good

gluteus
maximus

quadratus femorus

E

erector
spinae

Bad

F

push

rectus
abdominus

pull

erector
spinae

Figure 2-5

of necessity asymmetrical. Relatively symmetrical postures are used by players of most woodwind instruments, pianists, and percussionists. Those whose postures are significantly asymmetrical include string players, guitarists, brass players, and flutists. Instruments with playing postures that are intrinsically symmetrical pose fewer problems for the back; however, their players may quite unnecessarily adopt overtense or asymmetrical poses that should be consciously avoided. If standing, try to start from a stable posture with the weight taken equally on both feet. This does not mean that you should be rooted to the spot; in fact, changing position frequently is important as this ensures the load is not always carried by the same joints and muscles, but avoid spending long periods with the weight mainly on one leg, as this requires the spine to tilt to that side to bring the center of gravity over the foot. For wind players, extreme forward flexion or side-to-side movements of the trunk will also interfere with breath control by pushing the abdominal organs up into the thorax.

Among the woodwinds, the flute is particularly problematical for posture (fig. 2-6A). There are numerous hand and wrist problems associated with this instrument, which will be discussed in chapter 3, but playing posture may, in addition, cause problems in the shoulder region (Dommerholt 2000). In order to allow the right arm sufficient freedom to move, either the trunk or the neck (or both) must be rotated to enable the mouth to lie parallel with the lip plate. Any tendency to allow the trunk or neck to slump forward simply compounds the problem and should be avoided. This not only puts unnecessary strain on the back but also interferes with breathing. Students are often encouraged to hold the instrument horizontally at shoulder height,

Figure 2-5. A–C. Sitting posture. A. When we sit erect on a chair, the pelvis tends to rotate backward (dashed arrow) because the downward force of the trunk falls behind the point of contact of the pelvis with the seat (the ischial tuberosities). As a result, the degree of lumbar lordosis is reduced compared to that in erect standing. **B.** On a kneeling chair where the angle between the leg and the trunk is about 135°, the center of gravity of the trunk is brought into line with the point of contact of the pelvis with the seat. This minimizes the force rotating the pelvis backward and therefore the muscular effort needed to retain an erect posture. The degree of lumbar lordosis lies between that of erect standing and sitting, close to the form it takes up in the neutral state when no muscles are acting on it. **C.** In a reclining posture, the pelvis is strongly rotated backward because the center of gravity lies well behind the ischial tuberosities. The normal curvature of the lumbar spine is reversed (becomes kyphotic). **D–F. Pushing, pulling, and lifting. D.** When lifting an object, the power should come from the large, strong postural muscles of the leg, such as the quadratus femoris (which straightens the knee) and the gluteus maximus (which extends the hip joint). The back is kept straight; the erector spinae muscles only serve to stabilize it in this position so that the force acting on the body bears directly down onto the joints between the vertebrae. **E.** Lifting with a bent back is more dangerous. The power from the lift must come from the small, weak erector spinae muscles; the force on the spine acts across the plane of the intervertebral joints. The disks are squeezed strongly at the front, making a prolapse at the back that may cause compression of the spinal nerves or spinal cord. **F.** When moving a heavy object across the floor, it is better to push it than to pull it. When pushing, the reactive force of the object on the body extends the spine, causing it to bend backward. This is opposed by the strong rectus abdominus, which forms the front wall of the abdomen and acts with a large mechanical advantage on the vertebrae. When pulling, the reactive force flexes the spine forward. This is resisted by the weaker erector spinae muscles, which have a poorer mechanical advantage.

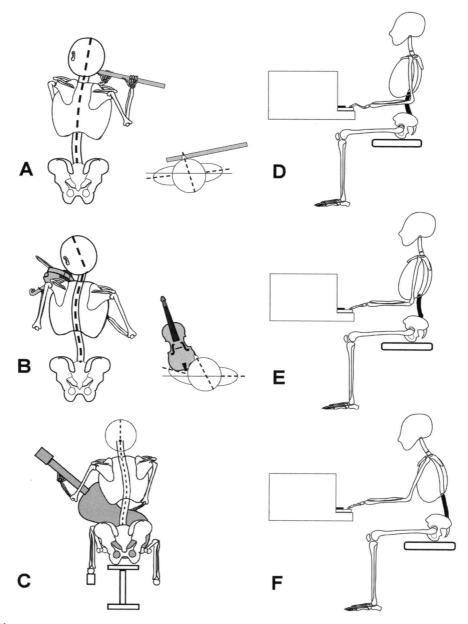

Figure 2-6

Figure 2-6.   A–C. Playing posture for the flute, violin, and guitar. (The postures are exaggerated to make the details more obvious.) A. Of the wind instruments, the flute requires the most awkward posture. The head and trunk are rotated to the left. The left arm is held across the body and the right arm is raised out to the side, which fatigues the muscles of the shoulders. This is often alleviated by tilting the trunk and/or the head to the right. B. A typical stance of violin players, showing the rotation of the head and tilt of the neck and the raised left shoulder, which produces a lateral deflection of the lumbar and thoracic spine. C. The guitar played in the seated position with the left foot raised onto a rest. The pelvis is tilted so that the weight is shifted toward the left ischial tuberosity. The shoulders also slope downward to the left, inducing a strong lateral curvature of the spine. To keep the head vertical, the neck must be deflected to the right. D–F. The effect of piano stool position on posture. The middle figure (E) shows the stool set at an optimal distance, which allows the upper arm to hang close to vertical and the forearm to be nearly horizontal when the fingers touch the keys. The sitting posture is fully erect with good lumbar lordosis, minimizing the amount of muscular effort needed to maintain the posture. In D the stool is set too close to the keyboard. To prevent the chest from projecting over the keyboard, lumbar lordosis is increased. The elbows now lie farther back relative to the trunk. This restricts arm movement, and the shoulders may have to be raised to keep the forearms horizontal, which may also restrict breathing. F. Here the stool is too far from the piano. Because the upper arm is extended, the entire weight of the arm must be supported by muscular effort, whereas when the stool is set at an optimal distance this is only true for the forearm. The trunk is flexed toward the piano, increasing the kyphosis of the thoracic spine, and the neck is extended. The normal lumbar curvature is reduced and may even be reversed. More muscular effort is required to maintain this posture as the center of gravity of the trunk is moved forward.

which requires that the upper arm be slightly elevated. This requires considerable activity in the supraspinatus muscle (see chapter 3). Prolonged contraction of this muscle can restrict its blood supply because the vessels within it are compressed (Dommerholt 2000); as the muscle consequently fatigues, the end of the flute starts to droop, the head is tilted to the right to maintain the correct angle with the head joint, and tension can be caused in the sternocleidomastoid muscle. A compromise in which the head is from the beginning allowed to tilt to the right by a small amount is used by many professional players.

Though it may not be immediately obvious to the observer, playing the trumpet, trombone, or French horn puts considerable asymmetrical strain on the shoulder and trunk musculature. In the first two cases, the instrument is held up and supported for long periods by the left arm. The problems this poses are exacerbated by the greater weight of modern instruments designed with larger bells to produce a bigger sound. The length of the trombone further serves to increase the leverage its weight can exert and a high, tense left shoulder is a common result. While the horn is not held so high, its weight (particularly if it is a double instrument) is considerable and can cause difficulties, especially for young players. One of the long-term physical consequences of playing such instruments is that the muscles that pull the shoulder upward (e.g., the trapezius and to a lesser extent the scalenes and levator scapulae—see chapter 3) are held under chronic tension during playing. The nerves running to the arm pass between the scalene muscles and can become compressed at this point. Because the shoulder and upper arms are extended forward in playing, the muscles that support them in this position (pectoralis major and the anterior fibers of the deltoid) become stronger. This tends to produce a shortening of the muscle fibers, pulling the humerus (the bone of the upper arm) forward in its socket. Muscles at the back of the shoulder that oppose this action and which are, in any case, smaller remain weak as they are used much less. This reduces the diameter of a small channel on top of the shoulder through which passes the tendon of the supraspinatus muscle, which raises the arm out to the side. Here it can become pinched, leading to shoulder pain in what is known as rotator cuff syndrome (see chapter 3). One remedy is to strengthen these weak muscles so that they draw the arm (and also the shoulder) backward to open up the channel again. If the upper arm is allowed to hang vertically and the forearm is held horizontally at a right angle to it, this can be achieved by rotating the arm outward and the shoulders backward against the resistance provided by an elastic exercise band. However, exercises for this type of shoulder problem must be chosen with care and after a proper analysis of the problem, as strengthening the wrong set of muscles may have the opposite effect to the one intended.

Asymmetric postures are unavoidable for players of stringed instruments. The consequences of holding the violin or viola under the chin are several (Kapandji 2000; Wynn Parry 1998). The left shoulder is often raised (hunched) and the chin pressed down into the chin rest. This causes fatigue in muscles, such as the trapezius (see chapter 3), that raise the shoulder. There is also often a tendency to rotate the left shoulder forward. Together these postures cause the thoracolumbar spine to curve to the right while the cervical spine is tilted to the left (fig. 2-6B). The cervical and thoracic regions of the vertebral column will be also be rotated in opposite directions in the horizontal plane. Over time the muscles on the left side of the trunk become stronger at the expense of those on the right, influencing posture even when not playing. The mild deformities of the spine that this produces in string players have been recorded by Bejjani, Kaye, and Benham (1996), who found that the left shoulder was chronically raised in many violinists and that harpists also had a particularly high incidence of scoliosis (29 percent in this sample).

It is important to minimize the deviation of the vertebral column from the normal erect position as much as possible. In the case of violin and viola players, the shoulders should be kept in line with the hips so that there is no torsion of the trunk. The shoulders should be kept down and the temptation to rotate the left shoulder forward resisted. If the instrument feels unstable, the shoulder and chin rests need to be adjusted. For the most part, the head faces forward (so that the neck is not twisted) with the instrument held out to the side. The music stand should therefore be straight in front of the body. It is also important to realize that we are not all identical in size and shape and that how the instrument is held and supported will vary between individuals. For example, the most ergonomically favorable angle at which the instrument is held out to the left will depend on arm length (Fischer 1998). Shoulder and chin rests are generally used to limit the degree to which the head must be tilted on the neck to stabilize the instrument, and tailoring one to suit will need some experimentation, both with different models and their fine adjustments.

The chin rest first appeared in the 1820s and its invention is usually attributed to Louis Spohr (Rabuffetti et al. 2007). It was a response to the greater freedom of movement that was required by the increased technical complexity of the nineteenth-century violin repertoire; however, there is no evidence that its design, either then or subsequently, was based on objectively determined ergonomic principles. With the exception of performers who play baroque music on period instruments, the use of chin rests today is almost universal. The origin of the shoulder rest is less clear, though the use of a pillow under the instrument was mentioned in *L'art du violon* by Baillot in 1834. Prior to this a chamois leather was often used to prevent the instrument from slipping. The expected effect of using a shoulder rest on the muscles involved in gripping the instrument has been confirmed using electromyography. It significantly reduces the activity in the trapezius (which raises the shoulder) and the sternocleidomastoid (which rotates the head to the opposite side and tilts it upward) (Levy et al. 1992). Activity is increased in the anterior fibers of the deltoid, which helps raise the arm out to the side, particularly when the arm is rotated outward as it may be when holding the violin.

When chin rests and shoulder rests are used in combination, it appears that the nature of the former is more significant than that of the latter in determining the degree of force used to hold the instrument (Okner, Kernozek, and Wade 1997). Though the design of the chin rest has a significant effect, it does not always follow the trend predicted. For example, Okner et al. found that a chin rest that was placed more centrally on the instrument, which was predicted to show the lowest loadings, in fact had the highest. There is currently insufficient information to know what aspects of chin rest design have most effect on chin pressure. However, the study found that playing more technically demanding music consistently led to the generation of higher pressures, but whether this was due to a greater requirement for support or the result of tension generated by psychological factors was not investigated.

Tall players with long necks often find that standard rests do not have a sufficient range of adjustment for comfort (Okner, Kernozek, and Wade 1997), and this contributes to the fact that they have a high incidence of posture-related problems, including spasms in the trapezius muscle, strain in other muscles of the neck, and pinching of nerve roots where they emerge from the spine. The consequences of changing the height of the shoulder rest on playing movements was examined in a group of fifteen violinists by Rabuffetti et al. (2007), though the analysis did not take into account the lengths of their necks. The height of the rest used could be adjusted over a range of 40 millimeters. Raising the rest had the beneficial effects of reducing the leftward rotation of the head and the elevation of the left shoulder, which was accompanied by a reduction in activity in the trapezius muscle, and also reduced the internal rotation of that shoulder. The violin was displaced forward and toward the right, but none of the changes affected the players' ability to maintain the correct angle between the bow and the strings. Any postural changes required of the right arm took place at the shoulder and so did not affect the wrist and hand posture used for holding the bow. Increasing the height of the rest did have some negative consequences for shoulder flexion and the degree of arm pronation; therefore, for any player the optimum rest height remains a compromise.

As many commercial shoulder rests have only a limited range of adjustment, it may be necessary to find specialist suppliers for these and for chin rests, or alternatively to invest in a customized support. This can involve having the surface of the rests molded to fit the player (Norris 2000) so that the force generated in holding the instrument is spread evenly over the entire contact area. The position of the chin rest on the instrument may also have to be adjusted in relation to arm length to allow full and free use of the bow. A discussion of some of these issues can be found in Lieberman (2000). It is important to note that young players whose bodies are growing rapidly may need regular adjustments in setup during their teenage years. Some of the postural consequences that may arise from problems with gripping the violin or viola and the effect of their resolution on postural symmetry are shown in animation 2-2. If you can access the commercially available video recordings of David Oistrakh (e.g., in Beethoven's Fifth Violin Sonata), you will see an excellent example of an ergonomic playing posture. Holding the violin under his chin hardly disturbs the symmetry of his head and shoulders, and the mobility of his head demonstrates that little tension is needed to grip the instrument. His fingers are relaxed so that even in the most rapid passagework, he appears to have plenty of time to make each movement.

Because of how the instrument is held, violin and viola players are susceptible to pain at the jaw joint (the temporomandibular joint) and in those who start at a very young age, the face may even become slightly asymmetrical as a result. A habit of exerting greater pressure than necessary is sometimes associated with a clenching of the teeth, which can lead to pain in the temporalis and masseter muscles that close the jaw (see chapter 6). Remodeling and wear of the surfaces of the joint may result, as well as excessive wear and even fracturing of the cusps of the molar teeth (Yeo et al. 2002). If it is consistent with the full use of the bow arm, moving the chin rest to the center of the instrument, so that it lies over the tailpiece, is one way of reducing the forces on the jaw (Blum and Ritter 1990). A common contributory factor to temporomandibular joint problems is stress, and nonplaying consequences such as nocturnal teeth grinding is often one result. As with many other problems encountered by musicians, treatment should address the underlying cause as well as the symptoms. While the use of plastic guards worn over the teeth to protect them from nighttime grinding may be appropriate to treat the symptoms, the ultimate resolution of the problem may also require modification of the shoulder and chin rest to reduce neck tension, as well as postural retraining and stress management.

The postural problems posed by the double bass are quite considerable and merit special mention. When standing, the player often has to lean to the right to allow the bow arm low enough access around the side of the instrument to the strings. This can be made a little easier by rotating the instrument to the right. Nevertheless, it is not unusual to see players whose right shoulder slopes sharply downward, while the left is almost horizontal. Furthermore, with such a large instrument, the height of the player is a significant factor for posture. Short players must hold the upper arm much higher out to the side to reach the top of the fingerboard, which leaves them prone to rotator cuff problems in the shoulder (see chapter 3). They may also experience problems reaching over the left side of the instrument to gain access to the lower end of the fingerboard. Playing seated (which is common in orchestras) can introduce its own problems. A player sitting symmetrically on the stool must lean far forward over the instrument in a position which is almost calculated to cause vulnerability to disk prolapse. For this reason it is more common to sit asymmetrically with one foot on the floor and one on the spar of the stool or on a footrest in order to minimize forward leaning.

In the normal playing position for the classical guitar, the left foot is often placed on a footrest so that the thigh can be raised to a suitable level to support the instrument. The trunk may be tilted to the left so that the weight of the body is shifted onto the left buttock, which in turn may lead to the right shoulder being raised and the left lowered, and the neck inclined to the left to keep the head vertical. As a result, the spine assumes an S-shaped curvature when seen from behind (fig. 2-6C). In addition, the player may hunch forward over the instrument to see the frets more clearly or because the back muscles are weak. This not only puts a strain on the back but also puts additional strain on the neck, as the head must be supported by muscular effort. It also results in the neck being bent backward to keep the head level, which tightens the throat and restricts breathing. Much of this can be corrected by careful attention to posture and by raising the music stand to a suitable level; however, the asymmetry caused by raising the left foot remains. One option is to keep both feet on the ground and place a firm, dome-shaped cushion on the left thigh to support and raise the instrument. This will help to reduce the lateral curvature of the spine. Other than this, avoidance of postural problems is best promoted by taking frequent rests to stretch and adjust posture during practice sessions (see comments by John Williams in Wynn Parry 1998).

SEATING

As many musicians mainly perform while sitting down, the question of seating is an important one, though it is only recently that it has begun to receive the attention it deserves (Horvath 2002, 2004). Not only do the postures required for playing different instruments vary considerably, but so do the dimensions of players. However, with the exception of providing high stools for double-bass players, this is rarely reflected in the seating made available to orchestras, which is usually in the form of a nonadjustable stacking chair of a standard size. In a typical orchestra of about one hundred players, it would not be surprising to find heights ranging from around five feet tall to well over six feet. To start with a rather extreme example, if a seated player is very short and cannot put the entire sole of the foot comfortably on the ground, significant pressure is experienced in the soft tissues of the back or thighs, which soon become uncomfortable (Keegan 1953). Tall players may have problems with the seat being too low, which reduces the lordosis of the lumbar spine. For wind players, this can have the secondary consequence of making it difficult to use full lung capacity. Occasionally one sees tall orchestral players sitting on a pair of stacking chairs to counter this problem, but this is a crude and unsatisfactory solution. For some instruments and players it is possible to play while sitting with the lower part of the back resting against a lumbar support (if the chair has one and the player has sufficient thigh length). Even if this is not the preferred playing position, the possibility of using the lumbar support to rest between bouts of playing provides considerable advantages. For the wind players in a symphony orchestra, this is a significant proportion of the time spent sitting on stage. For string players, who must spend most of the performance in the playing position, the question of posture and seating is perhaps most acute. Cellists and bass players in particular may find themselves in forward-leaning postures for long periods, which puts considerable strain on the back. Chairs that allow the flat surface of the seat to be tilted downward toward the front can be an advantage for these (and some other) players for the reasons outlined above. This posture can be adopted on normal chairs by sitting close to the front edge so that the thighs can slope downward or by placing blocks under the chair's back legs, a form of customization often seen on the stage.

The ideal chair should have adequate padding, adjustable seat height and tilt, and lumbar support. Is this an impossible dream? No—it is a description of the standard seating used by office workers, the only difference being that the musician's chair should not swivel or run on casters unless chaos is to ensue on the platform. The reason why office workers do not have to suffer the type of seating normally provided on stage is that health and safety regulations prohibit it. Why should musicians have to put up with less? There are indeed some chairs designed specifically with musicians in mind that include (or claim to include) many such features. Unfortunately, the easiest way to incorporate the degree of adjustability required is to use a design with a central pillar. This means the chair can't be stacked, which may not please the management. Some stacking chairs designed for musicians have much less adjustability while others do not deliver the levels of comfort they promise, so it is vital to try a variety of products with players of different sizes if you are considering these for your ensemble.

There is no single ideal sitting posture that can comfortably be maintained for long periods of time regardless of whether it promotes what is regarded as optimal lumbar lordosis. We frequently adjust our posture if the chair allows it, in order to redistribute the weight between the various load-bearing surfaces of the body. This ensures adequate blood flow to all of the tissues that are being compressed against the seat. This surface should not therefore be shaped in a way that restricts movement. Some of the more extreme "postural" designs such as kneeling stools may not allow much movement and may transfer some of the weight onto the less fleshy parts of the leg and knee. They may therefore not be comfortable for long periods. Sitting erect on a kneeling stool or on one with a saddle-shaped seat to optimize lumbar lordosis requires both more balance and, initially at least, more muscle activity than a slumped position (Gandavadi and Ramsay 2005), so being able to maintain an erect posture in a stool lacking lumbar support requires practice and fitness of postural muscles. The same is true for sitting erect at the front of the seat to achieve good posture, but the reward is a reduction in the risk of back pain. The solution is not just in the design of the chair; greater postural fitness will have other benefits for the quality of playing. In addition, a well-designed chair should have a padded sitting surface made of a material to which the performer is not liable to stick under warm conditions! While the chairs available during touring will be beyond the control of the ensemble, an investment in good seating in the orchestra's home venue is likely to have considerable benefits for the long-term well-being of the players, and will undoubtedly be reflected in performance quality. For touring, it may be worthwhile to consider portable accessories, such as cushions (wedge-shaped or otherwise), lumbar supports, and blocks for back chair legs, to cope with venues where the seating is traditional or unpredictable (Horvath 2002).

In general, it is recommended that long periods of sitting be broken up by periodic breaks of standing and walking, even if these last only a few minutes. This allows a redistribution of the nucleus pulposus of the intervertebral disks (McGill 2002) and relief for the compressed subcutaneous tissues of the buttocks. It can be followed by mild stretching involving pushing the hands up toward the ceiling and inhaling deeply, which gently and progressively extends the lumbar spine. These short breaks can easily be scheduled into rehearsals by understanding conductors who are likely to reap their reward in improved responsiveness from the players.

With instruments such as the piano or harpsichord, the fixed position of the keyboard makes not only the height of the seat but also its distance from the instrument critical. The design of the traditional piano stool at least makes it easy to regulate the height, which should normally be set so that the forearms are close to horizontal or slightly downward sloping during playing. If it is set too low or too high, the wrist joint may be overflexed or overextended, which affects the freedom of movement of the fingers (see chapter 3). Playing with hunched shoulders (whether developed as a mannerism or as a result of incorrect seat height) should be avoided as not only does this introduce tension in the shoulder and neck, but it also interferes with the recruitment of the muscles in these regions when they are actually required for playing (Brown 2000) (see animation 2-3). The stool should be placed in a position that allows the keys to be reached comfortably with the body held erect (fig. 2-6D–F, animation 2-3). If the stool is too close to the keyboard, the pelvis is rotated forward and the chest pulled back, leading to an exaggerated lumbar lordosis. This increases the muscular effort required and the possibility of developing low back pain, and it may also restrict breathing movements. It also means that the elbows are pushed backward so that the hands do not extend too far over the keys, restricting their freedom of movement from side to side. If the stool is too far from the keyboard, the pelvis tilts backward, straightening out the lumbar curvature and increasing the thoracic kyphosis (Kapandji 2000). The elbows straighten and greater muscular effort from the shoulders and upper arms is needed to support the hands above the keys. This increases tension in the shoulders, and because the center of gravity of the trunk is shifted forward, the erector spinae muscles of the back must work harder to support the spine.

If you modify your playing posture to make it more favorable, it will almost certainly feel strange at first because you are so used to the original one, no matter how awkward. Becoming acclimatized to the new posture will inevitably take time, but the long-term benefits will be considerable.

EXERCISES AND POSTURAL TRAINING

Beyond the mechanical fixes afforded by good seating, it is important to be able to make the most of the seat one is presented with by developing good posture. If one watches the string sections of a full orchestra, the range of postures displayed is often striking. Some look balanced and allow a natural movement of the body that appears to be part of the expressive nature of the playing, while others look so rigid and uncomfortable that it is hard to imagine that the sound being produced can be aesthetically pleasing. This is particularly noticeable in student orchestras, where inexperienced performers may be nervous or playing a second instrument with which they are not particularly experienced. However, it is often surprising to see that even among good professional players, poor and risky postures are quite common. This may be exacerbated by the setup of the instrument. For example, using an angled cello spike can provide advantages to some players, but it should not be seen as an excuse to allow the player to adopt a semirecumbent position! This will severely restrict movement of the arm and trunk and lead to a high probability of back pain. Janet Horvath (Horvath 2002) and Barbara Paull (Paull and Harrison 1997) describe a variety of simple exercises that can be used to relieve back tension and help build postural muscle strength as well as some clever exercises that can be employed surreptitiously to stretch trunk and other muscles even when on the platform. In rehearsal and practice, where the constraints are much less, regular stretching and rest between bouts of playing should be built into the sessions. These should not be seen as a luxury or fad but as a means of optimizing performance and limiting the risk of injury. Prevention is the most satisfactory and cost-effective way to treat injury.

Many players who are conscious of health issues have become interested in postural development programs such as the Alexander technique, Pilates and Feldenkreis systems, tai chi, and yoga. While the benefits of these programs have for the most part not yet been objectively assessed, the fact that they increase postural awareness, train important postural muscle groups, and increase flexibility is likely to be beneficial. There is also some evidence from properly designed and evaluated trials that the Alexander technique may have a positive effect on back pain (Ernst and Canter 2003). Many postural therapies also help to reduce stress, which is usually associated with excessive muscle tension, and contribute to reducing the impact of performance-related anxiety (see chapter 10). Maintaining a fixed posture for prolonged periods can lead to the development of some postural muscle groups at the expense of those that move the joints in the opposite direction. This leads to an undesirable reinforcement of the postural asymmetry, which can only be corrected by strengthening the weaker muscle groups. General exercises that involve symmetrical activity in postural muscles (e.g., walking, swimming, or involvement in some other form of sport) and maintenance of an acceptable body weight all contribute to good posture as well as provide many other health benefits.

REFERENCES

Adams, M. A., N. Bogduk, K. Burton, and P. Dolan. 2002. *The biomechanics of back pain.* Edinburgh: Churchill Livingstone.

Bejjani, F. J., G. M. Kaye, and M. Benham. 1996. Musculoskeletal and neuromuscular conditions of instrumental musicians. *Arch Phys Med Rehabil* 77 (4):406–13.

Blum, J., and G. Ritter. 1990. Violinists and violists with masses under the left side of the angle of the jaw known as "fiddler's neck." *Med Prob Perform Artists* 5 (4):155–60.

Brown, S. 2000. Promoting a healthy keyboard technique. In *Medical problems of the instrumental musician*, ed. R. Tubiana and P. C. Amadio. London: Martin Dunitz.

Dommerholt, J. 2000. Posture. In *Medical problems of the instrumental musician*, ed. R. Tubiana and P. C. Amadio. London: Martin Dunitz.

Ernst, E., and P. H. Canter. 2003. The Alexander technique: A systematic review of controlled clinical trials. *Forsch Komplementarmed Klass Naturheilkd* 10 (6):325–29.

Fischer, S. 1998. Technique and ease in violin playing. In *The musician's hand: A clinical guide*, ed. I. Winspur and C. B. Wynn Parry. London: Martin Dunitz.

Freemont, A. J., T. E. Peacock, P. Goupille, J. A. Hoyland, J. O'Brien, and M. I. Jayson. 1997. Nerve ingrowth into diseased intervertebral disc in chronic back pain. *Lancet* 350 (9072):178–81.

Gandavadi, A., and J. Ramsay. 2005. Effect of two seating positions on upper limb function in normal subjects. *Int J Ther Rehab* 12 (11):485–90.

Hall, S. J. 2003. *Basic biomechanics*. 4th ed. Boston: McGraw-Hill.

Harrison, D. D., S. O. Harrison, A. C. Croft, D. E. Harrison, and S. J. Troyanovich. 1999. Sitting biomechanics part I: Review of the literature. *J Manipulative Physiol Ther* 22 (9):594–609.

Horvath, J. 2002. *Playing (less) hurt: An injury prevention guide for musicians*. Minneapolis, Minn.: J. Horvath.

———. 2004. Stressing prevention. *Symphony* (March–April).

Kapandji, A. I. 2000. Anatomy of the spine. In *Medical problems of the instrumental musician*, ed. R. Tubiana and P. C. Amadio. London: Martin Dunitz.

Keegan, J. J. 1953. Alterations of the lumbar curve related to posture and seating. *J Bone Joint Surg Am* 35-A (3):589–603.

Levy, C. E., W. A. Lee, A. G. Brandfonbrener, J. Press, and A. E. Levy. 1992. Electromyographic analysis of muscular activity in the upper extremity generated by supporting a violin with and without a shoulder rest. *Med Prob Perform Artists* 7:103–9.

Lieberman, J. L. 2000. The importance of setup. *The Strad* (May/June).

McGill, S. 2002. *Low back disorders: Evidence-based prevention and rehabilitation*. Champaign, Ill.: Human Kinetics.

Norris, R. 2000. Applied ergonomics. In *Medical problems of the instrumental musician*, ed. R. Tubiana and P. C. Amadio. London: Martin Dunitz.

Okner, M. A. O., T. Kernozek, and M. G. Wade. 1997. Chin rest pressure in violin players: Musical repertoire, chin rests and shoulder pads as possible mediators. *Med Prob Perform Artists* 12:112–21.

Paull, B., and C. Harrison. 1997. *The athletic musician: A guide to playing without pain*. Lanham, Md.: Scarecrow Press.

Rabuffetti, M., R. M. Converti, S. Boccardi, and M. Ferrarin. 2007. Tuning of the violin-performer interface: An experimental study about the effects of shoulder rest variations on playing kinematics. *Med Prob Perform Artists* 22 (2):58–66.

Richardson, C. A., and G. A. Jull. 1995. Muscle control—pain control. What exercises would you prescribe? *Manual Therapy* 1:2–10.

White, A. A., and M. M. Panjabi. 1990. *Clinical biomechanics of the spine*. 2nd ed. Philadelphia: Lippincott.

Wynn Parry, C. B. 1998. The interface. In *The musician's hand: A clinical guide*, ed. I. Winspur and C. B. Wynn Parry. London: Martin Dunitz.

Yeo, D. K., T. P. Pham, J. Baker, and S. A. Porters. 2002. Specific orofacial problems experienced by musicians. *Aust Dent J* 47 (1):2–11.

Chapter Three

The Shoulder, Arm, and Hand

Structure and Problems

The upper limb is capable of a great range of movements, which is a reflection of its structure, the nature of its joints, and the action of its muscles. A knowledge of the anatomy of the upper limb and how it works is important to instrumental musicians for a variety of reasons. More than any other part of the body, it is the movements of the arm and the hand that are used to create music. Just as much as your instrument, these are the tools of your trade. By understanding how the movements are achieved, as well as their intrinsic limitations, the player will be better able to optimize performance without being tempted to demand what is not possible. Because of the range and repetitive nature of the movements required, the arm, hand, and shoulder are the most frequent sources of the pain and discomfort that can limit or even end the ability to play effectively. An appreciation of what may go wrong and how to reduce the risk of breakdown is the greatest assurance a player can have of a long and trouble-free career. The risk of injury cannot be eliminated entirely, however, so this chapter also explains the origin of some of the conditions that are most likely to limit performance. Their symptoms are described, together with the typical forms of treatment they may require. Among these symptoms are several that the player should recognize as warning signs that must not be ignored. This knowledge should provide the player with the confidence to seek help promptly and enable him or her to communicate effectively with the doctor or therapist. This chapter will also discuss some of the difficulties that may be experienced in diagnosing the primary source of an injury and promote an appreciation of the importance of following any prescribed treatment conscientiously.

ANATOMY OF THE UPPER LIMB

Most of what is covered in this chapter should be understandable without any previous knowledge of anatomical terminology (those of you who have this knowledge already may want to grit your teeth at this point!). In many places I have added the technical terms in parentheses as these will be useful if the reader wishes to explore

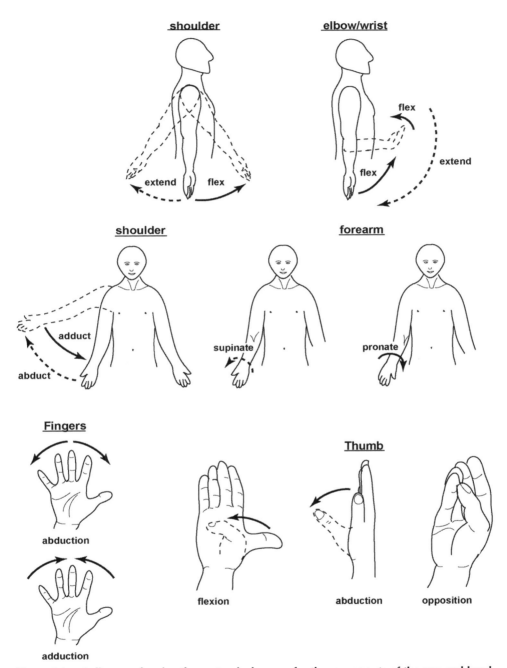

Figure 3-1. A diagram showing the anatomical names for the movements of the arm and hand.

any of the topics further. (For example, such information will be necessary to cope with many of the references at the end of the chapter.) Many of these terms are used because everyday language either does not provide an equivalent or cannot be used to describe important concepts with sufficient precision. This is nowhere more true than in descriptions of the movements of joints. For this reason the appropriate terms are explained in figure 3-1.

The Muscles and Joints of the Shoulder

The arm is relatively loosely attached to the trunk. Where two bones move against each other at a joint, they are said to articulate. The arm articulates with the shoulder blade (scapula), which in turn is braced against the breastbone (sternum) by a long lever formed by the collarbone (clavicle) (fig. 3-2). The collarbone is relatively narrow and provides the only bony connection between the arm and the trunk. If we fall on an outstretched arm it takes the full weight of the body, which is why it is prone to fracture under these circumstances. The shoulder blade is otherwise attached to the trunk only by muscles, which run both to the vertebral column (the spine) of the back and the neck, and to the chest wall (figs. 3-3, 3-4). The advantage of this arrangement is that it allows the shoulder blade to slide and rotate over the back of the ribcage, contributing to the great freedom of movement of the arm.

The shoulder blade has a complex shape (fig. 3-2A, B) but is basically a triangular plate with the apex pointing downward. The corner that points toward the arm ends in a flat oval plate that forms the socket (the glenoid) against which the upper bone of the arm (the humerus) articulates. A small bony process (the coracoid), shaped rather like a thumb, pushes forward from the glenoid and several muscles in the arm attach to it, the most familiar of which is the biceps. At the back of the shoulder blade, a long, ridgelike spine runs horizontally near the top edge. The spine ends in a flattened plate (the acromium) that lies horizontally above the shoulder joint, where the collarbone attaches to it. You can identify the acromium by running your finger along the collarbone to where it ends at the point of the shoulder. The largest muscle holding the shoulder blade in place is called the trapezius (fig. 3-3D). It has a triangular shape with its longest edge attached to the vertebral column and the back of the skull, and also to a ligament (the nuchal ligament) that runs between them. The muscle fibers run from here to the spine of the shoulder blade. The upper fibers run obliquely downward, forming the slope of the shoulders, and the middle fibers run horizontally, while the lower fibers run obliquely upward across the back. Consequently, depending on which fibers contract, the muscle can either raise the shoulder blade (as in shrugging), pull it downward, or pull it inward toward the spine. Underneath the trapezius are shorter muscles (the rhomboids) that pass from the vertical edge of the shoulder blade to the vertebral column, pulling the blade inward and upward. In this they are aided by the levator scapulae muscles, which pass more steeply upward to the vertebrae of the neck (fig. 3-3B). The muscles that support and move the shoulder blade are often a site of tension when we are under stress and are therefore a common target for massage. When the arm is raised, the point of the shoulder is rotated upward by the shoulder muscles, and so these are heavily used by string players. The shoulder blade is also attached to

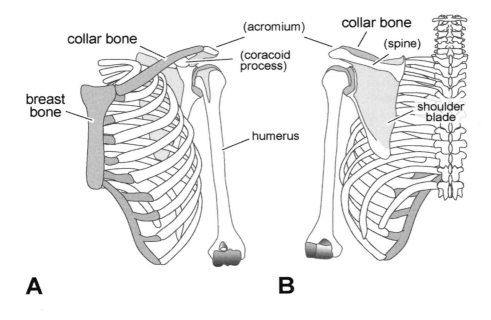

A   B

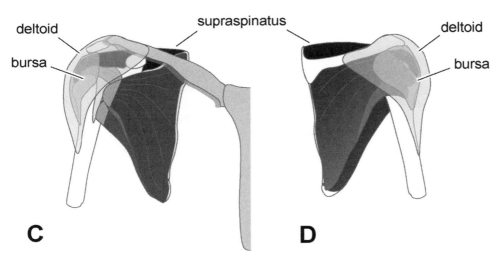

C   D

Figure 3-2.   The skeleton of the shoulder seen from the front (A) and the back (B). This shows how the humerus of the arm articulates with the shoulder blade. The structures named in parentheses are parts of the shoulder blade. The arm and shoulder are only attached to the body directly through the joint between the collarbone and the breastbone. The shoulder blade is otherwise supported only by muscles suspending it from the ribcage, spine, and skull. C, D: The bursa of the shoulder joint, revealed through the transparent deltoid muscle, as seen from the front (C) and back (D). The bursa (which is like an uninflated balloon containing a film of synovial fluid) allows the deltoid to slide smoothly over the underlying tissues, and as it extends under the acromium contributes to the smooth movement of the supraspinatus and infraspinatus tendons.

the rib cage by two other muscles. One is called the serratus anterior, and this runs from the side of the upper ribs, wrapping around the chest wall under the shoulder blade, to its vertical edge, which lies almost parallel with the vertebral column (figs. 3-3B and 3-4B). This muscle holds the shoulder blade against the back of the rib cage. The other muscle, the pectoralis minor, attaches the coracoid process to the front of the rib cage (fig. 3-4D) and assists the action of the serratus anterior.

The shallowness of the shoulder socket (glenoid) allows the arm a wide range of movement, but at the price of instability. For this reason, the top of the humerus must be held in position by muscles. Four muscles are involved (see animation 3-1). Two of these are found on the back of the shoulder blade on either side of its horizontal spine. One sits in the groove above the spine and is therefore called the supraspinatus. This raises the arm out to the side, a movement called abduction. The muscle below the spine (the infraspinatus) rotates the arm outward around its vertical axis (fig. 3-3C). The third muscle (the teres minor) is small and runs from the lateral edge of the shoulder blade to the back of the humerus, while the fourth (subscapularis) is a large triangular muscle that has its origin on the flat front surface of the shoulder blade. This also attaches the humerus and rotates the arm inward. The tendon of the supraspinatus must pass through a narrow gap that lies beneath the acromium to reach the humerus, and here it is vulnerable to being pinched if any of the tissues in this region become swollen (figs. 3-2, 3-4C, animation 3-2). This is a potential source of problems for string players in particular.

The shoulder joint is of the ball-and-socket type. The upper end of the humerus ends in a smooth hemispherical surface that allows the arm to rotate in many directions against the other face of the joint, which belongs to the shoulder blade. As with most moving joints, the surfaces that slide over one another are covered with a smooth, glassy, hard-wearing type of cartilage (hyaline cartilage—animation 3-1). In osteoarthritis, the surface of the cartilage becomes broken up and rough, restricting movement and causing pain. The joint is what is called a synovial joint, meaning that it is enclosed in a fibrous capsule or sac containing a lubricating fluid (synovial fluid) (animation 3-1). The socket of the shoulder joint is very shallow and the capsule quite loose. This allows the arm great freedom of movement, but this comes at a cost, as the joint is prone to dislocation. The stability of the joint is maintained largely by the broad, flat tendons belonging to the four muscles just described—supraspinatus, infraspinatus, teres minor, and subscapularis. These fuse with the joint capsule as they attach to the humerus just behind the ball-like articular surface that lies within the joint. The tendons therefore run behind, above, and in front of the joint, but leave the region below it (the armpit or axilla) unsupported (figs. 3-3C, 3-4C), which is why dislocation of the shoulder almost always occurs in the downward direction. Together the tendons form what is called the rotator cuff, and by acting in a concerted fashion, their muscles hold the head of the humerus in place (animation 3-1). Acting individually, they can rotate the arm around its long axis or contribute to holding it away from, or pulling it toward, the body.

Passing over the rotator cuff is the deltoid muscle, which arises from the shoulder blade (both from its spine and the acromium) and from the collarbone. The other end attaches to the lateral side of the upper part of the humerus. It therefore sits in a similar

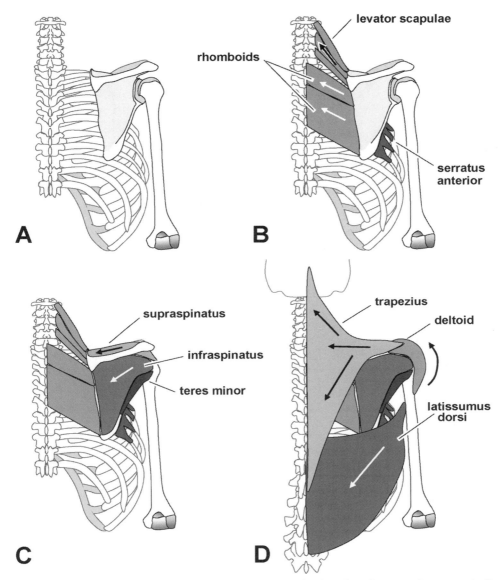

A

B

levator scapulae

rhomboids

serratus anterior

C

supraspinatus

infraspinatus

teres minor

D

trapezius

deltoid

latissumus dorsi

Figure 3-3.   Muscles attaching the shoulder blade to the back and to the arm. The arrows indicate the directions in which the muscles can move the shoulder blade. A. The skeleton. B. The rhomboids and levator scapulae pull the shoulder blade upward, while the serratus anterior holds it against the back of the chest. C. The rotator cuff muscles attach the shoulder blade to the arm. Their tendons deepen the socket of the joint to make it more stable. D. The muscle fibers of the trapezius fan out from the spine of the shoulder blade to the spine and the base of the skull. The upper fibers pull it upward, the middle fibers pull it inward, and the lower fibers pull it downward. The deltoid muscle links the spine of the shoulder blade to the side of the upper arm, which it helps to raise, while the latissimus dorsi pulls the raised arm downward.

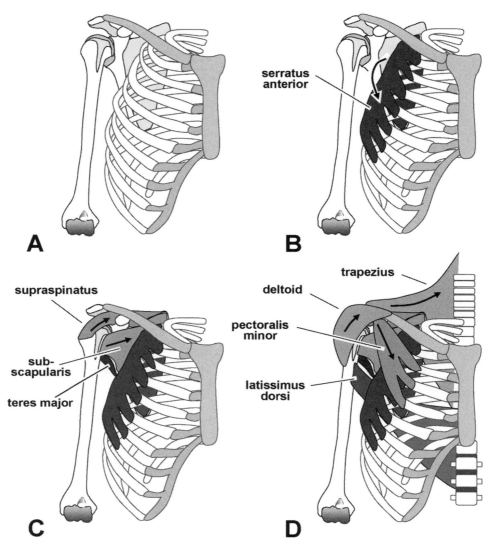

Figure 3-4. Muscles of the shoulder seen from the front. The arrows show the action of the muscles on the shoulder blade. A. Skeleton of the shoulder. B. The attachment of serratus anterior to the ribs. C. Muscles attaching the humerus to the shoulder blade. D. The pectoralis minor muscle, which pulls the coracoid process of the scapula toward the ribs.

position to an epaulet. This muscle raises the arm out to the side (abduction) and therefore aids the supraspinatus muscle. To enable the deltoid to slide smoothly over the rotator cuff tendons and the upper end of the humerus, it is separated from them by a thin-walled sac called a bursa (this is a Greek word meaning bag or purse) (fig. 3-2C, animation 3-2). The bursa extends under the acromium and also facilitates the smooth movement of the supraspinatus tendon within its channel. Normally the bursa contains a small amount of fluid, which allows the upper and lower surfaces of the sac to slide smoothly over one another as the deltoid and supraspinatus muscles contract, which they often do together as they have similar actions. There are several other bursae around the joint that contribute to the smooth movement of shoulder muscle tendons. If the surfaces do not slide smoothly and become stuck to one another (bursitis), pain and restriction of movement occurs (see below).

In most synovial joints there are no tendons running within the capsule, but the shoulder joint is unusual in this respect as a tendon belonging to the biceps muscle does enter the cavity. The biceps has two parts or heads (hence its name). As mentioned earlier, one is attached to the bony coracoid process of the shoulder blade that lies outside the joint; the other sends a narrow tendon into the capsule to reach its attachment site on the upper edge of the articular surface of the socket (the supraglenoid tubercle). The lower end of the biceps ends in the forearm, where it is attached by another tendon to a bone called the radius. The tendon is also attached to a sheet of fibrous tissue (deep fascia) that wraps around the muscles of the forearm. The biceps muscle has a number of functions; it flexes the shoulder and the elbow joints, but because of its attachment to the deep fascia it also helps to supinate the forearm (rotating the forearm so that when the elbow is straight, the palm faces forward). Supination is required for the playing of many instruments, for example, the left arm of the violin, viola, and flute.

The Muscles and Joints of the Elbow

The upper arm has only a single bone (the humerus—fig. 3-2), but at the elbow this articulates with the two bones of the forearm, the radius (which runs down the thumb side of the forearm) and the thinner ulna on the little-finger side (figs. 3-5, 3-6). The elbow joint is quite a complex affair. The main part is a hinge linking the humerus with the ulna; this allows movement in only one plane, but the joint also includes an arrangement that allows the radius to rotate. The ulna projects behind the end of the humerus (the point of the elbow). This provides an attachment site for the large muscle at the back of the arm, the triceps, which straightens (extends) the elbow (fig. 3-5A). The triceps has three heads, two of which arise from the humerus and one from the lateral edge of the shoulder blade, so like the biceps it also acts on the shoulder joint. The triceps is the only major muscle that extends the elbow; however, the biceps is aided in flexing the elbow by a number of other muscles including the brachialis, coracobrachialis, and brachioradialis, which run underneath and alongside it (fig. 3-5B, C).

The radius ends at the elbow in a round, disk-shaped head that articulates with the lower end of the humerus. Beneath the head is a narrow neck that is held in place by a tendinous ring (the annular ligament). This allows the radius to rotate around the ulna. If we hold the arm straight with the palm of the hand facing forward (supination), the radius and ulna lie parallel (fig. 3-6). When the palm of the hand is rotated to face backward (pronation), the ulna remains fixed and the radius rotates across it. This is brought about by pronator muscles that run between the radius and ulna. Keyboard instruments are played with both forearms pronated (i.e., with the thumb pointing toward the body), while the violin, viola, and flute are played with the right forearm pronated. Other woodwind and brass instruments such as the trumpet are played with the forearms in an intermediate position. Like the shoulder, the elbow joint is a synovial one and is

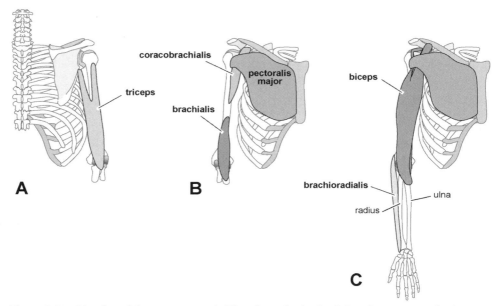

Figure 3-5. Muscles of the upper arm. A. View from the back of the triceps, a muscle that acts on the shoulder and straightens the elbow. B. View from the front showing the coracobrachialis, which acts on the shoulder joint to flex the arm. The brachialis and brachioradialis flex the elbow. C. The biceps acts on both the shoulder and the elbow.

associated with several bursae. One that lies beneath the skin at the point of the elbow is the most likely to become inflamed, for example, as a result of prolonged leaning on a desk (draftsman's elbow).

The Muscles and Joints of the Wrist

You may think of the wrist mainly as a hinge joint allowing up and down movements of the hand at right angles to its flat surfaces (as in waving); however, the curvature of the articular surfaces of the joint also allows movements from side to side in the plane of the hand. These movements are called radial or ulnar deviation (animation 3-5). Ulnar deviation is particularly important for violin and viola players as the left hand moves up the fingerboard toward the bridge. Pianists use both radial and ulnar deviation as their fingers run sequentially up or down the keyboard. The wrist is moved by two flexor and three extensor muscles running down each side of the forearm (figs. 3-8, 3-10). When both flexors or all of the extensors are active, the hand is simply drawn back (extended) or pulled forward (flexed), as in waving. Radial or ulnar deviation is caused when the flexor and extensor muscles on the same side contract together.

The Muscles and Joints of the Hand

The skeleton of the palm of the hand is made up of eight small bones (the carpals) together with five longer ones (metacarpals), each supporting one of the digits (fig. 3-7).

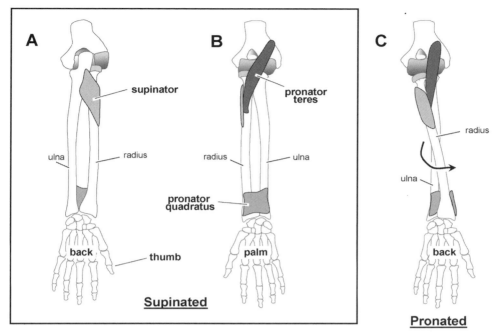

Figure 3-6. Supination and pronation of the forearm. If we stand with the arms straight and the palms facing forward, the two bones of the forearm (radius and ulna) run parallel. In this position, the thumbs point away from the body and the forearm is said to be supinated. Panel A shows this from the back of the arm and B, from the front. If the hand is then turned so that the palm faces the back and the thumbs point toward the body, the radius rotates across the ulna and the forearms are said to be pronated. The muscles responsible for these movements are indicated in larger typeface.

The small carpal bones are difficult to feel as separate entities, but the metacarpals can be easily appreciated by running a finger down the back of the hand from each finger or from the thumb. The radial and ulnar bones of the forearm articulate with three of the carpal bones. These are firmly bound by ligaments to the other carpal bones and to the metacarpals to form a fairly rigid framework for the palm. The heads of the metacarpals are also bound tightly together at the base of the fingers. The fingers themselves each contain three bones (phalanges). The metacarpal bone of the thumb has much more freedom of movement than those of the fingers. This is necessary to allow the thumb (which has only two phalangeal bones) to be brought into opposition with the other fingers to enable efficient gripping. We need not concern ourselves with the names of the carpal bones and their joints, but the names of the individual finger joints are important for delving deeper into the mechanism of finger action and its pathology. The knuckle is the metacarpophalangeal joint (sometimes abbreviated to MP), which is capable of flexion/extension, abduction/adduction, and circumduction (movement in an arc). The other two joints of the finger are hinge joints at which only flexion/extension is possible. The one nearest the knuckle is the proximal interphalangeal joint (PIP) and the last one, the distal interphalangeal joint (DIP).

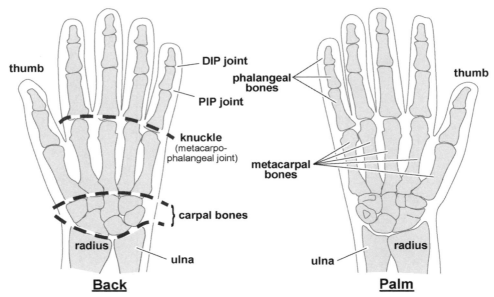

Figure 3-7.   Bones and joints of the hand. The skeleton of the base of the palm is formed from eight small carpal bones. The rest of the palm is made up of the five long metacarpals, while the fingers and thumb are supported by the phalangeal bones. The joint at the knuckle is called the metacarpophalangeal joint. The other two joints of the fingers are interphalangeal joints: the middle joint is the proximal interphalangeal joint (PIP) and the last one, the distal interphalangeal joint (DIP). Particular care is needed in treatment of injuries to the PIP to ensure that the full range of movement is retained.

Many players of stringed instruments believe that playing increases finger span and that this can be encouraged by stretching exercises; however, only a single study has examined this question rigorously. It compared the difference in span in the right and left hands, both between adjacent fingers and the total span between the index and little finger. The subjects were sixty-nine cellists, fifty-two guitarists, and eighty-three nonplaying control subjects, all right handed (Kloeppel 2000). The spreadability of the gap between several of the fingers was greater in the left hand in all three groups. The reason for this result in the control group is not known, but it has been speculated that specialization of the right hand for gripping may be a factor. The difference between the total finger span of the two hands was statistically significant only for cellists and appears to be the result of an increased flexibility at the metacarpophalangeal joints. However as the difference was only a few millimeters, its significance for playing would be quite minor. Differences in span were not associated with the age at which the instrument was taken up, though there was a significant correlation with current practice intensity.

The organization of the muscles used to move the fingers (or digits) is quite complicated and is a reflection of the degree of control we have over the individual joints. The muscles can be divided into two major groups, those that lie in the forearm (figs. 3-8, 3-10) and those that are found in the hand itself (figs. 3-9, 3-11, 3-12). The

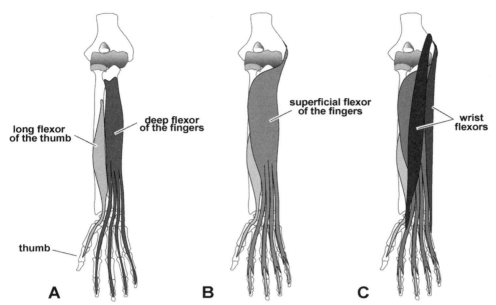

long flexor
of the thumb

deep flexor
of the fingers

superficial flexor
of the fingers

wrist
flexors

thumb

A   **B**   **C**

Figure 3-8. Muscles on the inner side of the forearm that flex the fingers and wrist. These muscles are shown in layers to make them easier to understand. A. The deep flexor muscles of the fingers and the long flexor of the thumb. The tendons of the deep flexors run all the way to the last joint of each finger. B. The superficial flexor muscles of the fingers. The tendons of the superficial flexor muscles do not act on the last finger joint. C. Flexors of the wrist.

forearm muscles are of course much larger and provide the power for finger movement and grip, whereas the muscles within the hand provide a more sophisticated and independent control over finger movement. We will start by considering the forearm muscles that flex (curl) the fingers. These of course lie on the side of the forearm that is continuous with the palm.

There are two layers of flexor muscles for the fingers, each with different actions. The more superficial layer (flexor digitorum superficialis) arises mainly from the ulnar (little finger) side of the humerus just above the elbow but is also attached to the ulna and radius (fig. 3-8B). Though named as if a single muscle, it is actually a fusion of several muscles that can be controlled separately, giving the individual fingers a considerable (though not complete) independence of movement. Superficial flexor tendons run down each of the four fingers, where they split into two and insert into the sides of the middle phalangeal bone (fig. 3-9C). This means that they flex only the knuckle (metacarpophalangeal joint) and the first (proximal interphalangeal) joint in the finger. To flex the last joint of the finger (the distal interphalangeal joint) requires the action of the deep flexor muscles (flexor digitorum profundus), as demonstrated in animation 3-3. This muscle arises mainly from the ulnar bone and again, one tendon runs into each of the four fingers, underneath the superficial flexor tendon (fig. 3-8A). Where the superficial tendon splits, the deep tendon emerges to attach to the last finger bone. The part of the muscle supplying the index finger is better separated

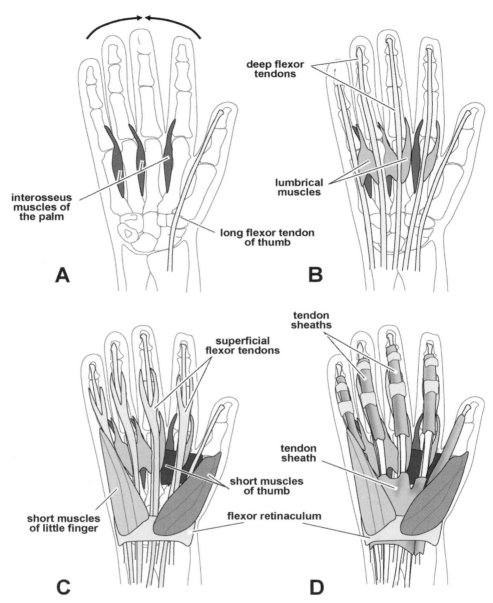

Figure 3-9. Muscles and tendons on the palmar side of the hand shown in layers. A. The palmar interosseus muscles. The direction in which they move the fingers is shown by the arrows. Also visible is the tendon of the long flexor of the thumb. This is sometimes linked to the deep flexor tendon of the index finger (Linburg-Comstock syndrome). B. The tendons of the deep flexor muscles of the fingers and their attached lumbrical muscles. C. At each edge of the hand are short muscles that act on the thumb and little finger to cause flexion, abduction, and opposition. The flexor retinaculum, which holds the flexor tendons down at the wrist, is also visible. D. The tendon sheaths (tenosynovia), which help to ensure free movement of the tendons under the retinaculum and the fibrous bands that hold the tendons down onto the fingers.

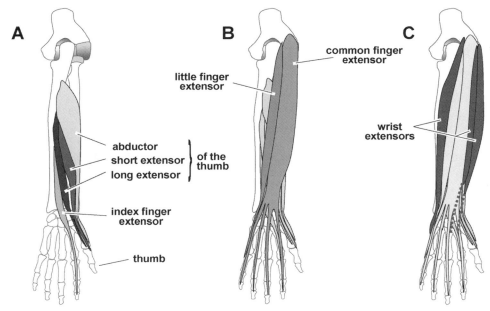

A

abductor
short extensor ⎫ of the
long extensor ⎭ thumb

index finger
extensor

thumb

B

little finger
extensor

common finger
extensor

C

wrist
extensors

Figure 3-10.   Muscles on the back of the forearm that extend the fingers and wrist. The muscles are shown in layers. A. The deepest muscles are those running to the thumb (two extensors and, farthest toward the radial edge of the arm, an abductor). Also in this layer is the extensor of the index finger. B. The next layer contains the common extensor for the four fingers plus the additional and separate extensor of the little finger, which contributes to its independence of movement. C. Extensors of the wrist.

than that to other fingers, giving the index finger a greater degree of independent movement. When a muscle contracts, it moves all of the joints between its origin and the place where its tendon is attached, so the deep flexor, in addition to moving the distal phalangeal joint, will flex the other joints of the finger and also contribute weakly to flexion of the wrist. Consequently, if the intention is to move only some of the joints, the movement of the others will have to be resisted by the action of antagonistic muscles. In this case, for example, wrist extensor muscles could be used to keep that joint straight.

The arrangement of the finger extensor muscles that lie in the forearm is rather different (fig. 3-10). There is only a single layer of common extensor muscle whose tendons run to the four fingers; however, in addition, there are entirely independent extensor muscles for the index and little fingers. All three muscles arise from what is called the common extensor origin on the radial (thumb) side of the humerus just above the elbow joint. The common extensor tendons become flattened where they attach to the three bones of the fingers. At the base of the first phalangeal bone of the finger, just beyond the knuckle joint, the tendon expands into a hood to which some small muscles of the hand also attach (figs. 3-11C, 3-12B, animation 3-3). On the back of the hand, the separate tendons of the common extensor muscle are linked to each other by a variable pattern of fibrous bands. In addition, some tendons run to a point

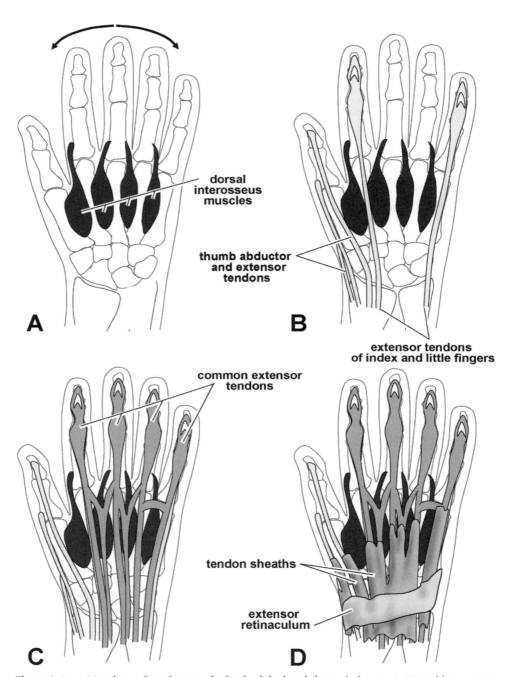

Figure 3-11. Muscles and tendons on the back of the hand shown in layers. A. Dorsal interosseus muscles. The direction in which they move the fingers is shown by the arrows. B. Tendons of the extensor of the index and little fingers, and of two extensors and a long abductor of the thumb. C. Tendons of the common extensor of the fingers. These are linked together by fibrous bands on the back of the hand that restrict their independence of movement. D. The tendon sheaths and the extensor retinaculum.

midway between the base of two fingers, where they divide to send one onto each finger. The tendon to the third finger is usually particularly tightly attached to that of the little finger. The consequence of this enslavement between fingers can clearly be observed in studies of the finger movements made by violinists (Wiesendanger, Baader, and Kazennikov 2006; Baader, Kazennikov, and Wiesendanger 2005). Often the enslaved finger does not make contact with its string; however, depending on the passage, this may not be critical and indeed, it may be possible to place this finger on a nonsounding string at a point that corresponds to the next note to be played upon it. A greater independence of the little and index fingers is, however, ensured by their separate extensor muscles. It has been proposed that cutting some of the fibrous bands linking the extensor tendons may benefit pianists by reducing the tension and thus limitation of these tendons, but there is absolutely no evidence to support this. One of the main factors in this is the limited degree to which the individual parts of the common extensor muscle controlling each tendon can be activated independently.

The ability to control the movement of the fingers individually is aided by a number of small muscles lying deep within the hand. Attached to the surfaces of the metacarpal bones are two sets of interosseus muscles, one in the palm and one on the back (dorsal surface) of the hand (figs. 3-9, 3-11, 3-12). Their tendons insert into the side of the first of the finger bones (the proximal phalanges) at the extensor tendon expansion. The dorsal interosseus muscles spread the fingers, and the palmar interosseus muscles draw them together. Another set of muscles deep within the palm are called the lumbricals because of their long, round, wormlike appearance. These arise from the deep flexor tendons and run to the extensor tendon expansion. Their action is complex, as the activity of the deep flexor muscles moves the tendons to which they are attached. Their main role is simultaneously to flex the knuckle and straighten the fingers by pulling on the extensor tendon expansions (fig. 3-12, animation 3-3). In this they are aided by the interosseus muscles. When the lumbrical and interosseus muscles are paralyzed, the hand assumes a clawlike form with the fingers curled in (i.e., the joints between the finger bones remain permanently flexed).

The Muscles in the Thumb and Little Finger

The little finger is controlled by some additional muscles within the hand that arise from the carpal bones and form a fleshy mass at the edge of the palm called the hypothenar eminence (fig. 3-9C). One of these is an abductor, whose role is similar to a dorsal interosseus muscle, drawing the little finger outward when the fingers are spread. In addition, there is a short flexor muscle that helps to curl the little finger into the palm. Finally, there is an opponens muscle that pulls the little finger over to meet the thumb to allow a prehensile grip.

The independent movement of the thumb is also important for gripping, and the long muscles that control it are quite distinct from those that move the fingers. On the front of the forearm there is a single long flexor of the thumb (flexor pollicis longus) (fig. 3-8A). On the back there are two extensor muscles (extensor pollicis longus and brevis) and an abductor muscle, which draws the thumb away from the hand (fig. 3-10A). The tendons of these muscles pass down the side of the thumb. Two run

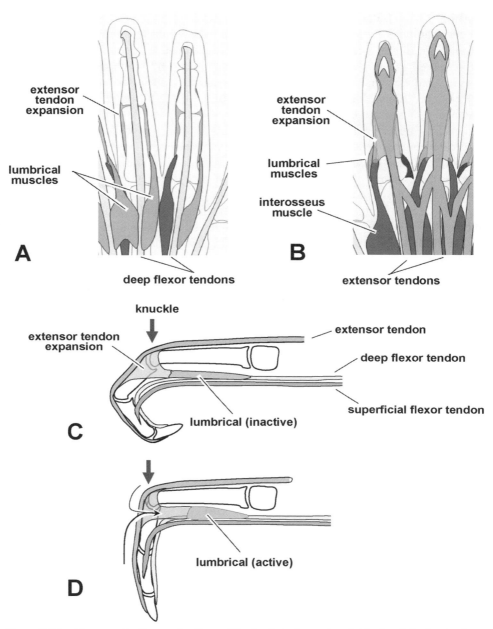

Figure 3-12. The organization and actions of the lumbrical muscles. A. The lumbricals arise from the deep flexor tendons but end in the extensor tendon expansion, forming a broad, hoodlike flap that attaches to the side of the finger just after the knuckle (B). C. The flexor muscles are active, curling the fingers, but the lumbrical muscle is relaxed. D. The lumbrical has contracted, pulling on the extensor tendon expansion. This straightens (extends) the finger, while the knuckle joint is flexed.

together, so when the thumb is stretched outward and backward, only two cords are visible, one representing the tendon of the long extensor and the other, the tendons of the abductor and the short extensor. The space between them is rather quaintly known as the "anatomical snuff box" because when snuff was a popular way to take tobacco, a pinch would be placed in this groove prior for sniffing. The thumb is also moved by muscles that form a mass that runs along the edge of the palm at its base (the thenar eminence). As with the little finger, this contains a short flexor, a short abductor, and an opponens muscle. In addition, there is a muscle (an adductor) in the web of skin between the thumb and index finger that pulls the thumb inward toward the palm (fig. 3-9C).

Tendon Movements in the Wrist and Hand

Many of the arm and hand problems of musicians involve places where tendons and nerves pass through restricted channels. This is most acute at the wrist. If the wrist is strongly flexed or extended, the long tendons that run to the fingers from the forearm will try to take the shortest route. If this was not restricted, they would rise above the surface of the wrist joint, raising the skin like a tent. In order to prevent this, the tendons are held down by strong bands of tissue called retinacula, which wrap around the wrist like a sweatband (figs. 3-9C and 3-11C, animation 3-4). The channel under the flexor retinaculum at the base of the palm is known as the carpal tunnel. Similar, smaller bands hold the tendons down onto the surface of each finger (fig. 3-9D, animation 3-4). The tendons are therefore confined to narrow channels beneath the retinacula. In order for them to be able to move freely, they are wrapped in tendon sheaths (figs. 3-9D, 3-11D) composed of two layers of synovial membrane forming a double cylinder (fig. 3-13A). The inner layer is wrapped around the tendon and, lubricated by the synovial fluid, this slides smoothly under the outer layer. The technical term for these tendon sheaths is tenosynovia. If the synovial membranes or the tendon become inflamed (tenosinovitis), movement becomes restricted and painful. This can create a vicious circle as the swelling caused by the inflammation results in more friction, leading to further damage and inflammation. The tightness of the spaces under the retinacula depends on the joint angle. For musicians, this is again most critical at the wrist. If the wrist is held straight, the cross-sectional area of the spaces beneath the retinacula are at their largest. If during playing the wrist is held strongly flexed or extended, or deviated in the ulnar or radial direction, the space is more restricted and the tendons are pushed together (see animation 3-5). In addition, when the wrist is deviated from the neutral position, the tendons of one set of muscles will be stretched, and this may limit the angle through which the finger joints can be moved by their antagonists. To demonstrate this, hold the wrist straight and make a tight fist. Now slowly flex the wrist, gradually forcing the hand farther downward; the fingers start to uncurl as the extensor tendons become taut. In other words, with increasing wrist flexion, the ability to flex the fingers is reduced. Clearly, then, if the wrist is in the neutral position, not only is the ability to move the fingers maximized but the movement of the tendons under the retinaculum is less likely to cause irritation or damage to it or its sheath due to friction. The player should therefore aim to develop a wrist posture as

Tendon sheaths and trigger finger

A) Tendon sheath normal

inner and outer layers of the sheath

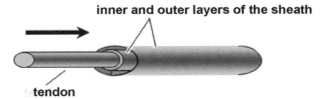

tendon

A film of fluid between the two layers of the sheath ensures that they slide smoothly over each other as the tendon moves inward

B) Trigger finger caused by swelling of the tendon

swelling on tendon

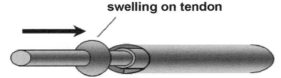

The tendon moves smoothly until the swelling encounters the entrance to the sheath

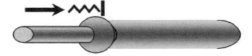

At this point the movement is blocked even though the muscle attached to the tendon continues to contract

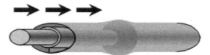

Finally the muscle tension reaches at level that forces the swelling rapidly into the sheath with an audible "pop"

Figure 3-13.   The tendon sheath and trigger finger.

close to neutral as is compatible with the playing of the instrument. In some cases this will be a simple question of playing posture, but if the difficulties cannot be resolved in this way, modifications to the instrument may make the difference between being able to continue playing and being forced to stop.

Limitations to Independent Finger Movement

The hand has evolved primarily for grasping, and though in man and other primates it has the added sophistication that the thumb can be opposed to the other fingers, the demands made of it in instrumental performance can push its design specifications to their limits. This is particularly marked in keyboard playing, though it also applies to some extent to string and woodwind players. The classical textbook description of the actions of the muscles controlling the hand can give a misleading picture of the degree to which the fingers can be controlled individually; however, there are several factors that mitigate against this. One is that it is often not possible to control the muscles that move the different fingers entirely independently. As has already been mentioned, the muscle bellies of the deep and superficial flexors and the common extensors of the fingers are partially fused, thus, contraction in any one of these is likely to produce some passive movement in the others. The degree of fusion varies between individuals and in the case of the flexors, slips of muscle may even cross between the deep and superficial muscle masses. Another important restriction to the independent control of finger movement is the degree to which the subdivisions of the muscle can be controlled separately by the nervous system. Studies of the deep flexors have revealed that in nonmusicians there is frequently a strong synchronization between the activity of motor neurons controlling the parts of the muscle acting on different fingers (Reilly, Nordstrom, and Schieber 2004). This is most noticeable for the bellies supplying adjacent fingers and is particularly strong between those of the ring and little fingers, whose tendons are also the most closely linked together. The degree of motor neuron synchrony appears rather less for the subdivisions of the common extensor of the fingers. You will be relieved to discover that studies of this muscle indicate that with practice it is possible to reduce the level of synchronization (Schmied, Ivarsson, and Fetz 1993; Schmied et al. 2000), which will allow the development of greater finger control.

Connections between tendons running to different fingers are also a significant feature of the hand. We have already encountered the extensive linkages between the tendons of the common extensor muscle; however, atypical connections are common and are rarely covered by standard anatomy textbooks. The common extensor tendon to the ring finger may be connected to the tendon of the separate extensor of the little finger, thus restricting its independent action (Allieu et al. 1998). One study has suggested that this may occur in up to 18 percent of individuals while in a further 34 percent, the separate extensor muscle of the little finger is entirely absent (Baker et al. 1981). What is less well appreciated is that within the carpal tunnel, extensive connections often exist between tendons of the deep flexor muscle running to the different fingers (Leijnse et al. 1997). These can be either fine tendinous linkages or adherent sheets of tenosynovium. Though the degree to which this affects finger movement during playing has not been assessed, tensions put on these structures during playing could make them potential sites of pain and inflammation. One study of music students revealed that the divisions of the deep and superficial flexor muscles supplying different fingers often show a considerable degree of dependence (Miller, Peck, and Watson 2002). Though this rarely affects the index finger, its incidence progressively increases for the second to fourth fingers, especially for the deep flexors. These were, however, asymptomatic in terms of discomfort or pain. Some attempt has been made to model the effect of such tendon linkages mathematically in the hope that it may ultimately be possible to identify the types of finger exercise that are capable of improving performance (Leijnse et al. 1992, 1993). Other exercises, which because of anatomical restrictions would be incapable of improving dexterity (and which might even cause tissue damage), could be discarded. For example, attempts to develop the ability to raise the fourth finger as high as the others despite the restrictions imposed by tendon linkages may be a particular source of injury (Brown 2000). Techniques that optimize the influence of the small intrinsic muscles of the hand (particularly the interosseus and lumbrical muscles), over which greater individual control can be exerted, may be useful for pianists and have been proposed by some teachers (Beauchamp 2003a).

Though the movements of the thumb are usually quite independent of those of the fingers, it is not unusual to find an anomalous linkage between the tendon of the long flexor of the thumb (flexor pollicis longus) and the deep flexor tendon of the index finger. This is known as Linburg-Comstock syndrome. Various studies have suggested an incidence of 20–35 percent in the general population, with about a quarter of cases showing the linkage in both hands. It is easy to demonstrate that this condition is quite common: ask a group of musicians to curl up their thumbs and to tell you if the index finger moves involuntarily (see video 3-1). Most affected individuals do not comment on it, as they assume that it is the norm. The degree of linkage varies considerably, and in a small proportion of instrumentalists it can lead to pain or difficulty in playing (Miller et al. 2003). This is one of the few tendon linkages where surgery is both feasible and generally beneficial (Allieu et al. 1998).

The considerable anatomical variation in the muscles and tendons in the hand is therefore an important factor in performance that should be both recognized and accepted by musicians and their teachers (Bergman, Afifi, and Miyauchi 2004). Certain muscles or tendons may be absent in some individuals, or their form or attachments may differ from the norm. The superficial flexor digitorum tendon to the little finger is missing in about 5 percent of hands (Miller et al. 2003). Variation is particularly common in the lumbrical muscles, where as many as 50 percent of hands do not show the standard pattern (Perkins and Hast 1993). The tendon of the third lumbrical muscle divides to insert into the ring and middle fingers in up to a third of the population, while in a few individuals there is no lumbrical insertion on the little finger at all. In addition, the range of movement of different joints in the hand varies, as does overall hand size. As a result, regardless of the degree of training, not all musicians are capable of moving the fingers in precisely the same way, and this should be reflected in a flexible approach to the teaching of playing technique in general and keyboard fingering in particular. Some practical examples of these problems and how they can be overcome are discussed by Beauchamp (Beauchamp 2003b).

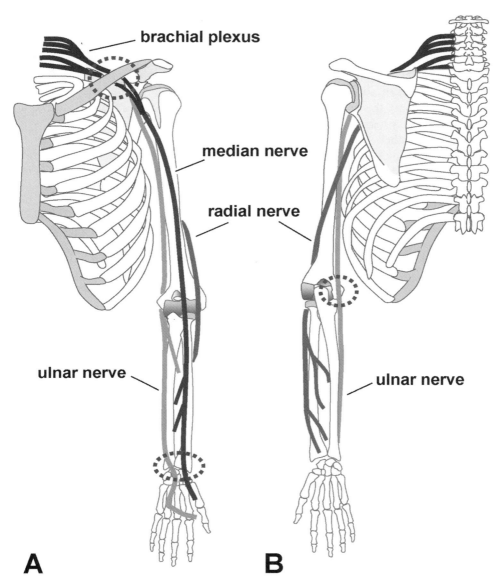

Figure 3-14. The paths of the radial, ulnar, and median nerves in the arm. These all arise from the brachial plexus, whose roots emerge from between the cervical vertebrae. A. View from the back. B. View from the front. The dashed circles show the most common sites of nerve compression or entrapment: the thoracic outlet where the nerves emerge from under the collarbone, the ulnar nerve at the elbow, and at the wrist, the median and, to a lesser extent, the ulnar nerves.

The Nerve Supply to the Arm and Hand

The nerves running to the arm originate from the cervical (neck) region of the spinal cord. They emerge from between the lower neck vertebrae as five nerve roots, which fuse and divide in a complex manner to form the nerves supplying the arm and shoulder. This cluster of nerve roots and their branches is called the brachial plexus. We will consider only the three largest nerves that emerge to supply the arm: the radial, medial, and ulnar nerves (fig. 3-14). To reach the arm, the nerves must pass through a narrow gap rather inappropriately called the thoracic outlet, which lies between the collarbone and the uppermost rib. As well as the nerves, this crowded space contains the main artery and vein supplying the arm and gives its name to a number of conditions (thoracic outlet syndromes) that can arise if either the nerves or the blood vessels become compressed here (see below).

The radial nerve spirals round the back of the upper arm, through the triceps muscle, which it supplies. When it emerges on the lateral side of the elbow, it crosses in front of the joint before turning to the back of the forearm to supply muscles there. It

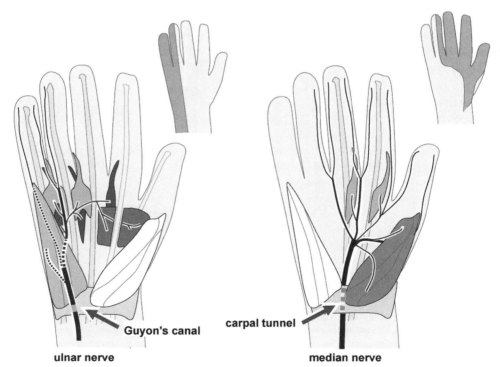

Figure 3-15.   The distribution of the ulnar and median nerve branches in the hand. The ulnar nerve supplies the muscles at the base of the little finger, the interosseus muscles, two of the lumbricals, and the adductor of the thumb. The median nerve supplies the muscles at the base of the thumb and the remaining lumbricals. The arrows indicate where the nerves may become trapped: Guyon's canal, a passage through the thickness of the retinaculum, for the ulnar nerve and the carpal tunnel for the median nerve. Nerve compression may produce tingling or numbness in the areas of skin supplied, indicated by the shaded regions in the small hand outlines.

therefore controls the extensor muscles of the elbow (triceps), wrist, and hand, which straighten the elbow and fingers and pull the wrist back. Of the three large nerves of the arm, the radial nerve is the least often damaged in musicians. However, because it wraps tightly round the humerus, it may be damaged if the bone is fractured.

The median nerve supplies mainly flexor muscles. It passes down the front of the upper arm underneath the biceps (though it doesn't supply it). Biceps and some associated muscles that flex the upper arm and elbow are controlled by the much smaller musculocutaneous nerve. The median nerve crosses in front of the elbow and between two parts of a muscle that pronates the forearm (pronator teres). This is an important relationship, as the median nerve can sometimes be entrapped and compressed by the muscle. The nerve branches extensively in the front of the forearm to supply flexor muscles of the wrist, fingers, and thumb. It enters the hand by passing under the retinaculum at the wrist (fig. 3-15). This narrow channel (the carpal tunnel) is one of the most common sites of median nerve compression. Within the hand, the median nerve supplies the pad of short muscles that move the thumb (the thenar eminence) and the lumbricals of the index and middle finger. It is also sensory to the skin on these two fingers, the thumb, and the side of the palm from which they arise. Compression of the nerve in the carpal tunnel may therefore produce a tingling or numbness in this area of skin and weakness or wasting of the muscles it supplies. The middle of the palm remains unaffected because the branch of the median nerve that provides it with sensation runs over the top of the retinaculum.

The ulnar nerve runs down the inside of the upper arm but supplies no muscles there. At the elbow, it passes behind the broad part of the humerus on the inner side just above the joint before passing into the front of the arm in a channel (the cubital tunnel) between the two heads of one of the wrist flexors (flexor carpi ulnaris). The ulnar nerve is very vulnerable here (as most of us know to our cost). If the elbow is struck forcibly against some object, the nerve may be pinched against the bone, which leads to pain and a tingling sensation in the little finger and the adjacent side of the ring finger, the region of the hand whose sensation is carried by this nerve. It can also become entrapped in the cubital tunnel (see animation 3-6). In the forearm it supplies one of the wrist flexors and contributes to the innervation of the deep flexor muscles of the fingers. At the wrist it passes under part of the retinaculum (Guyon's canal), where it is again vulnerable to compression, then supplies most of the small muscles of the hand (the short muscles to the little finger, all the interosseus muscles, the lumbricals for the fourth and little fingers, and the adductor of the thumb) (fig. 3-15). If the nerve is badly damaged at the elbow or in the hand, the resulting weakness in the lumbricals and interossei makes it difficult or impossible to straighten the little and fourth fingers, which curl into the palm as a result.

PLAYING-RELATED INJURY—YOU ARE NOT ALONE

The idea that certain precisely definable injuries are associated with particular professions is not a new one. For example, the Mad Hatter in *Alice in Wonderland* exhibits the symptoms of poisoning by the mercury compounds that were used in preparing fur for the cheaper varieties of top hats. Musculoskeletal problems associated with the maintenance of awkward postures or with repetitive movements were first recognized in a remarkable and wide-ranging study of occupational diseases by the seventeenth-century physician Bernardini Ramazzini (Franco 1999; Ramazzini 1964), though his findings were perhaps not generally appreciated by the medical community at that time, and certainly not widely acted upon for a further three hundred years. Over the last twenty to thirty years, there has been a growing awareness among orchestral managers and among some medical professionals that musicians are particularly vulnerable to performance-related injury. This awareness has arisen from the work of a few musicians who have risked their careers by publicizing their playing-related problems and by seeking to devise and implement practices in their own orchestras aimed at reducing the incidence of injury and promoting successful rehabilitation of injured players (Paull and Harrison 1997; Culf 1998; Horvath 2002, 2004). Awareness of these issues among players and managers has been aided by the emergence of arts medicine as a distinct discipline and the recognition that the treatment of musicians can be a specialized area for clinicians (Winspur and Wynn Parry 1998; Sataloff, Brandfonbrener, and Lederman 1998) in the way that sports medicine has long been. Indeed, the injuries experienced by musicians, as well as their treatments and prevention, have much in common with those of athletes. In the UK, schemes such as the Healthy Orchestra charter, developed by the Association of British Orchestras, the Musicians Benevolent Fund, and the British Association of Performing Arts Medicine, are being developed to promote musicians' health.

One of the seminal events that awakened interest in the medical problems of musicians was the publication in 1988 of the International Convention of Symphony and Orchestral Musicians Survey, which was based on questionnaires sent to over four thousand musicians (Fishbein et al. 1998). This was published in the newly formed journal *Medical Problems in Performing Artists*. There is, of course, always a danger with such surveys that the responders are a self-selecting population with injury problems that may not be typical of the whole population contacted. Also, many groups of musicians such as keyboard players, singers, and jazz or rock performers would have been underrepresented. Nevertheless, more than 55 percent of those contacted replied, which suggested that health issues were a major concern for these musicians. According to Wynn Parry (1998c), quoting summary data not in the original paper, the survey revealed musculoskeletal problems of the neck, shoulder, arm, or hand in over 66 percent of string players, 48 percent of woodwind players, and 32 percent of brass players. About half of these problems were rated "severe" by the players concerned. A large number of subsequent surveys of professional musicians and both school-age and university-level music students found incidences of performance-related pain or musculoskeletal problems of 34 to 87 percent, though in most cases severity was not assessed (Zaza 1998). Perhaps even more telling is a report of the experiences of a group of amateur musicians who went on a one-week performance course. The players who normally practiced only an hour a day played for six to seven hours daily for the week, and as a result 72 percent developed new and painful playing-related symptoms (Newmark and Lederman 1987). Although this is an isolated example, it is indicative of the consequences that can be expected from a rapid scaling up of playing intensity, a pattern of behavior that is likely to be common in musicians preparing for an imminent recital or audition (Newmark and Hochberg 1987) or among students on first entering the competitive environment of a music school. Nevertheless, most of the plethora of surveys of musicians' injuries rely on self-reporting of symptoms by the participants and therefore lack any objective medical assessment of the physical problems reported or, indeed, comparison with an age-matched control population of nonmusicians. They therefore take us little further in understanding the actual range and severity of playing-related injury.

Many musicians find it possible to continue to play in the face of upper-limb pain and may even accept it as an inevitable part of their profession. However heroic this may seem, it is ultimately counterproductive as, without diagnosis and treatment, the condition is likely to deteriorate until there is a clear loss of technique through tissue damage, muscle weakness, or an attrition of fine motor control (Fry and Rowley 1992). We have already seen in chapter 1 that pain is usually linked to inflammation, which exacerbates many of the injuries that musicians are likely to experience. In addition, changes in posture to compensate for loss of dexterity or restriction of movement frequently lead to difficulties at sites other than the original source of discomfort. This not only compounds the problem, but can make it much harder to diagnose the root cause. Symptoms such as extensive pain, loss of dexterity in the playing movements, tingling or numbness, muscle weakness, or any indication of changes in the shape or bulk of muscles in the arm or hand must be taken very seriously and help sought as rapidly as possible.

There may be many reasons why players stoically soldier on in the face of pain. First, in a few dark corners, the outmoded concept of "no pain—no gain" may still hold sway. The overview of pain in chapter 1 should have amply demonstrated that this is an inappropriate response. It certainly isn't applied to professional athletes, who are valuable commodities financially and whose teams therefore demand the most rapid and effective treatment for their injuries. Discomfort from exhaustion is one thing (and is probably what the old adage originally referred to), but pain as a result of tissue damage is quite another. Other reasons why musicians try to ignore pain may be a fear of revealing a physical weakness in a highly competitive profession, or a worry that they may be ordered to cease playing for a prolonged period or be encouraged to agree to a risky intervention such as surgery. Clinicians who are familiar with musicians' problems will be well aware of the psychological consequences of an embargo on playing. As to surgery, this is always a last resort and is appropriate in only a small proportion of cases. Treatment is more likely to involve a combination of less daunting therapies, and a central plank of this should always be reassessment of playing posture and technique, as well as a consideration of general health and fitness and an exploration of strategies to relieve stress, which is a major contributing factor to playing-related pain. Some of the treatment may even be directed at the instrument, to adapt it more closely to the body, or the physical limits of the player. Figure 3-16 provides a summary of the range and possible interactions of factors underlying performance-related problems experienced by a group of musicians who sought help at one well-known clinic specializing in performance-related problems.

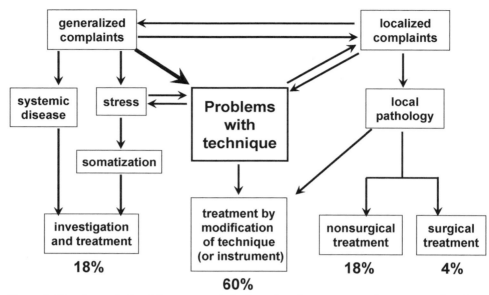

Figure 3-16. An analysis of the causes of playing-related symptoms and treatment of patients seen at a clinic run by Winspur and Wynn Parry (reproduced with permission from Winspur and Wynn Parry [1998], p. 38, fig. 2).

SEEKING HELP WHEN THINGS GO WRONG

Perhaps the most vital message to take on board about seeking help is to seek it early. The more established an injury is, the harder it will be to diagnose and treat, and the longer and more difficult will be the rehabilitation. It is also often important to seek out a clinician who is not only a specialist in the relevant medical discipline (e.g,. an orthopedic or neurological consultant), but also is familiar with these problems as they are manifested in the musician. The role of the general practitioner is to treat common ailments and to identify those that need the attention of a specialist, to whom the patient will then be referred. In most instances, the general practitioner will not be familiar with the specialist requirements of musicians, and it is unrealistic to expect this. In turn, hospital specialists, though undoubtedly possessing a detailed knowledge of a particular field of medicine, may see few musicians among their patients and may be more attuned to occupationally related limb problems among manual laborers or the elderly, if these make up the majority of their patients. A specialist will not ask a bricklayer with a suspected rotator cuff tear to bring in his hod, but someone with a knowledge of the upper-limb problems of musicians will certainly need to examine the patient with his or her instrument in order to understand the posture that player adopts and whether this needs correcting. If your doctor does not want to see your playing posture, you may wish to consult elsewhere. It is also vital that a detailed patient history is taken that takes into consideration all aspects of a musician's lifestyle. In a retrospective analysis of a group of over six hundred musicians presenting with upper-limb problems at a clinic specializing in musicians' problems, only 41 percent turned out to have a diagnosable physical condition (fig. 3-16). In 40 percent the symptoms arose from problems with technique, and in 19 percent the physical symptoms appeared to be a manifestation of stress and anxiety (Winspur and Wynn Parry 1998).

The specialist clinician will also apply a knowledge of the patient's instrument and lifestyle to devise a suitable treatment. This will take into consideration the importance of keeping any reduction in playing to the minimum that is compatible with a successful outcome. A well-planned rehabilitation program is not only important for therapeutic goals such as maintaining the mobility of affected joints, but also for retaining technical skills and ensuring the mental well-being of the patient. In addition, where surgical intervention is necessary, it is important that the way in which this is carried out has as little impact as possible on playing, and this may necessitate a rather different approach to that used for the same condition in a nonmusician (Winspur and Wynn Parry 1997). As will be seen from some of the later sections of this chapter, diagnosis of neuromuscular problems in the upper limb can be difficult and the symptoms are sometimes confusing, so unraveling the primary cause of the malady may require considerable insight. Furthermore, though the conditions seen in musicians occur quite frequently among nonmusicians, the symptoms may not be identical (Brandfonbrener 2003). Fortunately, clinicians with the necessary skills are increasingly to be found as arts medicine becomes an established discipline. The field is supported by a growing body of knowledge of the health problems of musicians that has come from research in a number of specialist centers that have arisen in Europe and the United States.

Fully resolving a playing-related problem is likely to involve a number of different therapeutic strategies. Your doctor will start the ball rolling by assessing and treating your immediate physical symptoms. This will often be followed by physiotherapy over a period of weeks or months to strengthen the muscles that give postural support to a joint that is causing problems, or to relieve pressure on a compressed nerve. Some of these exercises may be continued indefinitely to maintain muscle strength or joint flexibility. However, the primary cause also needs to be established, together with any factors that may have aggravated the original injury. If this is not done, it is likely to occur again, or at the very least, apprehension that it could limit or affect playing will remain. You may want to be a little less enthusiastic with your home-improvement or holiday pursuits if you think that these have been triggering factors, but even where there is an obvious starting point, you should reexamine your technique with your instrumental teacher or mentor and with a physiotherapist. This may result in some retraining during which a temporary reduction in the fluency of playing must be accepted for long-term gain. Remember that playing with good technique should ultimately improve performance! You may find it beneficial to use strategies such as the Alexander technique, Feldenkrais method, yoga, or tai chi to promote greater postural awareness and reduce stress, which is beneficial both for general emotional and physical well-being and for reducing chronic muscle tension.

Information on where to find doctors, physiotherapists, or dentists who specialize in the problems of musicians can be found in a number of places. In the UK, help can be obtained from the British Association for Performing Arts Medicine (BAPAM,

Totara Park House, Fourth Floor, 34-36 Gray's Inn Road, London WC1X 8HR; Tel.: 0845 602 0235, website: www.bapam.org). The equivalent organization in the United States is the Performing Arts Medical Association (Mary Fletcher, Executive Director, PAMA, P.O. Box 61228, Denver, CO 80206; Tel./Fax: 303-632-9255, e-mail: artsmed@comcast.net, website: www.artsmed.org). Many other useful sources can be found in the extensive resource list in Horvath (2002).

The details of treatment for individual conditions will vary according to your doctor's assessment of the symptoms and the precise diagnosis made, but the basic palette of treatments is explained here, though the list is far from exhaustive. This is done partly to avoid repetition in the following sections on specific ailments, but mainly to provide a general overview of the short-term consequences of seeking help. The object is to try to dispel unnecessary fears of how drastic treatment may be and the extent to which it may disrupt musical life, while still giving a realistic picture of what is likely to be involved. It is hoped that by clarifying these issues, players will be less resistant to seeking help in a timely fashion. The way these therapies are now applied owes a considerable amount to the development of sports medicine, which has played an important role in advancing the treatment of musculoskeletal and related problems. It is not only important to get athletes rehabilitated as rapidly as possible, but also to prevent a rapid recurrence of the injury. The same principles apply to the rehabilitation of musicians, even if they cannot command the same transfer fees!

Rest

Apart from the prospect of surgery, being advised to abstain from playing for a prolonged period of time may be the form of treatment most dreaded by musicians, for whom this may at best result in loss of facility through lack of practice, and at worst, loss of identity, self-esteem, and the ability to earn a livelihood. At one time, rest was the most commonly prescribed treatment for a wide range of musculoskeletal problems. The joint, tendon, or muscle was simply immobilized as much as possible until the condition resolved. While it remains true that for many conditions we still rely on the body to repair itself by its own internal mechanisms, rest is no longer seen as a panacea, and in most cases muscle wastage (which happens very rapidly), joint stiffness, and other consequences of immobility are positively disadvantageous for optimum recovery. Furthermore, after surgery to free tendons and nerves, it is particularly vital that physiotherapy and the control of inflammation start as soon as possible to prevent scar tissue from binding together structures that need to move relative to one another. The initial stages of treatment are aimed at reducing the acute symptoms (i.e., immediate symptoms of pain and inflammation that arise abruptly and may abate quite quickly). Nowadays, experienced practitioners dealing with musicians do not often advocate prolonged periods of complete rest; however, it is vital that the return to playing is carefully managed and that agreed timetables are strictly adhered to (Winspur 1998d). A musician with a serious problem may start playing again for as little as five minutes twice a day. Progress is carefully monitored and playing time increased accordingly. Following such a timetable may be frustrating initially, but it should be remembered that this will ultimately provide the quickest route to recovery. Though the periods of actual playing may be restricted, the player will benefit both musically and psychologically from perfecting the skills of mental rehearsal (see chapter 8) and in learning and analyzing scores that will be played on recovery. Of course, an even better approach is not to delay seeking help until the injury has developed to the extent that this is required. Practical advice for dealing with the period of rehabilitation can be found from a number of sources (Horvath 2002; Warrington 2003). The importance of a staged rehabilitation from injury is now recognized by some orchestras, which have put in place procedures that allow a progressive return to full playing (Horvath 2004). These are the orchestras that, even in a difficult financial climate, truly value their players and take a rational view of injury and its effect on performance. It is to be hoped that such practices will in time become the norm, as they are more likely to result in a full recovery and prevent an avoidable loss of career in injured musicians.

Treatment for Acute Pain and Inflammation

The acute symptoms of injury are often pain and swelling of the affected area. These two symptoms are related to a considerable degree, because the nerve endings that carry information on pain also release chemicals at the injury site that contribute to the inflammation (see chapter 1). Any restricted spaces within the tissue through which structures such as tendons or nerves must slide will become narrower, so that friction is generated by such movement. This creates a vicious circle in which further damage leads to more pain and inflammation. Rapid control of inflammation is therefore important. One anti-inflammatory treatment you will all have seen on the athletic fields is the application of cold packs. This constricts the blood vessels that are the source of the accumulating fluid, slowing the development of the inflammation. It is most effective when applied as quickly as possible after the injury or immediately when the swelling first appears. That is why injured athletes will apply an cold pack even when watching the remainder of the game in which they have been injured. A bag of frozen peas makes a good substitute for home use, as it can be molded to the shape of the injured region; however, if it is very cold, it may be necessary to put a cloth between the pack and the skin to prevent tissue damage. A typical strategy would be to apply the pack for twenty to thirty minutes every three to four hours. Inflammation can also be reduced by raising the swollen area to reduce the blood pressure that is driving the fluid into the damaged tissues. For the arm and hand, it is particularly effective if these can be raised above the head. Compression of the swollen region with elastic bandages will also help to prevent the fluid from accumulating. Oral drugs with both painkilling and anti-inflammatory properties (e.g., ibuprofen) may also be prescribed, while in more severe chronic conditions, such drugs may also be injected into the injury site by a skilled clinician.

Splinting

During rehabilitation from injury, splints may be employed to provide support or to transfer load from one part of the limb to another (see fig. 3-17). For example, in a clarinetist, a splint can be used to transfer the weight of the instrument from the last joint of the right thumb, where it is usually carried, to the base of the thumb, where it

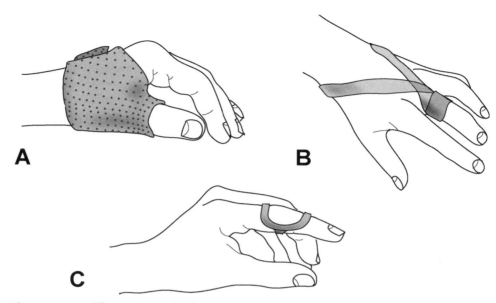

Figure 3-17. Different types of splints used on the fingers. A. Splint made from heat-molded plastic, which allows molding of the shape. This one supports the joint at the base of the thumb. B. A dynamic splint made from a flexible adhesive dressing, used to limit the degree of movement of the metacarpophalangeal joint. C. A ring splint made of plastic or metal used to support the finger joint at a fixed angle. This is useful where joint hypermobility might cause the finger joint to collapse under the loading experienced during playing.

exerts less leverage. Splints can also be used to keep an injured joint straight if there is a tendency for the damaged tissues to contract, which leads to chronic flexion. For the fingers in particular, the use of splints can greatly reduce the time needed to regain full extension of a joint after injury. Nowadays, rigid splints can take a variety of forms, some of which are shown in figure 3-17. Many are made of a stiff but thin thermo-plastic, which when warmed can be molded to the precise shape required. This is very useful for producing small, irregularly shaped splints to support the fingers, and also ensures a comfortable fit. Where it is necessary to fix or support a finger joint during routine playing as opposed to during rehabilitation or reeducation, ring splints can be worn. These are sets of metal or plastic rings, similar in thickness to thin jewelry rings, that are welded together so that when slipped onto the finger they lie round the bones on either side of a joint, holding it at a fixed angle. Dynamic splints (which serve to limit the range of movement of a joint) can be fashioned from adhesive tape to fix the end point of joint movement to help players learn new playing practices or to avoid a joint angle that may be risky (Stotko 1998).

Physiotherapy

Physiotherapy plays an important role in strengthening muscles and increasing joint flexibility, either to address directly the causes of a playing-related problem or as part of the process of rehabilitation after surgical or nonsurgical treatments. The muscles that are used in playing will be well developed but others that are important for posture may be less so and may need strengthening to increase hand or arm stability. When movement becomes restricted due to problems with tendons or joints, or because of nerve damage, muscles rapidly get smaller and weaker. Rebuilding them through a program of exercise is a much slower process, and it is important that this is carried out conscientiously. Similarly, regaining the full mobility of a joint that has been swollen or a tendon that has become tight in its sheath can also be difficult and sometimes painful, and a steady approach through physiotherapy is the only recourse. The boundary between physiotherapy, exercise, and body maintenance is a blurred one; activities such as the Alexander technique, Feldenkrais, yoga, and tai chi may start off in one role and end up in another. Equally, any aerobic exercise such as walking, jogging, or swimming can be viewed as physiotherapy, as these activities move joints and muscles in a different way from that required by playing an instrument. These forms of exercise will ultimately benefit your musical activities, not only through their specific effects on particular muscles and joints but also by improving general health through their conditioning effects on the cardiovascular and respiratory systems.

Surgery

For most conditions, surgery is the last resort, and it is important that before this course is decided upon, a most careful diagnosis is carried out to ensure that it is the most appropriate course of action. Under such review, surgical treatment is uncommon. In the above-mentioned sample of over six hundred musicians with upper limb problems, only 4 percent underwent surgery (see fig. 3-16) (Winspur and Wynn Parry 1998). As already mentioned, the surgical approach used for a particular condition in a musician may differ from that in a nonmusician. One important consideration is the site of the incisions that are to be made through the skin (Winspur 1998d). For example, these should not cross areas of skin used to close open holes on wind instruments or to hold down strings. Here the nature of the player's instrument must be considered carefully. For example, while in most wind instruments it is the pad of the last joint of the finger that is used to close the hole, in the bagpipe the skin on the middle joint is used in all but one finger. Similarly, incisions in any part of the finger or thumb that supports the weight of the instrument should be avoided if possible. It is equally important not to damage small nerve branches that carry sensory information from areas of the skin that contact the instrument.

The advantages of undergoing surgery under local anesthesia are increasingly familiar to us today. Patients are usually discharged on the same day as the operation, and the small degree of risk associated with general anesthesia is eliminated. In the case of operations on the musician's hand this approach has additional psychological advantages; for example, the patient can be kept informed and reassured as to the progress being made throughout the operation. To some extent the result of the intervention on active finger movement can also be checked before wound closure, if this is appropriate. All this gives the patient a greater feeling of control over what is happening, which can be very reassuring for those whose livelihood depends on a high level of hand function. Another very important consequence of hand surgery under local anesthesia is that the patient can, by placing the hand on the head, keep it well elevated from the instant the operation is completed. Though this may sound rather bizarre, it substantially reduces the degree of swelling and consequent pain that is experienced postoperatively, which considerably speeds recovery (Winspur 1998d). Unless the operation has been to repair traumatic accidental damage to tendons, it may be possible to start playing for a few minutes several times a day only four or five days after the operation. Musicians faced with the possibility of surgery of the arm or hand would do well to read a short paper by Winspur and Wynn Parry (2000) before assessing their options. The clinician should provide a realistic assessment of the risks as well as the benefits of surgery in the context of the high level of functionality required by today's professional musician. This will be very different from what is likely to be acceptable to most nonmusicians undergoing a similar treatment. Informed consent must be just that.

WHAT CAN GO WRONG?

Generalized Pain and Overuse Syndrome

One of the most common diagnoses given for pain among musicians (and indeed those in other professions requiring rapid repetitive movements over prolonged periods) is overuse syndrome. This term, which is commonly and perhaps sometimes glibly used, may often not really reflect the root of the problem. As a diagnosis it has been the subject of a considerable amount of debate among clinicians, which has tended to generate more heat than light. The usual definition given is of a condition arising as consequence of exceeding the biological or physical limits of the tissue (e.g., of a muscle, tendon, nerve, or joint). This doom-laden description suggests imminent physical collapse and the end of a career, but increasingly it appears that the definition probably misses the point. It is possible to play for years without problems and then start to experience pain. This does not generally mean that a body component has suddenly worn out; however, an injury to a tendon in the wrist, for example, no matter how it is acquired, is likely to be exacerbated by the constant rapid movement of the fingers that is the normal daily life of a musician. Perhaps "delayed treatment syndrome" might be a more illuminating term in many cases, as prompt recognition and diagnosis of the injury will go a long way to prevent the appearance of chronic symptoms. Overuse syndrome has sometimes been linked to repetitive strain injury (a term that will probably also be familiar to the reader), whose diagnosis at one time threatened to reach epidemic proportions. This name is now little used by clinicians, as it has become apparent that symptoms formerly associated with this condition are not necessarily caused by repetitive movements in themselves (for the reasons just given), nor by any form of strain (Wynn Parry 1998b).

The demands on the body experienced by musicians have many similarities with those of athletes, so let's illustrate this with a sporting analogy. Let us suppose that after keeping fit for years by running, you decide you want to get your exercise by rowing instead. You regard yourself as fit, so when you get in the boat or rowing machine, you are always pushing to achieve the same level of exercise you used to get from your daily five-mile run. Your performance in the boat improves in a gratifying manner over the first few sessions, then suddenly you start to get low back pain and feel discomfort in the middle of the back and one side of the chest. You put this down to the usual muscle discomfort associated with getting fit, but after a couple more sessions you have to admit that you have pulled a muscle connecting the shoulder blade to the ribs and must stop rowing. This and the back pain are technically overuse injuries, but only in the sense that you have exceeded the capabilities of the muscles at their current level of training. You don't imagine your sporting or even rowing days are over. There is no mystery about the source of the problem or its remedy. You realize that though your leg muscles are strong from years of pounding the pavement, those of your trunk and upper body are not at the same level. You let the injury heal, get some advice on technique, and return to rowing through a carefully monitored series of sessions, gradually increasing their length and the effort they require. This is not only for the benefit of the injured muscle, but also to ensure that your other upper-body muscles are not overstressed as they gradually increase in strength. In addition, you make sure you warm up thoroughly before you row strenuously. In this context you will recognize that the approach is simple common sense.

Now let's imagine a different scenario. You are a young musician and you have just entered a prestigious music school. You thought you were a pretty good player and are shocked to discover the standard of "the competition." Overnight you double your daily practice. Your arms are stiff when you wake up in the morning, and instead of improving, your playing gets worse because your fingers don't seem to want to respond the way you want them to. Not wishing to be defeated, you redouble your efforts and start to experience pain in the forearm and wrist, which finally makes playing almost impossible. The doctor gives the dreaded diagnosis of overuse syndrome (or perhaps some other condition with an even more impenetrable name). This no more means that your body can't cope with the life of a professional musician than was the case with the athlete. The remedy is likely to be similar to that of the previous example, but how much better it would have been to have avoided the breakdown by opting for a more measured approach to increasing practice. It is easy to say and hard to do, perhaps, but returning to full playing after injury takes time and may sap your confidence, so a carefully staged increase in daily practice will achieve your objectives more rapidly in the long run. From a psychological point of view, a good way to approach improving your level of skill in this situation is to set out a timetable with a regular series of goals. You can then pick them off one by one, and have confidence that after a given period of months you will have a good chance of achieving the level of performance you have set for yourself.

While there are many specific problems that arise in players of instruments that require rapid and sometimes forceful finger movements over prolonged periods of time, the underlying physical changes that result in overuse syndrome remain obscure. This situation is not aided by the fact that it has no widely agreed definition (Fry and Rowley 1992; Rozmaryn 1993; Brandfonbrener 2003; Winspur 2003). This is not a trivial problem, because a condition described only on the basis of a set of rather generalized symptoms may in fact represent a number of distinct conditions with different origins, each requiring a specific treatment. It is not even clear that it is actually the intensity of playing that is the problem, rather than the abrupt changes in patterns of practice. One's susceptibility to it may be strongly influenced by overall fitness, stress levels, and other lifestyle issues. A major contributory factor is likely to be posture. The one adopted, which should be tailored to your particular body shape, should minimize the chance of physical problems developing. Good posture in this sense will naturally form the basis of an efficient playing technique. A maintained high intensity of playing need not result in overuse syndrome as long as this is reached by gradual increments and if the technique is good, the lifestyle healthy and stable, and sensible practice and playing patterns including warm-up, stretching exercises, and periodic rest periods are adhered to (Horvath 2002; Lippman 1991). For a short, thoughtful account on overuse syndrome, the reader is referred to an excellent article by Wynn Parry (1998b).

The pain associated with overuse syndrome may initially be felt in the hand during playing but may later spread to the forearm and shoulder. One characteristic feature of this pain is that it is not restricted to any particular joint, tendon, or muscle group. As the condition deteriorates, pain may be experienced during movements involved in everyday tasks such as turning a door handle. Strangely, though the pain can be severe, its physical characteristics are often hard to pin down. For example, other than some slight muscle tenderness, there is usually no real muscle weakness or restriction of movement, and there may be no indication of tendonitis or loss of sensation. The condition has variously been attributed to biochemical changes in the muscle resulting from extreme fatigue (Wynn Parry 1998b), the breakdown products released from damaged, swollen muscles (Fry 2000), damage to the junction between the muscle and tendon (Lederman and Calabrese 1986), or inflammation of the synovial sheath of the tendon (Hochberg et al. 1983), which is actually tenosynovitis (see below). None of this confusion, however, detracts from the very real pain and disability that is experienced. Furthermore, chronic pain can cause long-term changes in the circuitry of the spinal cord, which may result in sensations that were previously innocuous becoming painful (chapter 1). This adds to the difficulties of resolving the problem.

Problems with Tendons

One specific problem that is sometimes linked to overuse is tendonitis. Though tendonitis literally means "inflammation of the tendon," in practice the symptoms may arise from inflammation of the synovial sheath of the tendon (the tenosynovium), in which case it should be known as tenosynovitis, or degenerative changes in the tendon even in the absence of inflammation. To make matters more confusing, many additional names are used to describe tendonitis of different types at particular sites in the upper limb (Rozmaryn 1993); as these are commonly in use by clinicians, several of the names will be employed in the following account. As with many apparently common conditions, vigorous debate continues as to the origin of the several forms of tendonitis. For example, though many consider that tendonitis can be a manifestation of repetitive strain injury, there is still a lack of objective evidence to support this

(Wynn Parry 1998e). Among musicians, tendonitis is not as common as one might expect given the repetitive nature of their playing movements, and when encountered in this group it often appears to have been triggered by a nonmusical activity (e.g., home-improvement project or sports), perhaps because these may involve short periods of intense physical effort of a type that the body is unused to. For example, it might be the consequence of a day spent putting up shelves or curtain track using a manual screwdriver, which involves maintaining a strong grip on the screwdriver coupled with repeated, forceful supination of the forearm against the resistance of the screw. Such activity might cause tendonitis in the shoulder, elbow, or wrist. Paint stripping and prolonged periods of vigorous sanding are also notorious for inducing tendonitis (Winspur and Wynn Parry 1998). Once it has developed, tendonitis is likely to be aggravated by the movements required for playing, though this in itself is not the primary cause. Nevertheless, prolonged practice of technically demanding pieces requiring rapid fingerwork can sometimes result in swelling and tenderness in the arm or hand of keyboard and string players. This may involve not only the tendon and tendon sheaths of the long flexor muscles of the fingers whose muscle bellies lie in the forearm, but also (and this is sometimes overlooked) those of the small intrinsic muscles of the hand, for example, the lumbrical and interosseus muscles (Silver and Rozmaryn 1998).

Problems with the shoulder are frequently seen in players of bowed string instruments because of the maintained elevated posture of the arm. If you watch the string section of almost any orchestra you will see that the frequency and degree of right-arm abduction in violinists and viola players, and of either arm in cellists, varies greatly between individuals. Discomfort may be experienced in the tendons of the rotator cuff muscles (rotator cuff syndrome), which connect the arm to the shoulder blade. This often originates from what is known as an impingement, in which the tendon becomes pinched against the bone. A common site of impingement is where the tendon of the supraspinatus muscle passes through the narrow channel under the acromium of the shoulder blade (animation 3-2). This may cause the tendon to swell due to inflammation, which only makes the impingement worse. The friction this generates can abrade and ultimately tear the tendon through completely. This is most likely to occur in people who are older or physically inactive, as muscles and tendons that are not used quickly become reduced in bulk and strength. Among musicians, rotator cuff problems are not only confined to players, but may also affect conductors. The chance of developing this and many other injuries is therefore reduced not only by good posture, but also by maintaining a reasonable level of general fitness, which helps maintain the muscles' integrity. This is important not only for muscles used directly in playing but also those that have a role in stabilization and support.

The extensor muscles of the fingers arise from a common flattened tendinous structure that attaches them to a lateral ridge on the lower end of the humerus, just above the elbow joint. This region is called the lateral epicondyle, meaning that it lies above (epi-) the articulation of the joint (condyle). Pain symptomatic of tendonitis in this region may occur after repeated forceful rotation of the hand and wrist, as in the example given above of using a screwdriver, or it may be associated with extension of the wrist while forcibly gripping the handle of something like a tennis racket or shovel. Though technically termed lateral epicondylitis, it is known more familiarly as tennis elbow.

Another common site of tendon pain is at the base of the thumb, where the tendons of the long abductor and extensor muscles of the thumb run in the walls of the anatomical snuff box. Tenderness in this regions may be a sign of de Quervain's syndrome, an inflammation of synovial sheaths of the tendons. It is sometimes seen in young female bassoonists and may also be present in other woodwind players who must support the weight of the instrument on the thumb (most commonly clarinetists). In keyboard players similar problems can be experienced in the flexor tendons of the fingers of either hand where they cross the wrist. In violinists and guitarists it is tendons of the left hand that are most commonly affected, particularly those of the middle and ring fingers (Winspur and Wynn Parry 1998). This may be accompanied by some transient numbness in the nearby skin. The tendon itself sometimes develops a nodule, which makes it difficult for the tendon to slide through the synovial sheath as the finger straightens (fig. 3-13). Nodules on tendons also arise due to rheumatoid arthritis or as a result of diabetes. When they occur in a flexor tendon, the finger tends to be held crooked as if round a trigger, which is why it is given the name "trigger finger." When a persistent attempt is made to extend the finger, the nodule presses against the entrance of the sheath until it finally forces its way in with a snapping sound.

Given time and a respite from inflammation, tendonitis will usually resolve itself. The symptoms can also be treated effectively by injections of anti-inflammatory drugs and local anesthetic into the tendon sheath, which usually provide dramatic and instantaneous relief. Such treatment is generally followed up by physiotherapy in the form of stretching and strengthening exercises (Winspur and Wynn Parry 1998; Silver and Rozmaryn 1998). Ring splints may also be utilized to restrict tendon movement, thus reducing the aggravation caused by the tendon continually passing through the trigger point. Though surgery is sometimes advocated to open the tendon sheath, this can carry particular risks for musicians. For example, in violinists, cutting open the sheath to provide relief for de Quervain's syndrome may leave the tendon prone to dislocation from its channel because of the flexed and radially deviated wrist posture that is sometimes required in either hand during playing (Winspur and Wynn Parry 1998).

Ganglion Cysts

Swellings under the skin of the wrist, called ganglion cysts, can cause inflammation of tendons. The cysts, which usually contain a mucuslike fluid, most often occur on the dorsal surface for the wrist. They are benign soft tissue tumors that sometimes arise from the sheath of a flexor tendon but more frequently derive from the capsule of the joints between the small carpal bones of the hand. They are more common in women and may cause dull, aching pain. Among instrumentalists, ganglia of the flexor sheaths are quite often seen in drummers and tympanists (Winspur and Wynn Parry 1998). If they do not affect playing they can be left alone; however, if they prevent full extension of the wrist or movement of tendons, or are compressing a nerve, they will require some form of treatment. This may be as simple as removing the fluid they contain with a syringe, though the result is likely to be temporary. Surgery is the ultimate option, though care must be taken to ensure that neither the tendons nor any small sensory nerves in their vicinity are damaged. Following surgery, physiotherapy is required to prevent internal scarring from causing attachments that limit tendon movement.

Dupuytren's Contracture

Dupuytren's contracture is not a disease of tendons, but of a tough fibrous sheet of tissue (the palmar aponeurosis) that extends across the palm of the hand, from the flexor retinaculum of the wrist to the base of the fingers. It forms a strong roof above the flexor tendons, giving them some protection from the compressive forces caused by gripping. In Dupuytren's contracture, the fibrous bands of the aponeurosis thicken and contract, causing the fingers to be drawn into a curled position. It usually starts with the little and ring fingers and is seen most often in men over fifty, but is almost exclusively a disease of northern Europeans (Winspur 1998a). It is genetically inherited and may have been spread initially by the Vikings, with the result that it is seen in many families in Ireland and the west coast of Scotland. It is perhaps most famous as "the curse of the MacCrimmons," who were a family of bagpipers from the island of Skye. The consequences for instrumentalists depend considerably on their instrument. It causes serious problems for bagpipers because of the importance of the little finger in playing. It is also troublesome in instruments that require a broad reach, such as the piano and bassoon, but is much less of a disability in string players, whose fingers are normally quite flexed during playing. Treatment requires surgery, which must be carefully managed to ensure a good result but need only entail a break from playing of one to three weeks with full schedule resuming after one to two months. For a fuller treatment of the history of this condition, and important guiding principles for surgery, the reader is referred to Winspur (1998a).

Problems with Joints

Joint Hypermobility

The range of movement that joints are capable of varies between individuals, and hypermobility is most obviously manifest in what is commonly called double-jointedness. This is frequently encountered among musicians and indeed may even improve playing facility in instruments where the ability to hold extreme joint angles is an advantage. Under these circumstances it may even reduce susceptibility to some other forms of playing-related injury (Rosety-Rodriguez et al. 2003). Historical examples of individuals with hypermobility include Paganini and Rachmaninoff, but it is actually more typical of women, especially in the early teenage years, and is particularly associated with those who have a tall, thin body type (Wynn Parry 1998e). It can cause considerable problems in joints that support the weight of the instrument or must remain fixed when strong forces are applied to them (e.g., the wrist in fortissimo piano playing). In order to reap the benefits without paying the penalty of tendonitis and sprains, it is important to build up the muscles that support the joints to resist the forces generated. Splinting may be useful if the muscles are not yet strong enough for this; for hypermobility of finger joints, ring splints (fig. 3-17C) may be very effective for guitarists and other string players.

Arthritis

There are two forms of arthritis, osteoarthritis and rheumatoid arthritis. Osteoarthritis is a disease of aging caused by physical wear of the joint surfaces, and joints that are used most intensively are likely to be affected first. It frequently manifests itself in older musicians as pain at the carpometacarpal joint, which lies at the base of the thumb. This problem is particularly serious for string players in either hand, and of course, in keyboard players. It also poses problems for the left hand of clarinetists, though this can be alleviated by using a strap or rod to support the weight of the instrument. There are a number of treatments that can help the musician cope with the condition (Winspur 1998c), for example, gentle stretching of the capsule of an affected finger or thumb joint or the control of inflammation by injection of anti-inflammatory drugs into it. If the joint cannot be held in a stable, pain-free position during playing, small splints may be used for this purpose; as a last resort the joint can be surgically fixed at an angle that allows playing.

Rheumatoid arthritis is an autoimmune disease in which the body's defenses against infection are turned inappropriately against the tissues of the joints. It first causes swelling in the membranes that secrete the lubricating synovial fluid but may then progress to a gradual destruction of the cartilages of the joint. The disease often progresses quite slowly with periodic flare-ups, allowing time to adapt the repertoire to the limitations it imposes or to alter playing technique to accommodate the resulting disability. The swelling can be controlled with anti-inflammatory drugs, and surgical treatment may be beneficial to free tendons that have been immobilized by chronic inflammation (Wynn Parry 1998d).

Bursitis

If the bursae associated with a joint become inflamed, the surfaces may not slide smoothly over one another, with the result that movement stretches the tissue, causing pain. This condition is known as bursitis (the ending "-itis" means inflammation, so tendonitis is an inflammation of the tendon, arthritis is inflammation of the joint, appendicitis is an inflammation of the appendix, etc.). In the upper limb, some of the most commonly affected bursae are those in the shoulder joint (animation 3-2). The pain may be particularly marked when the arm is raised, a movement required to some degree by a large proportion of instrumentalists. This movement is brought about by activity in the deltoid and supraspinatus muscles, both of which lie in contact with bursae. There are many bursae elsewhere in the body, for example, in the elbow and knee, and these can also exhibit bursitis. When it develops, movements that aggravate it should be reduced as much as possible and ice packs or drug treatment used to reduce the inflammation. If the injury is experienced repeatedly, recovery is likely to become slower, so techniques aimed at its prevention (such as warming up and stretching exercises) should be cultivated.

Frozen Shoulder (also Known as Adhesive Capsulitis)

The key to understanding this condition is in the second of its two names. The capsule of the shoulder joint is thin and loose to allow maximum freedom of movement. The wall of the capsule has folds and creases that can open out when the joint is held in extreme positions. If the capsule becomes inflamed or torn, scarring may result, which seals these folds together, restricting the movement of the joint. This may also happen if the shoulder has been immobilized as a result of another injury, or it may be associated with problems such as Dupuytren's contracture. For reasons that are unknown, it can be a consequence of metabolic disorders such as diabetes or thyroid conditions. Frozen shoulder may develop during recovery from conditions such as rotator cuff syndrome when the shoulder is immobilized, for example, with a sling, for long periods each day. It is therefore important that these periods are interspersed with gentle stretching exercises that take the arm through its full range of movement at the shoulder. Treatment for frozen shoulder becomes progressively more difficult the longer it is delayed. It generally involves physical therapy, ice treatment, and the use of anti-inflammatory drugs. Though surgery is sometimes advocated, this can sometimes be counterproductive as it may cause additional adhesions.

Damage to Finger Joints

The proximal interphalangeal (PIP) joint is the middle joint of the finger (fig. 3-7) and is not only quite prone to damage (generally as a result of nonmusical activities) but also does not recover well from the inflammation that follows injury. The problem is that if the joint becomes swollen, it does not remain straight but tends to become fixed at an angle of 20°–30°. Even when the original injury appears relatively minor (such as a sprain), this can be difficult to correct because the ligaments around the joint tend to contract over the first five to ten days after injury. It is therefore important to splint the joint straight for the first week or so, and subsequently to control the inflammation and carry out passive and active stretching of the joint in order to regain the full range of movement (Davies, Rogers, and Kember 1998).

Nerve Problems

Most problems related to the nerves of the arm result from compression, so we will first consider the structure of the nerve and how this affects its function. Nerves are composed of bundles of axons (the long, cablelike processes of nerve cells) that carry information to and from the spinal cord and brain. Some of the axons carry sensory information from the skin, muscles, and joints, and others run in the opposite direction and control the muscles. The axons are associated with nonneuronal cells called glial cells, which are vital for their normal function. One type of glial cell wraps around the larger-diameter axons to form what is called a myelin sheath. For reasons that we need not go into, this increases the rate at which information can flow along the axon. If the myelin sheath is damaged, the passage of information will slow or stop altogether. Depending on the type of axon affected, this will lead to either a loss of sensation or to muscle weakness or paralysis. If activity in the nerve is blocked, the muscles rapidly start to waste away, becoming noticeably smaller in a matter of weeks.

The axon bundles are surrounded by a fatty, elastic tissue that acts rather like bubble wrap, protecting them from compression. The entire nerve and its packing are wrapped in a tough outer sleeve that not only protects the softer tissue underneath from abrasion, but also adds tensile strength to the nerve. As a limb moves, the large nerves crossing the joints may slide 1–2 centimeters relative to the surrounding bones and, at certain points, may be stretched slightly around the bony projections of the skeleton. This is normal, and the elasticity of the nerve and the padding of fatty tissue around the nerve bundles protect the axons from damage. Sometimes, however, the nerve is compressed to a degree that compromises the ability of the axons to function normally. This may, for example, occur if a joint is held at an extreme angle for a prolonged period, which stretches it around a bony pulley (e.g., the ulnar nerve at the elbow). Where nerves run through narrow spaces, such as the carpal tunnel at the wrist, their ability to slide smoothly during joint movement may be reduced if the surrounding tissues swell sufficiently to trap the nerve. This can lead them to become compressed or overstretched or to rub against surrounding structures.

All tissues in the body require a blood supply, and nerves are no exception. One of the initial effects of nerve compression is that small blood vessels within the nerve collapse so that the cells within are starved of oxygen, blocking the flow of information along the axons. The initial consequence is numbness such as that experienced as a result of sitting for some time with one leg crossed over the opposite knee, a posture that compresses a nerve running down the back of the leg. Sensation rapidly returns when the legs are uncrossed; however, if the compression is maintained for a prolonged period, the myelin sheath may be damaged. Axons supplying muscles are generally most vulnerable, so some form of temporary paralysis is usually the main result, and a return to normal function may take several days. One example of this seen by many a world-weary general practitioner is "Saturday night palsy," which results when one falls asleep in a chair with one arm flung over the back, compressing nerves in the armpit. The name originates from less prosperous times when Saturday was the only night of alcoholic overindulgence, which not only made sleeping in a chair more likely (no doubt to keep the marital peace), but also provided the necessary anesthesia to prevent the victim being awakened by the discomfort. Though actual severing of axons is most commonly the result of traumatic injury, long-term nerve entrapment can sometimes also have this result (Lundborg and Dahlin 1994). This leads to long-term loss of sensation or motor control, which only resolves itself if the axons are able to regrow—a slow process which at best proceeds at a rate of about one millimeter per day.

One factor which can make precise diagnosis of nerve compression very difficult is that it is not unusual for it to occur at more than one site on the same nerve (Winspur 1998b; Lundborg and Dahlin 1994). The symptoms may reflect the two primary crush sites or be typical of only one. Relief of either crush site may (or may not) eliminate the symptoms of both. The prevalence of double compression suggests that pinching the nerve in one place makes a second compression more likely. The reasons for this are unclear, but one possibility is that the first compression induces some swelling in the nerve as a whole. Another is that trapping the nerve in one place increases the likelihood that it will be stretched at another place by joint movement. If entrapment of a nerve at the wrist indirectly results in compression of the nerve root where it leaves the vertebral column, the major symptoms may suggest only the problem in the neck. Surgical relief of this compression (which would be intrusive and risky) might then reveal the compression at the wrist. If the initial surgery had dealt with the wrist problem (a much more minor procedure), this might well have resolved the neck compression. Careful investigation of nerve compression before a definitive diagnosis is made is therefore very important. The first step involves noting the symptoms of altered sensation, muscle weakness, and clumsiness. The effects of applying pressure to the nerves at key points where they may suffer compression should also be determined. In addition, it is usual to test the speed at which signals run along the nerve (its conduction velocity) by stimulating it electrically at various points and recording from both the nerve and the muscles it supplies. This is achieved by placing electrodes on the skin over the nerve (a nerve conduction study) and recording from muscles using similar electrodes or by inserting fine wires into them (electromyography). Nerve compression may then reveal itself as a reduction in the speed of conduction. Though some patients may feel reluctant to undergo such tests, they use only low voltages and cause no damage. Though they can be a little uncomfortable, they are very important in identifying the presence and site of nerve compression and may prevent inappropriate surgery. It is important, however, that they be carried out by a clinician who is experienced in nerve conduction studies, as the results can be misleading if the tests are not set up properly.

In the arm, it is the median and ulnar nerves that most commonly suffer from compression, and only these will be considered here. The places where compression is most likely to occur are shown in figure 3-14. These are the thoracic outlet where the nerves pass under the collarbone, the ulnar nerve at the elbow, and the ulnar and median nerves at the wrist.

Thoracic Outlet Syndrome

The nerve roots that emerge from the brachial plexus at the root of the neck to supply the arm sometimes become compressed. This can either be caused by the muscles they pass between (the scalenes), by sheets of fibrous tissue that hold muscles and large blood vessels in place, or occasionally by the presence of an extra rib in the neck, which is found in about 1 percent of the population. The typical symptoms of thoracic outlet syndrome are spreading pain down the inner surface of the forearm accompanied by numbness in the little and third finger and a feeling of clumsiness or heaviness in the limb. These may be particularly associated with certain postures such as the arm being held out from the body either to the side or in front (Wynn Parry 1998e; Lederman 2003), which is a posture typical of many instrumentalists. It should be noted, however, that some of these symptoms are also typical of compression elsewhere in the arm. For example, the numbness in the little and third fingers is typical of ulnar nerve compression, so care must be taken in diagnosis. It is not uncommon to find that people with certain body types (or somatotypes) are prone to particular physical problems, and this is true of thoracic outlet syndrome, which is frequently seen in tall, thin individuals with sloping shoulders, in whom the thoracic outlet is likely to be narrow. It also appears to be more common in women than in men. The precise nature and incidence of thoracic outlet syndrome is highly controversial in medicine, yet it is one of the most common nerve compression problems diagnosed in musicians (Huang and Zager 2004; Lederman 1987). However, it remains uncertain whether it is genuinely a condition to which musicians are prone, or whether, because of the rather general nature of its symptoms, this diagnosis is often made when a more precise definition of the condition has not been achieved (Winspur 1998b). One of the most useful indications of genuine thoracic outlet syndrome is said by Wynn Parry to be a simple provocative test in which the symptoms are reproduced by applying pressure onto the roots of the brachial plexus at the base of the neck (Wynn Parry 1998b). A course of shoulder-raising exercises will often resolve the problem, and many musicians find that the Alexander technique is beneficial in improving posture in this regard. Initial treatment should always be conservative, the object being to strengthen muscles that resist the tendency for the shoulders to slump downward and compress the nerve plexus. Physiotherapy leads to a dramatic alleviation of the symptoms in most cases. The degree to which surgery is used varies considerably between clinics and is not necessarily linked to the incidence of successful outcome. Due to the anatomical complexity of the region, surgery is quite major and carries significant risks, though accurate data on how often important nerves or vessels are damaged are hard to come by (Lederman 1987).

Ulnar Nerve Entrapment

The most common site of entrapment of the ulnar nerve is where it wraps round the lower end of the humerus (the medial epicondyle). Here it lies in a groove in the bone called the cubital tunnel, where it is held in place by an overlying fibrous sheet (animation 3-6). When the elbow is bent the nerve slides within the channel by as much as a centimeter and is also stretched by several millimeters. The tunnel also becomes shallower during this movement, compressing the nerve. This is most marked when the arm is held out from the body and the wrist is extended (Verheyden and Palmer 2002), a posture that is not unusual in musicians (e.g., in violin and viola players). The compression is most likely to become a problem if the nerve is irritated and inflamed. The nerve can also be compressed just below in the upper forearm, where it passes between two parts of one of the flexor muscles of the wrist (flexor carpi ulnaris). In the early stages of the condition there may be a dull ache at the elbow, followed later by a numbness and tingling in the little and ring fingers and a loss of grip strength due to weakness of some of the flexor muscles in the forearm and of the small muscles within the hand. With the loss of their nerve supply, the muscles in the hand may start to degenerate. The most obvious sign of this is a flattening of the muscle mass that moves the little finger and lies along the edge of the hand. The most conservative treatment is to encourage postures in which the elbow is relatively straight, which, though impossible for many instrumentalists while playing, can at least be maintained at other times during the day, and when sleeping. In intractable cases, surgery is often successful; however, there are several surgical options whose merits need to be carefully compared. Compression of the ulnar nerve is also sometimes seen in the hand, where it runs through a narrow space between two carpal bones, called Guyon's canal (fig. 3-15). This may develop in flutists if the wrists (particularly the left) are habitually held in a strongly extended position (Wainapel 1988). Initial treatment involves splinting the wrist to maintain it in a posture that keeps the canal as open as possible; however, surgical release of the nerve may become necessary.

Median Nerve Entrapment

The most common of all nerve entrapments in the arm is carpal tunnel syndrome, which is a compression of the median nerve at the wrist (fig. 3-15, animation 3-5); however, it is also frequently misdiagnosed (Winspur 1998b). Among those who seek treatment, it is more than twice as common in women as in men (Dawson 1999). The carpal tunnel is the space under the retinaculum on the palmar side of the wrist and is crowded with tendons that slide back and forward in their synovial sheaths as the fingers are moved. Sitting on top of these, just below the retinaculum, is the median nerve. Inflammation of any of the surrounding structures or tissues can lead to compression of the nerve. This is sometimes associated with other conditions such as diabetes or pregnancy, presumably as a result of swelling in the tissue due to fluid retention. Pressure on the nerve is greatest during extreme flexion or extension of the wrist, particularly when coupled with finger flexion, a posture common during playing. In more than half of affected musicians, carpal tunnel syndrome is seen in both hands, but where this is not the case, it is the right hand that is more commonly affected, particularly in pianists and orchestral string players, who are the most vulnerable to carpal tunnel syndrome (Lederman 2003; Dawson 1999). This suggests that for string players, bowing technique may be a significant causative factor; however, another possibility is that carpal tunnel syndrome is more common in the dominant hand, perhaps because of its use in nonmusical activity (Lederman 2002).

Symptoms of carpal tunnel syndrome include tingling or disturbed sensation on the palmar surfaces of the thumb, index, and middle fingers (but not the palm itself). There can also be aching at night in the upper arm and shoulder. If the condition is allowed to progress, there may be a wasting of muscles in the hand supplied by the median nerve. The most dramatic indication of this is a thinning of the large pad of muscles called the thenar eminence, which controls the thumb. If the condition is of recent origin and not severe, treatment involves splinting of the wrist combined with anti-inflammatory drugs; however, in a considerable proportion of cases, surgery is necessary, though great care must be taken not to damage the nerve during this procedure.

Entrapment of Small Nerves in the Fingers

The main nerve branches that supply the fingers and the thumb run up their sides, where they may be vulnerable to compression in some instruments. For example, in the left hand of flutists the instrument rests partly on the side of the first segment (phalanx) of the index finger, just below the PIP joint, where it may rest on the digital nerve. Digital nerves may also be damaged when the side of the finger is used to pluck the string (e.g., in harpists or guitarists).

PREVENTING INJURY—
THE APPROACH TO PLAYING AND PRACTICE

Practice

For most musicians, a significant proportion of playing time is spent in the daily routine of individual practice, which is necessary to maintain concert levels of performance and to learn new repertoire. These periods are under the complete control of the player and can be carefully planned to develop and maintain a technique that is not only effective at producing the required musical results, but will also limit the chance of injury. There should be no conflict of interest between these aims because the two are usually synonymous. Useful information on many aspects of practice and posture and minimizing tension is available from several sources (Wynn Parry 1998a; Warrington 2003; Horvath 2002; Culf 1998; Paull and Harrison 1997). The first stage is to warm up the muscles to be used, something which is done without the instrument. This is particularly important in the morning when muscles are stiffer and tighter after the hours of inactivity spent in sleep. Warm-up is best followed by the playing of some easy pieces or exercises concentrating on accuracy, at the same time settling into a comfortable and sustainable posture (about which, more below). The room should be at a reasonable temperature; if this is not possible, the arms and hands need to be kept warm by wearing appropriate clothing in order to maintain the temperature and suppleness of the muscles. This is particularly important for the forearms, which contain the large muscles moving the hand and fingers. Some players may find it useful to wear fingerless gloves though even with these, cold fingers may tend to slip on the keys because of the lack of moisture on the pads from sweat.

Prolonged periods of practice should be split up into short sessions of perhaps thirty-five to forty-five minutes separated by intervals of a few minutes during which it is beneficial to do some stretching exercises for the playing (arm and hand) and postural (back, neck, and shoulder) muscles. After finishing playing, a further period of stretching is useful as a way of preventing the asymmetries of playing posture being carried over into normal life. During this period you will probably want to concentrate on the postural muscles that have been active but produce relatively little movement—those in the back, neck, shoulders, and upper arm. The demands of playing are similar to those of more traditionally recognized athletic pursuits, the only difference being that many of the muscles most actively employed are relatively small. In order to prevent strain, they should be given the same attention as those used in sports. The athletic analogy applies equally to how you approach an increase in practice intensity. An athlete switching from speed to strength training or vice versa will make the transition gradually. Similarly, if as a musician you intend to increase the amount of time you play each day, this must be built up gradually. If you have been on holiday for a couple of weeks during which you did little or no playing, it is not sensible to return immediately to the same schedule you were following immediately before the break. This is even more relevant if you are returning to orchestral or group playing after injury. We can all see that this would be common sense for a soccer player or runner, but it somehow it appears less obvious for musicians, though it is just as relevant.

The demands made of the body may also change if you switch to a new instrument. Changing from a flute with a C foot joint to one with a B foot joint will significantly increase the weight you must support, as will exchanging a single French horn for a double. Among string players, quite small increases in bow weight can create significant arm problems if the change is not managed carefully, while instruments such as violas can vary considerably in their dimensions. Perhaps after learning your craft as a woodwind player on a modern instrument, you decide to explore the baroque repertoire with a period instrument. Though the instrument itself will be lighter, it may require a greater finger spread. In all of these situations, it is sensible to transfer to the new instrument gradually to give yourself time to adapt physically to the change of loading on the limbs. It is usually advisable to return to quite simple repertoire during the initial period of adjustment.

Many players attribute great importance to mental rehearsal (see chapter 8), which means going through a piece from the score or from memory while away from the instrument, rehearsing mentally the movements of the fingers and arms (Fischer 1998; Warrington 2003). Mental rehearsal is also common among athletes who perform complex body movements, such as divers, gymnasts, or high jumpers, and more will be said about this topic in the chapter dealing with the control of motor activity by the brain. For musicians the advantage of mental rehearsal is that it allows familiarization with the structure of the piece, virtual practice of movements, and even the development of interpretation when access to an instrument is not possible and without the risk of physical strain. It may also help to reveal sources of muscle tension, which may be perceptible during mental rehearsal of some note sequences even in the absence of full playing movements of the fingers.

In an orchestral or ensemble environment, the player has less control over the structure of the playing sessions than when practicing alone; however, even in the group setting, discreet stretching exercises and judicious strategies for resting overtaxed joints can be practiced in the intervals between bouts of playing. An extensive range of rest and stretching techniques developed for use on stage and off has been compiled by Janet Horvath, a professional cellist who has suffered from and overcome severe overuse problems (Horvath 2002).

Posture and Movement

The details of correct posture for the whole gamut of orchestral and nonorchestral instruments are beyond the scope of this book; however, we will here deal with the general anatomical principles that underlie good arm posture. Back posture is dealt with in chapter 2, and information relevant to individual instruments is found elsewhere (Horvath 2002; Wynn Parry 1998a; Paull and Harrison 1997).

Over the last two decades, there have been a considerable number of studies directed at analyzing the postures and movements that underlie the playing of keyboard and string instruments. For bowed stringed instruments in particular it has proved much easier to collect data than to find a useful way of analyzing them and applying the results, which may explain the high proportion of "preliminary studies" in the literature. Though equipment is now available to quantify the complex three-dimensional movements required in string playing, analyzing sufficient numbers of individuals with different levels of experience and different body types to determine what might be optimal strategies remains highly challenging. Almost all of the published literature sets out with the stated aim of providing information that will help players to avoid injury (Visentin and Shan 2003, 2004; Shan and Visentin 2003; Turner-Stokes and Reid 1999), but this remains a distant goal. The range of variables relevant to this type of analysis is daunting and many, such as the dimensions of the players themselves, have yet to be considered. The best way forward may be to focus on relatively narrow but well-defined questions of likely biomechanical or clinical significance, such as the angle or loading of a particular joint. One of the earliest investigations into the physiology of string playing published in English is that of Szende and Nemessuri (Szende and Nemessuri 1971), which concentrates mainly on providing an accurate description of which muscles are active during various playing movements. Given the technology of the day this was a considerable achievement, and in addition it showed a general awareness of the roots of performance-related injury well ahead of its time. There have been few attempts to record muscle activity during playing since, though two brief papers by Koehler (1995, 1996) suggest that this type of information might be useful in biofeedback strategies for optimizing muscle activity.

One of the joints in the arm most critical in terms of posture is the wrist. It is vulnerable because so many tendons and nerves cross it in the narrow channels that lie beneath the restraining bands of the retinacula. This space available is greatest (and the potential friction on tendons least) when the wrist is held in a neutral position as a straight extension of the arm. In this position it is neither extended or flexed, nor deviated to the radial (thumb) or ulnar (little finger) side. When playing an instrument requiring rapid finger movement, the wrist should be kept close to this position as often as is possible. One group of instrumentalists who are particularly prone to hold both the left and the right wrists in a hyperflexed position are guitarists (fig. 3-18). One reason for this may be that they are often self-taught, but it is not difficult to avoid this playing posture. Players of bowed string instruments also need to guard against maintaining a strong flexion of the wrists in either hand, though it is unavoidable at the farthest reaches of the fingerboard, where strong ulnar deviation is also necessary. In pianists both extreme flexion and extension of the wrist are sometimes seen as a result of using a piano stool that is either too low or too high (animation 2-3). If set at a height that allows the forearms to lie close to the horizontal, the wrist will return to the neutral position. The shoulders should be kept relaxed as much as possible, though tension may be used periodically to create certain effects during playing. The pianist should also guard against excessive radial and ulnar deviation of the wrist (fig. 3-19). Avoiding this may periodically require the player to extend the arm away from the body, to lean to one or other side, or even to move along the stool for complex passages at the extreme ends of the keyboard. For most wind instruments the wrists naturally lie in the correct position; however, in the flute there is often a tendency to hyperextend the left wrist and to flex the right wrist. Extension of the left wrist can be reduced by clipping a support such as a Bo-Pep onto the instrument. If you need to convince yourself of the advantages of the neutral wrist position, try this experiment, suggested by Janet Horvath (2002). Spread and straighten the fingers, first with

Good   # Bad

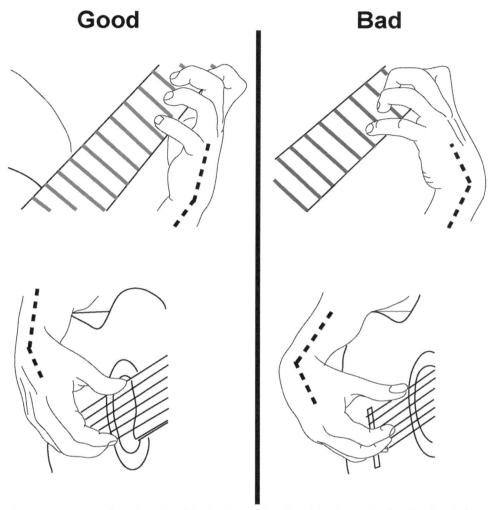

Figure 3-18. Examples of good and bad wrist and hand position in a guitarist. Good technique involves reducing wrist flexion to a minimum. In the poor posture, both wrists are strongly flexed, which may compress the tendons and median nerve.

the wrist fully extended (cocked up), then with the wrist fully flexed (drooping), and finally in the correct horizontal position. The difference in the degree of comfort and in the force required for the movement is quite remarkable.

When developing good technique, the ultimate aim should be to eliminate any unnecessary muscular activity from playing. This has been investigated in a study that compared the forces applied to the keys by amateur pianists (who played less than one hour a day) and expert players (who practiced four hours or more a day) (Parlitz, Peschel, and Altenmuller 1998). Interestingly, in the photograph showing the equipment used to monitor key force, the hand of the pianist exhibits extreme wrist extension. One hopes that this belonged to a member of the amateur group! Several of the

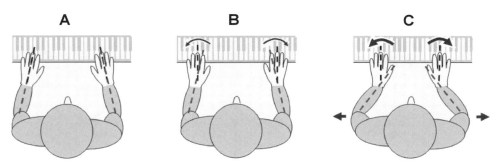

Figure 3-19. Ulnar deviation of the wrist in pianists. **A.** When playing in the center of the keyboard, the forearms point inward and the fingers do not lie parallel to the keys. **B.** To bring the fingers in line with the keys, the wrist must be rotated outward (ulnar deviation). This may restrict the movement of finger tendons in the carpal tunnel. **C.** If the elbows are held away from the body, the misalignment of fingers leads to an even more pronounced ulnar deviation.

tasks (taken from Dohnanyi studies) on which the comparison was based required one or more keys to be held down while the remaining fingers played a repeating pattern of eighth notes as in a very slow trill. The expert players applied a very light and unvarying pressure to the keys of the sustained notes, while the pressure applied by the amateurs was many times greater and fluctuated with the movement of the moving fingers. The amateurs were largely unaware of the force they were exerting, which appeared to form part of a strategy aimed at stabilizing the stationary fingers. This was not necessary for the experienced pianists because they had developed a much more independent control of the fingers; however, even among such players a continuing reduction in finger force with the number of years of playing has been found (Wolf et al. 1993; Jabusch 2006). In more difficult tasks of a similar nature set by Parlitz et al., the expert players did increase the force on the stationary fingers slightly. Although this time there was less difference between the two groups in the magnitude of the pressure applied by the moving fingers, the experts applied this for much shorter periods during each key strike. When playing passages with a regular rhythm, for example, sixteenth-note scales, the variability in the time between each note strike declines markedly with experience, though this may require many years to develop (Wagner, Poingek, and Teckhaus 1973).

The forces acting on the individual joints of the fingers are affected by the posture of the hand. They are at a maximum when the hand is held flat with the fingers extended straight out. When the fingers are curved so that the last joint lies perpendicular to the key, the forces on the last finger joint (distal interphalangeal joint or DIP; fig. 3-7) and on the tendon of the flexor digitorum profundus muscle (which moves that joint) are at a minimum (Wolf et al. 1993). A little self-experimentation will reveal that one negative consequence of curving the fingers is to make abduction and adduction at the metacarpophalangeal (knuckle) joint (i.e., spreading the fingers and drawing them together again) more difficult (Bejjani et al. 1989), as is circumduction (moving the finger in an arc). In this, the index finger is least affected. Hand positions that theoretically minimize the force applied to all of the finger joints involve moderate flexion of the metacarpophalangeal joint (Harding, Brandt, and Hillberry 1993), which would necessitate considerable extension of the wrist. Optimizing hand position will always therefore remain a compromise (Harding, Brandt, and Hillberry 1998).

Joints are usually moved by pairs of antagonistic muscles; for example, there are muscles that flex the fingers, and this movement can be opposed by muscles that extend them. The differences seen between the two groups of pianists mentioned above may partly have been the presence in the amateurs of a significant degree of simultaneous activity (co-contraction) in antagonistic muscle pairs controlling the fingers. One might imagine that when the flexors are contracting, the extensors would be relaxed and vice versa; however, this is often not the case. To take an extreme example, if a weight lifter holds a barbell above his or her head, the flexors and extensors of the wrist contract simultaneously to hold it straight, thus preventing the weight from turning the joint in either direction. Where movement is required, co-contraction can still be helpful in promoting joint stability. For the fingers of a pianist, for example, this would apply when the keys are struck forcibly in very loud passages. However, in most playing situations, it is neither necessary nor helpful and simply slows finger speed and responsiveness. Increasing the pressure on a string or on the key of a woodwind or brass instrument above the level needed for a firm contact is pointless. If you are unsure of the notes you are playing, however, you may find you are co-contracting opposing finger muscles, perhaps in unconscious readiness to move the finger in the opposite direction if a mistake is made. In order to relax them, the notes may have to be relearned securely. Without constant vigilance, this habit can become ingrained. Whatever its reason, co-contraction makes moving the joint in the correct direction harder, as it is necessary to overcome the opposing muscle to do so. It may also cause the fingers to rise higher than necessary when taken off the key, as a greater initial force is needed to overcome the continuing flexor muscle activity. This extends the minimum period before the finger can be brought back into contact with the key, slowing playing speed. As you become more familiar with a piece of music, co-contraction is likely to decline (Fry 2000); nevertheless, a conscious effort to relax antagonistic muscles should be maintained at all times so that only the minimum force is used. Not attempting to play complex passages at full speed until the notes are fully secure may also help eliminate co-contraction and in the long run shorten the time required to play these passages fluently.

Stress or anxiety also induces inappropriate muscle tension. If you are grinding your teeth at night when you are asleep, you are probably co-contracting your finger muscles by day as well as experiencing tension in your shoulders and arms. Under such circumstances, playing becomes very tiring! This is one reason why stress, which is basically a psychological factor, can produce the physical symptoms of overuse injury.

Instrument Ergonomics

The shape and form (the somatotype) of the human body varies greatly between individuals; however, for reasons dictated largely by acoustics and tradition, most instruments come in one size only. Musicians generally choose to play a particular instrument for emotive reasons related to the quality of the sound it produces, and only rarely alter their choice because it does not suit their physical attributes. Of course, through thousands of hours of playing the body will probably become modified to a considerable degree to accommodate the requirements of the instrument. Development of increased breath control, physical strength and stamina, and neuromuscular coordination are all part of learning to play an instrument well. Ultimately, however, hands or arms do not grow larger or bodies taller because a pianist or cellist requires it. By developing great technique, some players can compensate wonderfully for what appear to be major physical disadvantages; however, there are obvious limits to this process. In attempting to achieve mastery over the instrument, temporary gain may be acquired only as the result of adopting postures or habits that are in the long term unsustainable. The physical challenges posed by the instrument are not restricted only to playing. Many instruments are bulky or heavy (particularly in their protective cases), and some of the most awkward, such as the harp, are traditionally played by the smaller members of the orchestra. The risk of injury when moving an instrument may be alleviated by something as simple as adding wheels to the case. While this may be standard for very large or awkward instruments, smaller or younger players should consider installing these for instruments such as the cello or horn, for which they may currently be less common.

It is a strange anomaly that many musical instruments do not appear to have been designed with the human body in mind but more in accordance with certain aesthetic principles. Sometimes even the posture used in playing is influenced by art! Prinner in 1677 advised players to hold the violin firmly with the chin in order to increase the dexterity of the left hand, which as a result could be released from having also to support the instrument. Apparently some players of the time rested the instrument against the chest or arm, not because they felt that this was more comfortable or produced better results, but in imitation of a painting of an angel playing to St. Francis (Manze 2003). The picture in question is probably one by Guercino (1591–1666), now housed in the Gemäldegalerie of Dresden, showing an angel in just such a posture, which is more akin to that used for the viola da braccia.

Other problems arise when instruments evolve from a form that was once quite manageable to one that now puts considerable strain on the body. The early clarinet, which was made of boxwood and had a relatively simple set of keys (Baines 1977), weighed only about 10.5 ounces (300 grams). A good modern instrument made of Grenadilla wood, with the Boehm key system, or indeed a plastic student instrument, weighs 1.75–2 pounds (800–900 grams), but the player is still expected to support the weight on the end of the right thumb. This is frequently a source of discomfort. No one would dream of attempting to play one of the larger woodwind instruments such as an alto saxophone or bassoon while supporting the instrument solely in this way, but until recently there appears to have been little impetus to develop alternatives for smaller instruments such as the clarinet or oboe. Fortunately this is beginning to change (Markison 1990, 1998; Wynn Parry et al. 1998), and a variety of supportive devices have been invented by players and instrument makers. These include neck slings, supporting rods, or modifications of the existing support to spread the weight over a larger area or to transfer the weight to the metacarpophalangeal joint at the base of the thumb. Such supports may be of particular interest to older players, as the joints of the thumb are frequently among the first to be affected by arthritis. Even in the absence of physical problems, many players find it useful to employ such supports and indeed may use a range of them in various circumstances. A full discussion of the ever-increasing range of such supports is beyond the scope of this book, but a review of some of these can be found in Rosset i Llobet and Odam (2007). I will illustrate the principles behind ergonomic woodwind design by considering a progressive series of adaptations that are used in the flute, which, among woodwind instruments, is one of the most problematical for posture. Much of the difficulty stems from the necessity of holding the instrument horizontally out to the right. This requires that the right arm be held abducted and the left hand, strongly supinated. In order to align the mouth with the lip plate, the head and trunk must be rotated to the left, with the result that the left arm is held across the body. In the alto flute, the head joint doubles back on itself in a "U" shape so that the right arm can comfortably reach the keys, and similar head joints for the standard flutes may be useful for children. Those interested in what effect this has on the acoustics of the instrument are referred to Coltman (1984). Other options include changing the angle of the head joint relative to the body of the instrument so that the right arm lies lower, or in the most extreme case, so that the body of the instrument runs vertically like that of other woodwind instruments, though this may create other ergonomic problems. A number of less extreme modifications can be made to the instrument to ease the position of the left wrist and hand. Though in many instruments the keys played by the first three fingers of the left hand lie in line (fig. 3-20A), most manufacturers now offer an offset G option (fig. 3-20B) that reduces the degree of supination required to place the ring finger on its key. Some players find it useful to extend the length of all of the keys played by the first three fingers, though this is not a standard configuration (fig. 3-20D). An inexpensive plastic saddle can also be clipped to the instrument to reduce the pressure needed to support it by the left hand, reduce the extension of the left wrist, and allow the index finger to adopt a less cramped position (fig. 3-20C).

The major postural problems posed by brass instruments stem largely from their weight. Over the last few decades this has increased considerably for many instruments due to changes in design in response to the demand for a greater volume of sound. In the last chapter we saw how this can cause problems for the muscles of the shoulder and the roots of the brachial plexus as they emerge from between the scalene muscles. A set of support devices (Ergobrass) are available that are based on telescopic rod supports fixed to the instruments. These run either to the floor, to the seat of the chair between the player's legs, or to a sling that can be worn discreetly under the jacket. These supports may also be useful for young players, as, by freeing them from the need to support the instrument, they will be able to adopt a good playing posture. They can be gradually weaned off the support as they develop physically.

String players may be more resistant to tampering with the structure of their instruments than wind players; however, they may want to bear in mind that many of the priceless historical instruments now in circulation are far from their original state. That Stradivarius cello you covet did not acquire its spike until the nineteenth century, but the thought of gripping the cello between the shins in the pursuit of authenticity is not an idea that many modern players would relish and would impose a severe limit on the use of vibrato. Cellists and double-bass players also have an option for bows

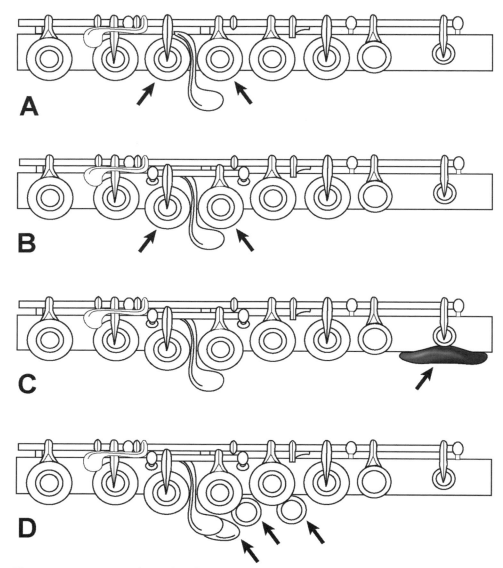

Figure 3-20. A progressive series of ergonomic modifications of the flute. A. In-line G keys (arrows) require maximal supination of the left wrist so that the upper of the two can be covered by the pad of the ring finger. B. By offsetting the G keys, the requirement for supination is reduced. C. Addition of a support for the basal segment of the index finger (e.g., a Bo-Pep) reduces wrist extension and index finger flexion. D. Extending the keys operated by the little, ring, and middle fingers can further reduce wrist supination.

between the more commonly used French type (which is similar to the modern violin bow) and the German type. The German bow has several advantages for those experiencing arm problems. It requires less inward rotation of the shoulder and flexion or pronation of the wrist and reduces the force transmitted through the basal joint of the thumb (fig. 3-21A, B). Though ergonomic factors are not the sole concern for players, this may provide a solution if problems with these joints prove otherwise intractable.

If you are lucky enough to be the owner of a seventeenth- or eighteenth-century violin or viola and are playing in a conventional orchestra, your instrument will have undergone an even more drastic transformation to increase the volume of sound it produces. The original neck will have been replaced by one that is longer and thinner and has been reset at a greater angle relative to the body. If this is the case, the original scroll may have been grafted back on. It will have acquired a new, longer fingerboard, the bridge will be higher, and even the bass bar that lies on the inside of the belly will have been replaced by one that is thicker and longer than the original. The strings, some of which are now overwound, are at higher tension, and the instrument is played with a different type of bow. In addition, a chin rest and shoulder rest will have been added. From this perspective, a few further changes from the traditional design may not seem so sacrilegious if you are in the market for a modern instrument. Remember, if the instrument is more user friendly, not only will you reduce your susceptibility to injury, you are also likely to play better. The physical challenges for the player are greater in the viola than the violin due to its larger (and more variable) size. Recently a number of approaches have been proposed to improve its ergonomics. Otto Erdesz created some instruments in which the upper bout on the treble side was cut away to improve access to the fingerboard (fig. 3-21E), and recently more radical solutions have emerged from the designs of David Rivinus. These have addressed not only the ergonomics but also the acoustics of the instrument. The least extreme of these displaces and tilts the fingerboard toward the treble side to improve the access of the left hand (fig. 3-21D). In Rivinus's Pellegrina viola, however, the symmetry of the body of the instrument has been sacrificed to improve ergonomics and sound quality, and though the result may seem to owe more than a little to Salvador Dali, it is clearly an instrument designed with the body of the player in mind (fig. 3-21F). The fingerboard is again displaced and canted, and the rib height on the bass side is higher than that on the treble. In addition, the body of the instrument is distorted asymmetrically so that the area of the belly is increased without affecting access to the fingerboard or increasing the distance from the button to the peg box. The result of these and other modifications is to produce an instrument that sounds like a large viola, but which is ergonomically more friendly than a small one.

Notwithstanding some flirtations with 7/8-size keyboards (Wristen et al. 2006), the options for pianists are limited, as the dimensions of piano keys are necessarily standardized, though players of baroque music benefit not only from the narrower keys of the harpsichord, but also from music that demands less in terms of hand extension and in finger force, which in these instruments plays no role in dynamics. However, the weight of the action will vary from instrument to instrument, and though for recital purposes one must accept the piano provided, the player's own piano used for the long hours of daily practice at home is another matter. This can be regulated and

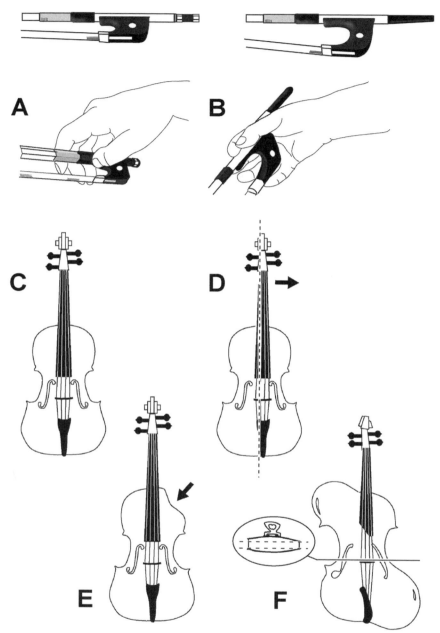

Figure 3.21. The two types of cello bows and the different hand grip used for each. A. French type. B. German type. Note that the hand is pronated and the wrist flexed for the French bow, but supinated and straighter for the German. C–F. Ergonomic modifications to the viola. C. A normal viola. D. Design by David Rivinus; the shape of the body is unchanged but the neck is moved to one side to improve the access of the left hand to the upper parts of the fingerboard. E. Design by Otto Erdesz; the upper bout is cut away to improve left-hand access. F. The Pellegrina viola is a radical ergonomic redesign by David Rivinus (www.rivinus-instruments.com/) in which the symmetry of the body of the instrument is sacrificed for practical aims. The ribs on the bass side (inset) are also higher than those on the treble side.

maintained to ensure that the action is both light and even across the keyboard, which will help to reduce the chances of injury.

REFERENCES

Allieu, Y., K. Hamitouche, J. L. Roux, and Y. Beaton. 1998. Unique surgical conditions. In *The musician's hand: A clinical guide*, ed. I. Winspur and C. B. Wynn Parry. London: Martin Dunitz.

Baader, A. P., O. Kazennikov, and M. Wiesendanger. 2005. Coordination of bowing and fingering in violin playing. *Brain Res Cogn Brain Res* 23 (2–3):436–43.

Baines, A. 1977. *Woodwind instruments and their history*. London: Faber and Faber.

Baker, D. S., J. S. Gaul Jr., V. K. Williams, and M. Graves. 1981. The little finger superficialis—clinical investigation of its anatomic and functional shortcomings. *J Hand Surg (Am)* 6 (4):374–78.

Beauchamp, R. 2003a. Curved fingers—and tension. *Music and Health*, at www.musicand health.co.uk/articles/tension.html (accessed April 23, 2008).

———. 2003b. Examples of passages that may cause problems due to tendon linkages or absences. *Music and Health*, at www.musicandhealth.co.uk/linkages.htm (accessed April 23, 2008).

Bejjani, F. J., L. Ferraram, N. Xu, C. M. Tomaino, L. Pavlidis, J. Wu, and J. Dommerholt. 1989. Comparison of three piano techniques as an implementation of a proposed experimental design. *Med Prob Perform Artists* 4:109–13.

Bergman, R. A., A. K. Afifi, and R. Miyauchi. 2004. *Illustrated encyclopedia of human anatomic variation*, at www.anatomyatlases.org/AnatomicVariants/AnatomyHP.shtml (accessed April 23, 2008).

Brandfonbrener, A. G. 2003. Musculoskeletal problems of instrumental musicians. *Hand Clin* 19 (2):v–vi, 231–39.

Brown, S. 2000. Promoting a healthy keyboard technique. In *Medical problems of the instrumental musician*, ed. R. Tubiana and P. C. Amadio. London: Martin Dunitz.

Coltman, J. W. 1984. Enhanced power from a recurved flute. *J Acoust Soc Am* 75:1642–43.

Culf, N. 1998. *Musician's injuries: A guide to their understanding and prevention*. Guildford, UK: Parapress.

Davies, A. T., G. Rogers, and J. Kember. 1998. The physical therapist's contribution. In *The musician's hand: A clinical guide*, ed. I. Winspur and C. B. Wynn Parry. London: Martin Dunitz.

Dawson, W. J. 1999. Carpal tunnel syndrome in instrumentalists: A review of 15 years' clinical experience. *Med Prob Perform Artists* 14 (1):25–29.

Fischer, S. 1998. Technique and ease in violin playing. In *The musician's hand: A clinical guide*, ed. I. Winspur and C. B. Wynn Parry. London: Martin Dunitz.

Fishbein, M., S. E. Middlestadt, V. Ottati, S. Straus, and A. Ellis. 1998. Medical problems among ICSOM musicians: Overview of a national survey. *Med Prob Perform Artists* 3 (1):1–8.

Franco, G. 1999. Ramazzini and workers' health. *Lancet* 354 (9181):858–61.

Fry, H. J. H. 2000. Overuse syndrome. In *Medical problems of the instrumental musician*, ed. R. Tubiana and P. C. Amadio. London: Martin Dunitz.

Fry, H. J., and G. Rowley. 1992. Instrumental musicians showing technique impairment with painful overuse. *Md Med J* 41 (10):899–903.

Harding, D. C., K. D. Brandt, and B. M. Hillberry. 1993. Finger joint force minimization in pianists using optimization techniques. *J Biomech* 26 (12):1403–12.

———. 1998. Minimization of finger joint forces and tendon tensions in pianists. *Med Prob Perform Artists* 4:103–8.

Hochberg, F. H., R. D. Leffert, M. D. Heller, and L. Merriman. 1983. Hand difficulties among musicians. *JAMA* 249 (14):1869–72.

Horvath, J. 2002. *Playing (less) hurt: An injury prevention guide for musicians.* Minneapolis, Minn.: J. Horvath.

———. 2004. Stressing prevention. *Symphony* (March–April).

Huang, J. H., and E. L. Zager. 2004. Thoracic outlet syndrome. *Neurosurgery* 55 (4):897–902; discussion 902–3.

Jabusch, H. C. 2006. Movement analysis in pianists. In *Music, motor control and the brain*, ed. E. Altenmuller, M. Wiesendanger, and J. Kesselring. Oxford: Oxford University Press.

Kloeppel, R. 2000. Do the "spreadability" and finger length of cellists and guitarists change due to practice? *Med Prob Perform Artists* 15:23–30.

Koehler, W. K. 1995. The effect of electromyographic feedback on achievement in bowing technique. *Proceedings of the Second International Technological Directions in Music Learning Conference*, at music.utsa.edu:16080/tdml/conf-II/II-Koehler.html (accessed April 23, 2008).

———. 1996. Physiological mapping of bowing: Six case studies. *Proceedings of the Third International Technological Directions in Music Learning Conference*, at music.utsa.edu/tdml/conf-III/III-Koehler/III-Koehler.html (accessed April 23, 2008).

Lederman, R. J. 1987. Thoracic outlet syndromes: Review of the controversies and a report of 17 instrumental musicians. *Med Prob Perform Artists* 2:87–91.

———. 2002. Neuromuscular problems in musicians. *Neurologist* 8 (3):163–74.

———. 2003. Neuromuscular and musculoskeletal problems in instrumental musicians. *Muscle Nerve* 27 (5):549–61.

Lederman, R. J., and C. H. Calabrese. 1986. Overuse syndromes in instrumentalists. *Med Prob Perform Artists* 1:7–11.

Leijnse, J. N., J. E. Bonte, J. M. Landsmeer, J. J. Kalker, J. C. Van der Meulen, and C. J. Snijders. 1992. Biomechanics of the finger with anatomical restrictions—the significance for the exercising hand of the musician. *J Biomech* 25 (11):1253–64.

Leijnse, J. N., C. J. Snijders, J. E. Bonte, J. M. Landsmeer, J. J. Kalker, J. C. Van der Meulen, G. J. Sonneveld, and S. E. Hovius. 1993. The hand of the musician: The kinematics of the bidigital finger system with anatomical restrictions. *J Biomech* 26 (10):1169–79.

Leijnse, J. N., E. T. Walbeehm, G. J. Sonneveld, S. E. Hovius, and J. M. Kauer. 1997. Connections between the tendons of the musculus flexor digitorum profundus involving the synovial sheaths in the carpal tunnel. *Acta Anat (Basel)* 160 (2):112–22.

Lippman, H. I. 1991. A fresh look at overuse syndrome in musical performers: Is "overuse" overused? *Med Prob Perform Artists* 6:57–60.

Lundborg, G., and L. B. Dahlin. 1994. Pathophysiology of nerve compression. In *Repetitive motion disorders of the upper extremity*, ed. S. L. Gordon, S. J. Blair, L. J. Fine, and K. N. An. Rosemont, Ill.: American Academy of Orthopaedic Surgeons.

Manze, A. 2003. Biber violin sonatas (sleeve notes). *Harmonia Mundi*, HMX 2907344.45.

Markison, R. E. 1990. Treatment of musical hands: Redesign of the interface. *Hand Clin* 6 (3):525–44.

———. 1998. Adjustment of the musical interface. In *The musician's hand: A clinical guide*, ed. I. Winspur and C. B. Wynn Parry. London: Martin Dunitz.

Miller, G., F. Peck, A. Brain, and S. Watson. 2003. Musculotendinous anomalies in musician and nonmusician hands. *Plast Reconstr Surg* 112 (7):1815–22; discussion 1823–24.

Miller, G., F. Peck, and J. S. Watson. 2002. Pain disorders and variations in upper limb morphology in music students. *Med Prob Perform Artists* 17:169–72.

Newmark, J., and F. H. Hochberg. 1987. "Doctor, it hurts when I play": Painful disorders among instrumental musicians. *Med Prob Perform Artists* 2:93–97.

Newmark, J., and R. J. Lederman. 1987. Practice doesn't necessarily make perfect. Incidence of overuse syndromes in amateur instrumentalists. *Med Prob Perform Artists* 2:93–97.

Parlitz, D., T. Peschel, and E. Altenmuller. 1998. Assessment of dynamic finger forces in pianists: Effects of training and expertise. *J Biomech* 31 (11):1063–67.

Paull, Barbara, and Christine Harrison. 1997. *The athletic musician: A guide to playing without pain*. Lanham, Md.: Scarecrow Press.

Perkins, R. E., and M. H. Hast. 1993. Common variations in muscles and tendons of the human hand. *Clin Anat* 6:226–31.

Ramazzini, B. 1964. *Diseases of workers*, *History of medicine series, 23*. New York: Hafner Publishing.

Reilly, K. T., M. A. Nordstrom, and M. H. Schieber. 2004. Short-term synchronization between motor units in different functional subdivisions of the human flexor digitorum profundus muscle. *J Neurophysiol* 92 (2):734–42.

Rosety-Rodriguez, M., F. J. Ordonez, J. Farias, M. Rosety, C. Carrasco, A. Ribelles, J. M. Rosety, and M. Gomez del Valle. 2003. The influence of the active range of movement of pianists' wrists on repetitive strain injury. *Eur J Anat* 7 (2):75–77.

Rosset i Llobet, J., and G. Odam. 2007. *The musician's body: A maintenance manual for peak performance*. London: Guildhall School of Music and Drama; Burlington, Vt.: Ashgate Publishing.

Rozmaryn, L. M. 1993. Upper extremity disorders in performing artists. *Md Med J* 42 (3):255–60.

Sataloff, R. T., A. G. Brandfonbrener, and R. J. Lederman. 1998. *Performing arts medicine*. 2nd ed. San Diego: Singular Publishing Group.

Schmied, A., C. Ivarsson, and E. E. Fetz. 1993. Short-term synchronization of motor units in human extensor digitorum communis muscle: Relation to contractile properties and voluntary control. *Exp Brain Res* 97 (1):159–72.

Schmied, A., S. Pagni, H. Sturm, and J. P. Vedel. 2000. Selective enhancement of motoneurone short-term synchrony during an attention-demanding task. *Exp Brain Res* 133 (3):377–90.

Shan, G., and P. Visentin. 2003. A quantitative three-dimensional analysis of arm kinematics in violin performance. *Med Prob Perform Artists* 18:3–10.

Silver, J. K., and L. M. Rozmaryn. 1998. Overuse tendinitis of the intrinsic muscles. *Orthopedics* 21 (8):891–94.

Stotko, L. 1998. Dynamically splinting the musical hand. *Med Prob Perform Artists* 13:109–13.

Szende, O., and M. Nemessuri. 1971. *The physiology of violin playing*. London: Collet's.

Turner-Stokes, L., and K. Reid. 1999. Three-dimensional motion analysis of upper limb movement in the bowing arm of string-playing musicians. *Clin Biomech (Bristol, Avon)* 14 (6):426–33.

Verheyden, J. R., and A. K. Palmer. 2002. Cubital tunnel syndrome. *E-medicine*, at www.emedicine.com/orthoped/topic479.htm (accessed April 23, 2008).

Visentin, P., and G. Shan. 2003. The kinetic characteristics of the bow arm during violin performance: An examination of internal loads as a function of tempo. *Med Prob Perform Artists* 18:91–97.

———. 2004. An innovative approach to understand overuse injuries: Biomechanical modeling as a platform to integrate information obtained from various analytical tools. *Med Prob Perform Artists* 19:90–96.

Wagner, C., E. Poingek, and L. Teckhaus. 1973. Piano learning and programmed instruction. *J Res Music Educ* 21 (2):106–22.

Wainapel, S. F. 1988. The not-so-magic flute: Two cases of distal ulnar nerve entrapment. *Med Prob Perform Artists* 3:63–65.

Warrington, J. 2003. Hand therapy for the musician: Instrument-focused rehabilitation. *Hand Clin* 19 (2):vii, 287–301.

Wiesendanger, M., A. P. Baader, and O. Kazennikov. 2006. Fingering and bowing in violinists: A motor control approach. In *Music, motor control and the brain*, ed. E. Altenmuller, M. Wiesendanger, and J. Kesselring. Oxford: Oxford University Press.

Winspur, I. 1998a. Dupuytren's contracture. In *The musician's hand: A clinical guide*, ed. I. Winspur and C. B. Wynn Parry. London: Martin Dunitz.

———. 1998b. Nerve compression syndromes. In *The musician's hand: A clinical guide*, ed. I. Winspur and C. B. Wynn Parry. London: Martin Dunitz.

———. 1998c. Osteoarthritis. In *The musician's hand: A clinical guide*, ed. I. Winspur and C. B. Wynn Parry. London: Martin Dunitz.

———. 1998d. Surgical indications, planning and technique. In *The musician's hand: A clinical guide*, ed. I. Winspur and C. B. Wynn Parry. London: Martin Dunitz.

———. 2003. Controversies surrounding "misuse," "overuse," and "repetition" in musicians. *Hand Clin* 19 (2):vii–viii, 325–29.

Winspur, I., and C. B. Wynn Parry. 1997. The musician's hand. *J Hand Surg (Br)* 22 (4):433–40.

———. 1998. *The musician's hand: A clinical guide*. London: Martin Dunitz.

———. 2000. Musician's hands: A surgeon's perspective. *Med Prob Perform Artists* 15 (1):31.

Wolf, F. G., M. S. Keane, K. D. Brandt, and B. M. Hillberry. 1993. An investigation of finger joint and tendon forces in experienced pianists. *Med Prob Perform Artists* 8:84–95.

Wristen, B. G., P. Jung, A. K. G. Wismer, and M. S. Hallbeck. 2006. Assessment of muscle activity and joint angles in small-handed pianists: A pilot study on 7/8-sized keyboard versus the full-sized keyboard. *Med Prob Perform Artists* 21 (1):3–9.

Wynn Parry, C. B. 1998a. The interface. In *The musician's hand: A clinical guide*, ed. I. Winspur and C. B. Wynn Parry. London: Martin Dunitz.

———. 1998b. Misuse and overuse. In *The musician's hand: A clinical guide*, ed. I. Winspur and C. B. Wynn Parry. London: Martin Dunitz.

———. 1998c. The musician's hand and arm pain. In *The musician's hand: A clinical guide*, ed. I. Winspur and C. B. Wynn Parry. London: Martin Dunitz.

———. 1998d. Rheumatoid arthritis. In *The musician's hand: A clinical guide*, ed. I. Winspur and C. B. Wynn Parry. London: Martin Dunitz.

———. 1998e. Specific conditions. In *The musician's hand: A clinical guide*, ed. I. Winspur and C. B. Wynn Parry. London: Martin Dunitz.

Wynn Parry, C. B., S. Fischer, J. Williams, B. Gregor-Smith, C. Grindea, and J. Kember. 1998. The interface. In *The musician's hand: A clinical guide*, ed. I. Winspur and C. B. Wynn Parry. London: Martin Dunitz.

Zaza, C. 1998. Playing-related musculoskeletal disorders in musicians: A systematic review of incidence and prevalence. *CMAJ* 158 (8):1019–25.

Chapter Four

Breathing in Singing and Wind Playing

Even though we all breathe constantly without being aware of it and can also readily bring this under conscious control, the events that take place during inspiration (breathing in) and expiration (breathing out) are far from intuitive. The reasons for this will become clear later on in this chapter, but the consequence for singers and wind players is that they often have misconceptions about breath control, which are reflected in the language they use to describe the respiratory mechanisms that they believe underlie singing and wind playing.

This chapter does not seek to describe an optimum strategy for respiration in musicians. Research into the physiological processes that are involved has much further to go before it can provide comprehensive and objective guidance. In the meantime, it must be left to singers, wind players, and their teachers to decide on the best approach, which will be determined by each performer's experience and aesthetic goals and, as we shall see, may also be influenced by that individual's particular body type. Instead, this chapter has two main objectives. The first is to provide an accurate description of the activity of respiratory muscles and the movements they produce during normal respiration. This is an essential starting point for all singers and wind players and will allow them to communicate and discuss aspects of their technique accurately and unambiguously. The second objective is to review the results that have been obtained from the scientific analysis of respiratory activity underlying singing and wind playing. It will be clear from this section that the small body of knowledge that currently exists is still quite rudimentary, not least because it is based on studies of only a few individuals. Furthermore, in order to make such investigations practical, the number of parameters measured in each study must be quite restricted. The musical tasks the subjects are asked to carry out must also be both few and simple so that they are readily repeatable and comparable between individuals and generate an amount of data that can realistically be analyzed. The published studies of singers focus predominantly on those who are classically trained. To a large extent this is because the respiratory demands made on them are greatest, as they perform without amplification and may have to make themselves heard over a full orchestra. As we shall see, this has a major effect on the nature of the sound they produce. Finally, of course, we cannot

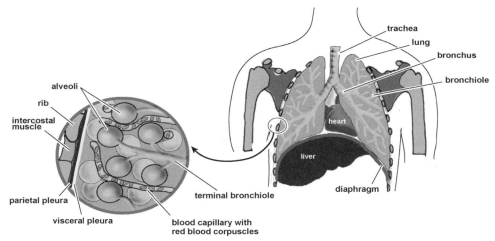

Figure 4-1. Lung structure. The trachea divides into two bronchi, one entering each lung. Like the trachea, these are held open by rigid rings of cartilage. They divide into progressively smaller-diameter airways called bronchioles, which lack cartilaginous rings. The narrowest of these are the terminal bronchi, which end in alveoli. Here oxygen passes to the red blood corpuscles, while carbon dioxide diffuses out of the blood plasma in the opposite direction. The lungs are covered with a sheet of visceral pleura, while the inner surface of the chest is lined with a sheet of parietal pleura. These are held in contact by the surface tension of a film of watery fluid that prevents the lungs from collapsing.

hear the voices of the participants in these studies and so we cannot assess whether we find the outcome of the different approaches used to be to our particular tastes. Despite these limitations, the information that is currently available may at least provide some food for thought and a basis for personal experimentation.

THE STRUCTURE OF THE LUNGS

During inspiration, air passes through the larynx into the trachea (windpipe), which divides into two tubes called bronchi, one of which enters each lung (fig. 4-1). The trachea and the bronchi and their major branches in the lungs are held open by a series of rings made of cartilage. Once inside the lung, the bronchi continue to divide repeatedly into smaller and thinner-walled tubes, ending in fine branches known as respiratory bronchioles. These lack any cartilaginous scaffolding and terminate in large numbers of small sacs called alveoli, where the air is brought into close contact with very narrow, thin-walled blood vessels known as capillaries. Here, oxygen and carbon dioxide need travel only a short distance as they diffuse into and out of the blood, making the process very efficient. Oxygen diffuses from the alveolar air into the capillaries and binds to the hemoglobin contained within the red blood cells. Carbon dioxide produced by the tissues of the body dissolves in the blood plasma, the watery fluid that carries the red blood cells, and on reaching the lungs diffuses out in the opposite direction into the alveoli. The structure of the lungs is designed not only

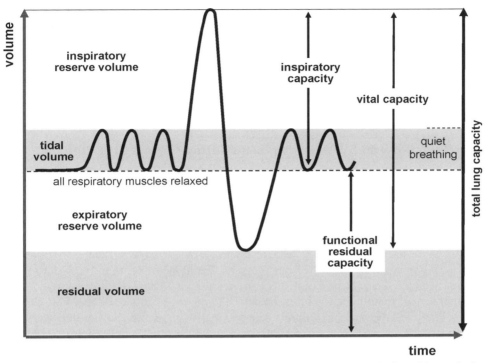

Figure 4-2.   Diagram showing lung function parameters. During normal quiet breathing only the tidal volume is used. With a maximal intake of breath the inspiratory reserve volume is used. If the breath is then driven out completely, we pass through the tidal volume band into the expiratory reserve volume. This exhalation uses all of the vital capacity. This leaves the residual volume which cannot be expelled because the chest has a rigid outer wall on three sides. As the outer surface of the lungs is held in contact with this, they cannot collapse completely.

to bring the respiratory and blood systems very close together, but also to pack within a small volume an enormous surface area for gaseous exchange. There are about 300 million alveoli in each lung, and their total surface area is approximately 100 square meters. The composition of air taken into the lungs is approximately 21 percent oxygen and 79 percent nitrogen. The nitrogen is inert and plays no role in respiration. In exhaled air the oxygen concentration falls to 17 percent, while the carbon dioxide that has diffused out of the blood makes up 4 percent. If we hold our breath, it is the buildup of carbon dioxide in the bloodstream that is the stimulus that ultimately forces us to breathe again. During singing or wind playing, the lungs are used not only for respiration but also as a reservoir for the air that is used to set up the vibration of the larynx, lips, or reed. The limitation to the length of the breath is generally determined by how quickly the available volume of air in the lungs flows out. In some instruments such as the oboe, however, the flow rate is very slow and so the buildup of carbon dioxide can become the limiting factor, requiring the remaining air to be quickly exhaled before the air in the lungs is exhausted, and a new breath is taken. The amount of carbon dioxide dissolved in the blood affects its acidity (or pH), which in turn influences its other properties, such as the ability of the hemoglobin to bind oxygen. If we breathe very rapidly when not physically exerting ourselves, then too much carbon dioxide may be lost from the plasma. This can be caused by performance anxiety (Widmer et al. 1997) or an unsuitable breathing strategy. One of the immediate consequences of this may be dizziness due to a constriction of blood vessels in the brain and an increase in heart rate. Consequently it is important not to overbreathe when using the lungs as bellows during singing or wind playing.

Muscle Action and Skeletal Movement during Normal Breathing

During normal quiet breathing (i.e., when we are sitting passively and neither speaking nor carrying out any physical activity) only about one-tenth of our total lung capacity is used (fig. 4-2). This is called the tidal volume and is typically of the order of about 500 milliliters. Tidal breathing uses only the muscles of the chest, and each breath ends when all of the respiratory muscles are relaxed. At the end of a quiet breath, more air (the expiratory reserve volume) can be expelled using the muscles of the abdominal wall. If we fill our lungs as full as possible, then blow out all the air that we can, the volume exhaled constitutes the vital capacity of the lungs. About 1.5 liters of air remains in the lungs because the rib cage cannot collapse completely; this is known as the residual volume. The residual volume plus the expiratory reserve volume make up the functional residual capacity. The total lung capacity is the vital capacity plus the residual volume. Singing and wind playing require much larger volumes of air than we need for quiet breathing and for most wind instruments this must be delivered at much higher pressures. For both activities, we often take breaths that use a large percentage of our vital capacity and end well below the level of our functional residual capacity. Though it is intuitively obvious that vital capacity and the pressure that can be achieved will vary with body size, the extent of normal range may come as a surprise. From our own observations of a group of college wind players aged between eighteen and twenty-one and in good health, it is clear that a woman with a height of five feet two inches (157 cm) may have a vital capacity of only 3.5 liters, while that of a six-foot two-inch (188 cm) man may approach 7 liters! Clearly this needs to be fully appreciated by singing and instrumental teachers.

Respiration involves the action of muscles in both the chest (the thorax) and the abdomen, the two large chambers that form the trunk. The thorax contains the lungs and heart, and its side walls are formed by the rib cage. Beneath the thorax lies the abdomen, whose walls are muscular and which contains the liver, gut, and other major visceral organs. The boundary between the thorax and abdomen is formed by a horizontal sheet of muscle called the diaphragm (figs. 4-1, 4-3, 4-4). Though this plays a key role in respiration, its action is often misunderstood.

During inspiration, expansion of the lungs results in a transient reduction in their internal pressure. As a consequence, air from the atmosphere flows in through the trachea until the pressure inside and outside the lungs is equalized. During expiration, the lungs are compressed, increasing their internal pressure and airflows out until the internal and external pressures are once more equal. Lung tissue itself contains no muscle, so changes in lung volume are brought about indirectly by the movement of the walls of the thorax. Each lung is covered by a thin, transparent membrane that forms a sac (the visceral pleura) that is attached to its surface (fig. 4-1). The inside of the thorax is also lined by a similar sac (the parietal pleura). These two layers of pleura lie in contact, and during respiratory movements they slide smoothly over each other. They can do this because they are lubricated by a thin film of fluid that lies between them. If the two layers briefly stick to each other, as sometimes happens with lung infections such as pleurisy, then a sharp pain is experienced in the chest when a breath is taken in. The layer of fluid also holds the two layers of pleura in contact by surface tension. This is the same principle we use to stick a plastic toll pass holder to a car windshield. If the two layers of pleura did not adhere in this way, then expanding the chest wall would not expand the lungs. If the chest wall is punctured and air gets into the space between the visceral and parietal pleura, the lung (which is elastic and is stretched when in contact with the chest wall) collapses away from the ribs and becomes useless for respiration. This is extremely dangerous as the lung cannot be inflated again until the air between the two layers of pleura is removed.

Normal respiratory movements mainly involve the muscles of the thorax and of the abdomen (figs. 4-3, 4-4). The lateral walls of the thorax are formed by the ribs, which are hinged from the spine (vertebral column) at the back and are attached by stiff cartilage to a flat bone called the sternum (breastbone) at the front. Several sets of muscle move the ribs during respiration. Between adjacent ribs run the intercostal muscles (fig. 4-3), of which there are three sheets in each rib space; the outermost sheet is formed by the external intercostals, whose main action is to swing the ribs upward and outward when air is drawn into the lungs. The inner two layers (the intermediate and internal intercostals) pull the ribs downward to force air out of the lungs. The floor

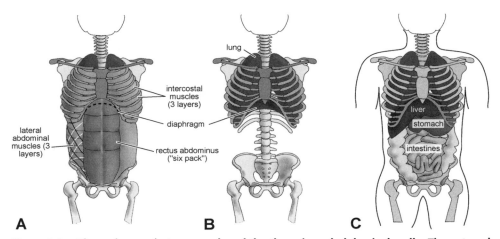

Figure 4-3. The major respiratory muscles of the thoracic and abdominal walls. The external intercostal muscles that run between the ribs are muscles of inhalation. A. The lateral abdominal wall muscles and the rectus abdominus muscle are involved in exhalation. There are three layers of lateral abdominal muscles whose fibers run in different directions (indicated by the lines). B. The diaphragm forms the floor of the chest cavity and is attached to the liver. C. Contraction of the lateral abdominal walls during exhalation compresses the viscera and pushes the diaphragm upward.

of the thorax is formed by the diaphragm, which is a sheet of muscle covered with parietal pleura. The liver is attached to the underside of the diaphragm, and when the diaphragm is at rest, the liver pushes it up into the thorax as a dome (figs. 4-3, 4-4). The muscles of the abdominal wall also play a major role in respiration. The anterior wall of the abdomen is formed by the rectus abdominus. This is a large, vertically running muscle divided into segments that when well developed are popularly known as a "six-pack." The side walls of the abdomen are made up of three overlapping layers, the internal and external obliques and the transverse abdominal muscles (we will refer to these as the lateral abdominal muscles). Though each sheet is thin, their fibers run in different directions so that together they form a strong muscular wall. The development of these muscles is a major goal of the Pilates exercise system. Several other muscle groups are also involved in respiration; however, the ones described above are the most important, and the mechanics of respiration can be readily understood on the basis of their actions. We will therefore consider how these operate first.

The abdomen is effectively a sealed chamber, while the space in the chest that contains the lungs is open to the outside via the trachea and mouth. The chest and abdomen are separated by the muscular diaphragm, which at rest, as we have seen, is pushed upward into the chest by the abdominal organs. During inspiration, the diaphragm contracts and therefore flattens, causing the liver to be pushed downward like a piston (fig. 4-4). At the same time, the external intercostal muscles raise the chest. The joints between the ribs and the spine allow the ribs to swing outward and upward, which increases both the width of the thorax and the distance between the vertebral column and the sternum, as well as lifting the rib cage upward. The combined action of the diaphragm and external intercostal muscles is to increase the volume of the thorax and reduce the pressure of the air within the lungs. Air then flows in through the mouth and nose, until the pressures inside and out are equalized. When we breathe very energetically (for example after vigorous exercise), movements of the thorax may be aided by muscles in the neck that attach to the upper two ribs or to the collarbone (clavicle), but under normal circumstances, these muscles are not much used.

The abdomen is supported at the back by the incompressible bony pillar formed by the lumbar spine, but its lateral and anterior walls are purely muscular, so when the diaphragm contracts and descends, these walls must bulge outward. The extent and effectiveness of the movements of the diaphragm are influenced by posture. If a sitting player or singer is slumped forward, the contents of the abdomen are forced farther upward into the thorax than when standing. The walls of the abdomen are also less free to expand, and a more forceful action of the diaphragm is necessary for full inspiration. This will force the body into a more upright position. If the performer is reclining, the abdominal organs slump back against the spine when the diaphragm descends. The muscular wall of the abdomen does not bulge outward and the rib cage does not fall so far passively during expiration. In both situations the result is a reduction in vital capacity—the amount of air available for singing or wind playing.

To expand the thorax, the inspiratory muscles have to overcome not only the effect of gravity in raising the ribs, but also the natural elasticity of the lungs and the rib cage. When the intercostal muscles relax during expiration, these forces cause the rib cage to fall passively toward the rest position. The diaphragm relaxes and the muscles

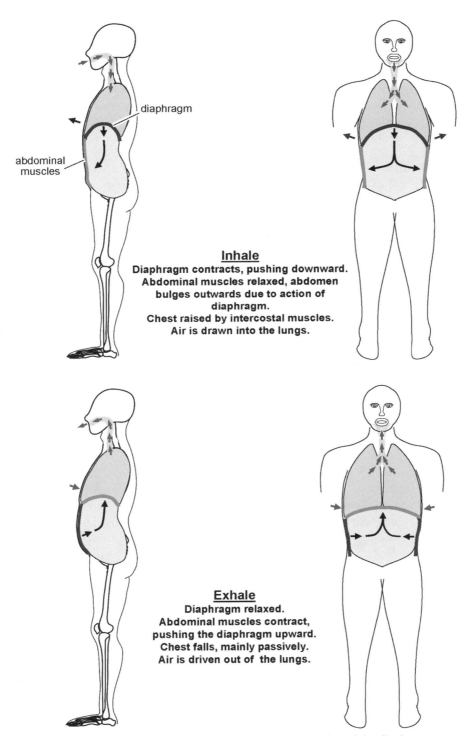

Inhale
Diaphragm contracts, pushing downward.
Abdominal muscles relaxed, abdomen
bulges outwards due to action of
diaphragm.
Chest raised by intercostal muscles.
Air is drawn into the lungs.

Exhale
Diaphragm relaxed.
Abdominal muscles contract,
pushing the diaphragm upward.
Chest falls, mainly passively.
Air is driven out of the lungs.

Figure 4-4.   A summary of respiratory movements and the action of the diaphragm.

of the abdomen wall contract. Because the abdomen is a sealed chamber, compressing its muscular walls forces it to elongate. There is no scope for extension at its lower end, which is blocked off by the floor of the pelvis, so the contents of the abdomen push the relaxed diaphragm upward into the thorax, again like a piston (fig. 4-4). The contrasting roles of the diaphragm and the abdominal muscles are explained in animation 4-1 and shown running continuously in animation 4-2. Because they are the main active component of expiration, the abdominal muscles make an important contribution to controlling the breath during singing. In addition, they are the primary means by which the high air pressures needed to initiate and maintain the vibrations of the reed or the lips in wind players are generated. The pattern of activation in the main inspiratory and expiratory muscles is shown schematically in figure 4-5. This shows a preparatory breath followed by a breath-supporting vocalization and ends with a second silent breath. The breath pressure sustained during singing, which must induce the vibration of the vocal folds of the larynx, is considerably higher than the pressure generated in a silent breath.

The activity of respiratory muscles during singing and wind playing is more complicated than has been described above. This is because of the requirement for very precise control of the pressure and flow rate of exhaled air to regulate the volume, pitch, and temporal structure of the notes. If we fill our lungs to capacity and exhale passively using just the elastic forces of the thorax, the result is a sigh, which empties them in a few seconds. The effect of the elastic forces on breath pressure is indicated by what is labeled the relaxation line in figure 4-5. In order to prolong the breath or maintain a constant breath pressure when the mouth is open, we have to resist the elastic recoil of the thorax when it is high, at the beginning of the breath. This is called respiratory braking and explains why the intercostal muscles remain active after the onset of expiration during singing (fig. 4-5). With the descent of the ribs thus controlled, we can further reduce or stop the flow of air by contracting the diaphragm. However, in some singers, this may only be used for specific vocal effects of short duration (see below). Later during the exhalation, the elastic forces fall below the level necessary to maintain the required breath pressure and so the expiratory muscles of the abdomen and the inner intercostal muscles are recruited. The lateral abdominal muscles and the inner intercostals contract first. The rectus abdominus muscle makes its contribution only toward the end of the breath to force the last of the air from the lungs should this be necessary. As the rectus muscle runs from the rib cage to the front of the pelvis, strong contractions pull the trunk forward and so this muscle is rarely contracted in singing or wind playing.

Auxiliary Respiratory Muscles

In addition to the diaphragm, the intercostal muscles, and the muscles of the abdominal wall, a number of other muscles have been implicated in respiration, at least under certain circumstances. These are known as auxiliary respiratory muscles and some among them feature prominently in certain schools of vocal pedagogy. Most of the muscles discussed in this section are shown in figure 4-6. Some act directly on the ribs but others exert their effects indirectly via the shoulder girdle or upper arm. The

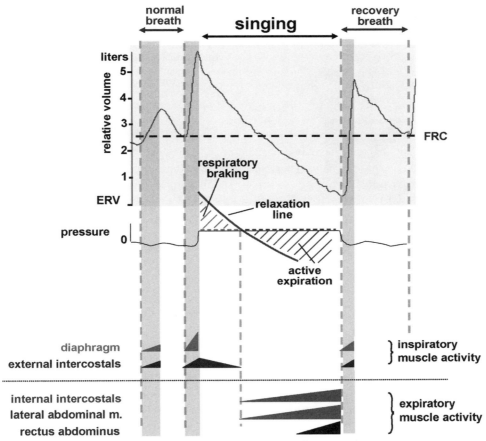

Figure 4-5. Respiratory muscle activity during singing or speaking. This diagram demonstrates in an idealized format the pattern of activity of the major respiratory muscles underlying an episode of vocalization. The changing level of activity of the muscles is indicated by the slopes of the triangles (Ladefoged, 1967).

principal roles of most of these muscles are quite unrelated to respiration, and some may only be able to make a significant contribution to breath control when certain postures are adopted or when the arm or shoulder blade is held fixed either by the action of other muscles or by leaning the arms on a stationary surface.

The first set of auxiliary respiratory muscles we will consider are associated with the trunk. These are the serratus posterior muscles, the latissumus dorsi, the pectoral muscles, and the subclavius. There are two groups of serratus posterior muscles. The serratus posterior superior muscles typically run obliquely downward from the last vertebra of the neck and the upper thoracic vertebrae and attach to the second to fourth ribs, which they are said to draw upward during forced inspiration. The serratus posterior inferior muscles run from the last thoracic and upper lumbar vertebrae to the lowest four ribs, which they pull downward. Considerable controversy has surrounded the possible role of both sets of muscles in breathing. A comprehensive review of the

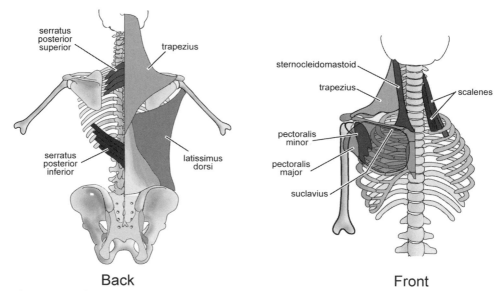

Figure 4-6. The muscles shown are suggested to play an accessory role in respiration, though they are best known for other unrelated actions.

available literature (Vilensky et al. 2001) suggests that these muscles probably have no significant respiratory role but that the sensations generated when they are stretched may influence the activity of muscles that are actively involved in breathing. The serratus posterior inferior muscles might, for example, contribute to the sensations in the lower back during inspiration that are referred to by some singing teachers.

Some singing schools make considerable play of the role of the latissimus dorsi muscle in breathing (Miller 1997). On the face of it, this is rather surprising as the main function of this muscle is to move the arm. At one end it is attached to the lower thoracic vertebrae and, indirectly through a broad, tough sheet of tissue, to the lumbar vertebrae and the hip girdle. At the other end it attaches to the humerus (the bone of the upper arm) just below the shoulder and thus forms the back wall of the armpit. Its main action is to pull the arm downward. As a consequence, it is very well developed in swimmers, who use it to pull themselves through the water. The suggestion that it plays a role in respiration arises because of its attachment to the lower three ribs, which it might conceivably raise during inhalation; however, this would only be effective if the upper arms were held rigidly immobile, which is not normally the case in singers. Physiological studies of the muscle (Orozco-Levi et al. 1995) show it can be used to aid respiration but usually only when the breath is drawn in through the mouth against considerable resistance (i.e., the subject has to suck hard to inhale). Consequently, it is highly unlikely that this muscle plays any significant role in breathing movements underlying singing. The other possibility is that it helps maintain a posture that is optimal for the supported voice; however, this has yet to be investigated.

Campbell (1970) considers that the pectoral muscles (pectoralis major and minor) may also be brought into play during forced inhalation but not in normal breathing.

The pectoralis major is attached at one end to the breastbone and the cartilages that link this to the ribs and to the adjacent part of the collarbone. From these regions it runs to the humerus of the upper arm. Its main action is therefore on the arm, but if this is held fixed it will pull the upper ribs outward and upward. The pectoralis minor runs from the third to fifth ribs to a spur (the coracoid process) that projects forward from the shoulder blade. Its action is usually described as stabilizing the shoulder blade or pulling it downward, but if the shoulder blade is held fixed by other muscles, the ribs would be pulled upward; however, this muscle's role in respiration has not been investigated in any detail. The subclavius is a small muscle that holds the collarbone against the junction of the first rib with the breastbone. It, together with the pectoral muscles and the trapezius (see below) might be brought into play in so-called clavicular breathing (Miller 1997), in which the chest is raised as a consequence of lifting the shoulders; however, this strategy is frowned upon in most schools of singing and is likely to have a number of consequences that do not favor good vocal performance. Without the engagement of these muscles, the shoulders can be readily lifted without raising the chest or having any significant effect on breathing.

Many of the muscles of the neck are also multifunctional; their involvement in breathing, though important for singers, is often viewed as a secondary role by anatomists. The primary function of muscles with an accessory respiratory function is to stabilize or rotate the head (sternocleidomastoid muscle), tilt the head from side to side (the scalene muscles), or raise the shoulders or pull them toward the spine (trapezius). The neck also contains other muscle groups that do not play any obvious role in respiration. Singers often experience neck pain or tension that probably results from stress and can interfere with performance (Pettersen and Westgaard 2005), and so understanding the action of these muscles and reducing their activity where possible is important in vocal teaching.

The actions of the trapezius muscle are complex. Though their most commonly cited action is the raising of the shoulders in a shrugging movement, this is brought about only by the upper part of the muscle, whose fibers run upward to the cervical spine and the underside of the skull. The fibers of the middle part run horizontally and draw the shoulder blades toward the spine, while the fibers of the lower part run obliquely downward and pull the shoulders in that direction. Only the upper part is generally referred to in the context of singing. In standard texts dealing with respiration, it is generally said that the trapezius can aid inspiration by raising the shoulder girdle. As the shoulder is attached to the thorax by the muscles described previously, this pulls the rib cage upward (Campbell 1970). In singing, however, the trapezius appears to be involved in expiration, during which it may compress the thorax by pulling on the shoulders and rotating the shoulder blades toward the spine (Pettersen and Westgaard 2004). The degree to which it is active varies greatly among singers, but tension in the muscle is said to be greatest among those who are relatively inexperienced. It is well established that contraction of the trapezius is often linked to emotional stress, and under these circumstances it may serve no physiological function (Waersted, Bjorklund, and Westgaard 1994). Reducing shoulder tension is generally regarded as beneficial to voice production. When singers are trained to do so through biofeedback techniques, no compensatory changes are seen in the activity of other respiratory muscles, suggesting that the activity of the trapezius is superfluous to most vocal tasks (Pettersen and Westgaard 2002, 2004).

As activity patterns of the sternocleidomastoid and scalene muscles during singing have many similarities, we will deal with them together. One sternocleidomastoid muscle runs on each side of the neck, from the skull just behind the ear to the breastbone (sternum) and the adjacent part of the collarbone (clavicle). If the muscle contracts only on one side, this turns the head upward and to the opposite side, but when both sides act together this thrusts the head forward. If the head is held in a fixed position, the two muscles pull the sternum upward, which helps draw air into the lungs. There are three scalene muscles on each side of the neck. They run from the sides of the neck vertebrae to the first and second ribs. If the neck is free to move, the scalenes bend the neck to the side they are on, but if the neck is held straight by other muscles, the combined action of the right and left scalenes is to pull the ribs they attach to upward, aiding inhalation. Interpreting the activity of the sternocleidomastoid and scalene muscles during singing is complicated by the fact that they are involved not only in breathing, but also in positioning and stabilizing the head, which in turn has an effect on the height of the larynx. The sternocleidomastoid muscles are generally not involved in quiet breathing not related to singing, but there is often activity in the scalenes. With deeper breaths they are progressively brought into play, and activity in the scalenes increases (Campbell 1970; Pettersen and Westgaard 2005). As singers often take breaths close to 100 percent vital capacity, it is common to find marked activity in both sets of muscles, particularly toward the end of inhalation. There is often a brief peak of activation that coincides with start of phonation and more irregular bursts of activity during sung phrases, which may reflect a role in resisting (and therefore giving greater control over) expiratory movements (Campbell 1970; Pettersen and Westgaard 2005). This activity was particularly marked in a study in which performers were asked to sing glissandi that rose to the uppermost part of the range and then fell again (Pettersen et al. 2005). In most of the singers studied, the lowest part of the thorax contracted first, while the upper part was kept expanded until the highest tone was reached. A burst of activity then occurred in the sternocleidomastoid and scalene muscles at the transition point where the upper part of the thorax began to fall. Patterns of muscle activity during inhalation are nevertheless idiosyncratic, and some singers appear to make little use of these muscles under most circumstances. This may be related to the overall respiratory strategy used; for example, in one singer who showed no peak of activity at the turning point of the glissando, the upper and lower parts of the thorax fell in parallel during its entirety. More will be said later about the variability in respiratory patterns exhibited by different individuals.

Among some singing teachers of the German school, contraction of the muscles of the buttocks and pelvic floor is sometimes invoked as a component of breath support (Miller 1997). It is, however, difficult to justify this on anatomical grounds. The primary function of the largest muscle of the buttock, the gluteus maximus, is to stabilize or extend the thigh (draw it backward, e.g., during walking or running) and to rotate it outward. However, in standing, when the foot is planted firmly on the ground, it can be used to rotate the pelvis backward and hence contribute to holding the trunk erect. Clearly this erect posture will contribute to efficient breathing, though the gluteus maximus is only one of the muscles responsible and makes only a relatively small contribution to this. The muscles of the pelvic floor, the most prominent of which is the levator ani, block off the lower opening of the abdomen and also contribute to the sphincters (or seals) of the anus, urethra (the channel for urine), and vagina. Singers may be encouraged to tense this muscle while clenching the buttocks during passages or phrases that require strong breath support by requests to "sit on the breath" or "squeeze the dime" (Miller 1997). There is, however, no anatomical rationale to explain why this might produce a significant benefit for singers. The muscles of the pelvic floor can be weakened by damage during childbirth or as a consequence of age, and as a result a sudden increase in abdominal pressure due to sneezing or even laughter may cause leakage of urine (stress incontinence). It is possible that this has led to the misguided notion that clenching the buttocks and tensing the pelvic floor is needed to support the breath; however, the pressures produced in the chest and abdomen in the explosive action of sneezing far exceed those generated during singing. Any signs of stress incontinence in singers should first be addressed by exercises designed to strengthen the pelvic floor, which should obviate any requirement to clench during performance.

The Concept of Support

The control of the diaphragm and intercostal muscles in combination with the contraction of the expiratory muscles of the abdominal wall constitutes a significant part of what is usually called "support." However, also embodied in this concept are greater voice resonance, clarity, and range, which arise partly from other manipulations of the vocal tract. Despite its importance, there is no single and unambiguous definition of support, and the word has different shades of meaning for different singers and teachers (Griffin et al. 1995). The terms *Atemstütze* and *appoggio* refer approximately to the same phenomenon. Distinctions are made in some schools between singing with "no support," "chest support," or "diaphragm support" (Winckel 1952); however, these concepts are based on subjective sensations that can be misleading and may reflect an incomplete understanding of the mechanics and anatomy of respiration (Watson and Hixon 1985). In addition, it is almost impossible to assess subjectively all that is going on physically during singing, not only because many muscles in the vocal tract and respiratory system are being activated simultaneously, but also because some key muscles (most crucially for the present discussion, the diaphragm) have a relatively poor sensory nerve supply, meaning that we are not generally aware of when they are active. There is, however, little disagreement on the beneficial effects of support to the quality of the voice and a high degree of consistency in the recognition of supported singing among those professionally involved with singers (Sand and Sundberg 2005).

In some schools of singing, the role of the abdominal muscles in support is emphasized (Thorpe et al. 2001), but it is only recently that objective analyses of the activity of different muscle groups during singing and wind playing have been attempted. Even in studies with this aim, the actions of the muscles are often inferred only indirectly from measurements of thoracic or abdominal dimensions or pressure levels in different parts of the vocal tract. This may be due to the understandable reluctance of experimenters and their subjects to use invasive techniques such as placing electrodes directly into the muscles themselves. In its most general sense, support is the regulation of air pressure and the velocity of airflow in the respiratory system during expiratory episodes underlying singing or wind playing and is generated by a dynamic interaction between expiratory and inspiratory muscles. Changes in air pressure below the glottis (the opening between the vocal folds of the larynx) are largely driven by the movement of the contents of the abdomen (i.e., the visceral organs) as they are pushed up by the abdominal muscles. Their mass gives them considerable inertia, and obtaining precise control of their movement requires, as we have seen, the concerted actions of both the expiratory muscles of the abdominal wall and the inspiratory muscles of the diaphragm and thorax. At certain stages of the respiratory cycle these may even be active simultaneously, the strength of contraction of the antagonistic muscles being continually adjusted to produce precise movements in the abdominal mass and control changes in subglottic pressure (Leanderson, Sundberg, and von Euler 1987).

The concept of support is rather different for wind players, and its precise nature depends to a large extent on the type of instrument. In the flute and recorder, the control issues most closely resemble those discussed for singers, as the mouth is either fully open or the resistance to airflow very low. For these instruments, sound can be generated using elastic recoil forces alone when the lungs are fully inflated (see below). In reed and brass instruments, where the air column in the pharynx is stopped at the embouchure, the pressure required to produce the sound is much greater than can be generated by elastic recoil and always requires the involvement of the abdominal muscles. For players of these instruments the word "support" will therefore refer exclusively to the action of the expiratory muscles. As the abdominal and intercostal muscles contain many sensory nerve endings, we are well aware when they are active. The lack of sensation from the diaphragm may partly explain why breath support is often inappropriately linked to this muscle. The word "diaphragm" is often used when what is actually meant are the muscles of the abdominal walls, which, of course, have the opposite action.

MUSCLE ACTIVITY DURING SINGING OR WIND PLAYING

It is not possible to obtain a detailed understanding of how the chest and abdominal walls move during breathing by following their movements visually or by relying entirely on subjective sensation. This information can be obtained, however, with a device known as a plethysmograph. There are many designs of plethysmographs, but one of the most straightforward to use (the inductive plethysmograph) employs elastic bands that are placed around the chest and abdomen to monitor their movements. The bands contain open coils of wire whose resistance changes as they expand and contract, providing a measure of the changes in their circumference. The bands are light and comfortable and do not interfere with the movements they are measuring. Demonstrations of how these can be used to analyze singing and wind playing are shown in videos 4-1 and 4-2, and a number of the studies referred to below use variants of this technique. The traces generated have a sawtooth contour, with a rapid upward movement representing inhalation and a more gentle slope seen during the exhalation that underlies singing or playing. The most useful information that can be drawn from plethysmography is provided by the angles of the slopes of the traces from the bands on the chest and abdomen and their relationship in time. This is difficult to assess visually; however, the chest movement can be plotted against the abdominal movement to create what is known as a Konno-Mead diagram (fig. 4-7), which is relatively simple to interpret intuitively (Konno and Mead 1967), even for those with no background in respiratory physiology. The practical application of Konno-Mead diagrams to breathing in singers and wind players is demonstrated in videos 4-3 and 4-4. In the idealized examples shown in figure 4-7, the movement of the abdomen is represented along the horizontal axis and that of the thorax on the vertical axis. Two types of reference lines are often shown on the traces. The first are isovolume lines, which are obtained from inspiratory and expiratory movements made with the mouth and glottis closed. Any slope on the diagram that is parallel to these lines represents complementary movements of the chest and abdominal wall that result in no overall change in lung volume. The other reference is the relaxation line, which represents the passive falling of the chest and recoil of the abdomen in the absence of any muscular activity, for example, during a sigh. It is important to note that the graph has no time dimension, so the duration of each phase of respiration cannot be determined from these diagrams. You will see from the section of the videos showing the lines being generated in real time that some segments of the traces are drawn rapidly (e.g., during inhalation) and others more slowly. Konno-Mead diagrams have been quite extensively used for studying respiration in singers, but so far appear in only one paper on wind playing (Cossette, Sliwinski, and Macklem 2000). They have great potential for providing an objective analysis of breathing patterns between singers of different types and players of the same or different instruments, and we are currently performing extensive studies using this technique at the Royal Welsh College of Music and Drama and at Cardiff University.

If we return to an examination of the idealized Konno-Mead diagrams in figure 4-7, we can see that at the beginning of an inspiration, the contraction of the diaphragm pushes the contents of the abdomen downward, causing its wall to bulge outward. This may induce a brief decline in thoracic volume as the contraction of the diaphragm pulls the lower edge of the thorax inward, followed by the engagement of the intercostal muscles that raise the ribcage, rotating the ribs outward, while the diaphragm continues to contract. At the transition between inspiration and expiration, the abdominal muscles contract, which initially pushes the chest wall farther out. This does not necessarily involve a change in lung volume, as it may run nearly parallel to the isovolume line; however, for loud singing or speech, some reduction in volume is usually present. The movement represents what is called "prephonatory posturing," which may optimize the position of the chest wall for the start of vocalization, initiating the support mechanism and raising lung pressure sufficiently to drive the vocal cords, lips, or reed at a level sufficient to generate the note to be produced. Expiration then begins with a continued contraction of the muscles of the abdominal wall together with the downward rotation of the ribs driven by the elastic forces released as the external intercostal muscles relax.

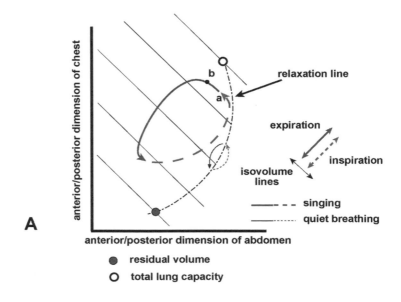

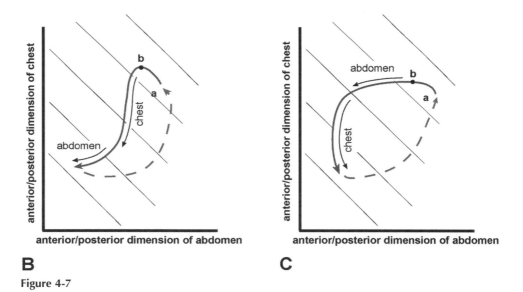

Figure 4-7

Three different strategies for expiration can be distinguished using Konno-Mead diagrams. In the first, the abdomen and the chest move inward proportionately at the same time, resulting in an almost straight diagonal line running downward and to the left (fig. 4-7A). In the second, the chest falls first and the abdominal wall only moves inward later (fig. 4-7B), while in the third, the order is reversed so that abdominal movement precedes that of the chest (fig. 4-7C).

Figure 4-7. Konno-Mead diagrams can be used to illustrate the changing dimensions of the chest and abdomen during breathing. Idealized diagrams for three different breathing strategies are shown here. The vertical axis represents the horizontal depth or circumference of the chest (depending on method) and the horizontal axis, the same dimension for the abdomen. The oblique parallel lines are isovolume contours; that is, movements parallel to these lines produce no overall change in lung volume. The relaxation line represents the change in the dimensions when the chest wall is allowed to fall passively. During quiet breathing the movements of the chest and abdomen are very small and lie close to the relaxation line. During singing, the movements are much larger. At the start of exhalation (a) there is initially no change in chest volume; the line between (a) and (b) runs parallel to the isovolume line. This is called prephonatory posturing and is required to increase the air pressure in the lungs before singing. The voice is produced from (b) onward. The first phase of inspiration is mainly due to the outward movement of the abdominal wall as its muscles relax and the diaphragm is pushed downward, but the contribution of the chest progressively increases as the external intercostal muscles pull the ribs upward and outward. Note that the Konno-Mead diagram has no time dimension, so it is not possible to deduce from it how long each phase of the cycle lasts. A. Comparison of the changing dimensions of the chest and abdomen seen during quiet breathing with that during singing. During the vocal phase of exhalation, the line runs almost diagonally, indicating that the walls of the chest and abdomen are moving inward at the same time. The same phase in B is at first entirely due to an inward movement of the chest (i.e., the trace falls vertically); when this ends, contraction of the abdominal muscles takes over. In C, the opposite occurs: the first part of the exhalation is entirely due to abdominal muscle activity (indicated by the horizontal direction of the trace) but then switches to chest movement. Konno-Mead diagrams are further explained in videos 4-3 and 4-4.

Singing

In objective studies of respiration in singers, one feature emerges strongly, namely, that patterns of chest and abdominal movements and of muscular activity vary widely between individuals. This may in part reflect different schools of singing pedagogy, but there are clearly other factors at work as well. In some singers, the changes in thoracic and abdominal dimensions run in parallel as in figure 4-7A (Thorpe et al. 2001), while others are taught to hold the rib cage out as the muscles of the abdominal wall contract (fig. 4-7C). The dramatic effects of different strategies can be seen in video 4-3. The variability in relative contribution of chest and abdominal movements may also reflect differences in posture or the biomechanical properties of the thorax and abdomen in different individuals for whom one or another strategy may be more suited (Wilder 1983; Hoit and Hixon 1986). Individuals can be classified into three broad categories according to body type (somatotype): endomorphs, who are plump; ectomorphs, who are slight; and mesomorphs, who are muscular (fig. 4-8). A preliminary study of tidal breathing and breathing during speech suggests that individuals with different somatotypes may use quite different respiratory strategies (Hoit and Hixon 1986). Unfortunately, this work is based on data obtained from only twelve subjects. The categorization of these three discrete somatotypes is now also outdated, given the ease with which we can obtain information on a wide range of parameters reflecting body composition. Given the potential importance of the concept that optimal breathing strategies (and perhaps other aspects of technique) might be related to somatotype in singers (and indeed in other performers), a proper analysis of this question should be given a high priority.

Body type	Breathing Strategy
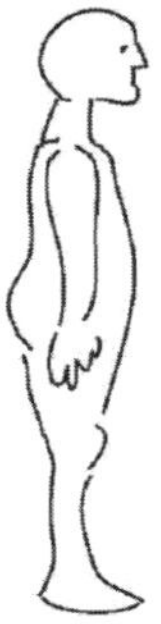	**Endomorph** (plump build) Tidal breathing: deep and slow Speech breathing: Expiration is driven predominantly by abdominal activity, which is sometimes sufficient to cause a paradoxical upward movement of the chest wall. This use of abdominal muscles may be in order to counteract the downward pull of the abdominal organs on the diaphragm during expiration. Movement of chest wall makes a smaller contribution. This is typical of the "pear-shaped up" breathing posture.
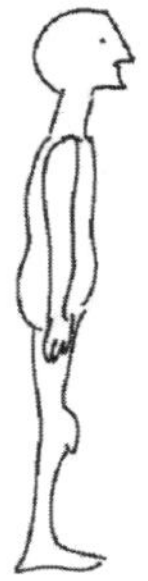	**Ectomorph** (slight build) Tidal breathing: shallower and faster than endomorph Speech breathing: Inspiration is predominantly brought about by raising the chest wall and expiration by a falling of the chest wall, with smaller contributions from abdominal muscles. Paradoxical upward movement of chest during expiration is not seen. This is typical of the "pear-shaped down" breathing posture.
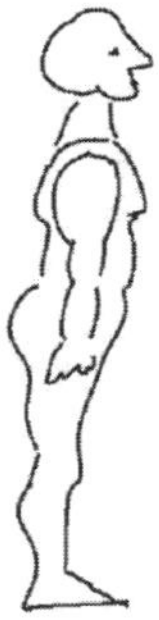	**Mesomorph** (muscular build) Tidal breathing: shallower and faster than endomorph Speech breathing: Mechanism lies between the extremes of those used by endomorphs and ectomorphs. Both chest and abdominal mechanisms are active.

Figure 4-8.   The differences in respiratory patterns between individuals with different body types as proposed by Hoit and Hixon (1986).

If the conclusions of Hoit and Hixon are correct, it is likely that the more demanding breathing strategies required by singing will show similar variability. They concluded that endomorphs use longer and slower breaths during normal quiet breathing and appear to employ predominantly abdominal mechanisms for breathing during speech (fig. 4-8). This would have some similarities with what is sometimes called the "pear-shaped up" breathing posture in singers (fig. 4-9), in which the abdomen is strongly distended at the end of inhalation, while the chest is kept high for as long as possible

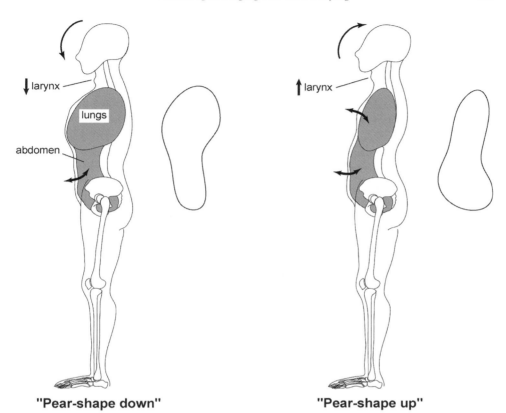

"Pear-shape down"   **"Pear-shape up"**

Figure 4-9. **Two breathing strategies sometimes described in singers. In the "pear-shape down" posture, the chest is held high, and the aim is to exhale mainly through contraction of the abdominal muscles. When seen from the side, the cavities of the chest and abdomen have the shape of an upside-down pear (see outline). The chin is held down, allowing the larynx to descend. In the "pear-shape up" posture, the chest also falls during expiration. The singer leans back and raises the chin, which tends to pull the larynx up. The consequences of these strategies for the voice are discussed in chapter 5.**

during the exhalation (Titze 2000). This should produce a Konno-Mead trace similar to that in figure 4-7C. With this strategy the contraction of the abdominal muscles during exhalation may cause a paradoxical upward movement of the chest wall (in the direction normally seen during inhalation). The greater use of the abdominal muscles, coupled with the longer breaths, pushes the diaphragm upward into the thorax farther than during shorter, shallower breaths, or where inhalation is predominantly driven by raising the chest wall. The result is a greater stretching of the diaphragm in its passive state, which may make it more effective in increasing the volume of the thorax when it contracts during inhalation. It is generally accepted that individuals develop the breathing strategies that are energetically most cost effective for them, so the predominance of abdominal mechanisms in endomorphs presumably suits those with large body mass. This might be necessary because of the greater mass of the visceral organs (especially the liver, which hangs from the underside of the diaphragm) and the more substantial oxygen demands of a larger body. The ectomorphs take shorter, shallower breaths during normal quiet breathing and make much less use of abdominal volume changes during speech breathing, in which most of the change in lung volume is brought about by the rising and falling of the chest wall (fig. 4-7B). This would resemble the "pear-shaped down" strategy of some singers, in which both chest and abdomen work together (fig. 4-9). Mesomorphs use breathing strategies that lie somewhere between those of the endomorphs and ectomorphs.

Despite the fact that many singers favor the "pear-shaped up" posture (which is probably equivalent to the "noble" posture described by some singers), direct measurements from performers suggest that changes in the dimensions of the chest wall always make by far the greatest contribution to changes in lung volume (Thomasson and Sundberg 2001b). In this study, the contribution of the abdominal wall varied considerably between three male singers (all baritones), but the question of body type or breathing strategy was not addressed. However, even if the movement of the abdominal wall is relatively small, the degree of tension in the muscles that form it will be a significant factor in ensuring that the fall in the chest wall drives air efficiently through the larynx. What actually takes place during "pear-shaped up" and "pear-shaped down" breathing and the possible advantages of the two strategies therefore remain uncertain (Titze 2000). As will be seen in chapter 5, one significant factor may be the effect that these postures have on laryngeal height.

As can be seen in figure 4-10, singers use most of their vital capacity when required to sing long phrases while even for shorter ones, lung volumes decline well into the zone of the functional residual capacity. However, the breath intake is matched to phrase length so that excess air does not have to be exhaled at the end, which would be a waste of both energy and time, delaying the onset of the following phrase and possibly inducing the effects of hyperventilation. In quiet speech, lung volumes tend to stay mainly above the line marking the functional residual capacity, while in declamatory speech at the intensity used by actors in live theater, the pattern begins to resemble that used in singing. One prominent feature of the lung volume traces for declamatory speech and singing is a sharp decline immediately before the onset of the sound. This represents prephonatory posturing, which is necessary to raise lung pressure to a level appropriate to generate the vibration of the vocal folds for the succeeding note (see videos 4-1 and 4-3).

Physiological studies of respiratory activity during singing reinforce the idea that different singers employ quite distinct strategies to achieve the same goals (Griffin et al. 1995; Thorpe et al. 2001), though the respiratory pattern in a given individual asked to repeat the same exercise is highly consistent (Thomasson and Sundberg 2001a). This is nowhere more true than in the use of the diaphragm. In some singers it is active not only during inhalation, but remains so during the initial stages of exhalation when lung volume is high. Its activity then declines progressively as the lungs deflate during singing. By pushing the floor of the chest cavity downward, it reduces the change in volume caused by the elastic recoil forces of the lungs and rib cage. In other singers there is no evidence of any diaphragmatic activity during phonation. These individuals presumably rely solely on the intercostal muscles to slow the fall of the thorax. There are several factors that might support a greater role for the

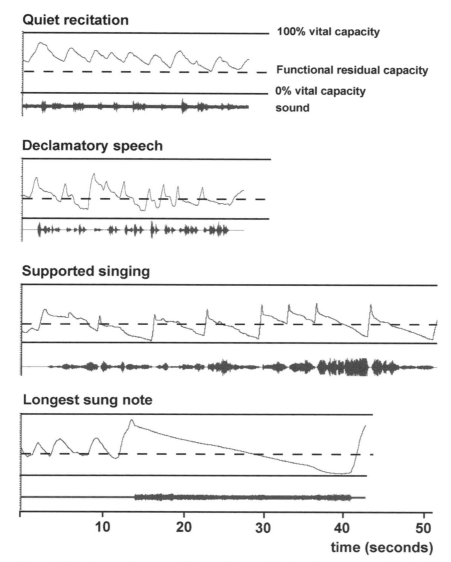

Figure 4-10. Lung volumes used in speaking and singing the same text (the Welsh hymn "Cwm Rhondda," heard in video 4-2). In the upper part of each figure, changes in lung volume obtained using plethysmography (expressed as a percentage of vital capacity) are shown during the passage, which requires several breaths. During quiet recitation, the respiratory trace remains above the functional residual capacity (FRC) line, which represents the level at which all respiratory muscles are relaxed. With declamatory speech at a volume appropriate for a stage performance, the trace dips frequently below the FRC into the range where the abdominal muscles are engaged. In supported singing using the projected voice, this extends almost to the lower limit of vital capacity. As the sung phrases for this piece are relatively short, inhalations do not approach 100 percent vital capacity. This does occur, however, when the singer is asked to produce the longest note possible (bottom trace). In the traces for declamatory speech and singing, each exhalation starts with a sharp reduction in lung volume that precedes phonation (prephonatory posturing). This raises the air pressure in the lungs to a level appropriate for the onset of the vocal fold vibration.

intercostal muscles over the diaphragm in respiratory braking. First, the thoracic wall has a much larger area of contact with the lungs (about 75 percent) compared to the diaphragm, and so to produce the same pressure change, the movement of the ribs can be much smaller than that required of the diaphragm. Second, the ribs are raised by a series of short intercostal muscles (one set in each rib space) that will allow greater control and range of contraction than the diaphragm, which is a single sheet of much longer muscle fibers. Third, when the singer is upright, particularly when standing, the viscera pull the diaphragm down passively anyway (Watson and Hixon 1985), which may render significant contraction of the diaphragm unnecessary. Furthermore, using the diaphragm in this way eats into vital capacity in a way that braking using the intercostals does not. Finally, as previously mentioned, there is little subjective sensation of diaphragm contraction, so its effects can only be appreciated indirectly through tension changes in the thoracic or abdominal wall. This may reduce the level of precision possible in its control.

Because of the controversy concerning the role of the diaphragm and the importance attributed to it by many singing teachers, several studies have been designed to gain a detailed objective assessment of how it operates during singing. One experiment, in which a group of highly trained singers were asked to repeatedly sing the unvoiced consonant "p" followed by the vowel "a" (pa, pa, pa, pa, pa, pa . . .), exemplified the different patterns of diaphragmatic activity that are used by different individuals to create an apparently similar effect (Leanderson, Sundberg, and von Euler 1987). In one singer, the diaphragm remained inactive throughout the expiration. In a second, there was a tonic contraction of the diaphragm to counter elastic recoil of the thorax at the beginning of the breath. In a third, the diaphragm was active only phasically at the beginning of the breath, during the vowel element, reducing subglottal pressure transiently. The diaphragm then relaxed (allowing subglottal pressure to rise) during the occlusion of the lips for the "p," thus emphasising the explosive transition between the "p" and the "a." In a fourth singer, the activation of the diaphragm was similar to the third, except that this time the peaks of its contraction coincided with the "p," which would decrease its explosive character but reduce breath expenditure. We are of course left wondering whether the results of these four strategies (particularly the ones involving phasic activity of the diaphragm) sound different to the listener, something a written report cannot tell us, but as they appear to be properties of the individual techniques of the singers concerned, they may have contributed to the individuality of each singer's vocal character. On the other hand, they might equally reflect a slightly different interpretation of what was being asked for in the task.

Differences in strategy were again apparent when three of the same singers were asked to sing alternating notes an octave apart (fig. 4-11). In two of the singers, the diaphragm contracted to reduce subglottal pressure as the pitch dropped almost instan-taneously from the high note to the low (fig. 4-11A). This effect was most marked at the beginning of the breath, when thoracic recoil pressures were high. One subject, however, who used his abdominal wall musculature to raise abdominal pressure to a much higher level than the others, contracted the diaphragm most strongly during the high notes (fig. 4-11B), presumably counteracting this with a considerable increase in abdominal muscle activity! One explanation suggested for this behavior is that under

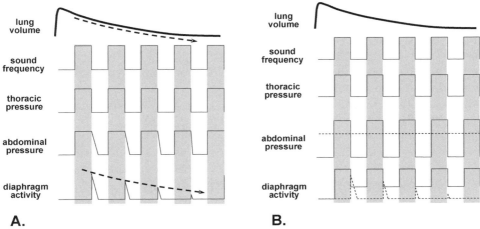

A.   **B.**

Figure 4-11.   Different ways of using the diaphragm during singing. The diagrams are idealized representations of actual traces shown in Leanderson et al. (1987). Singers were asked to alternate repeatedly between two notes an octave apart. Some singers use the strategy shown in A, where the diaphragm contracts rapidly at the end of the high note to produce a rapid drop in thoracic (lung) pressure. As the lungs gradually deflate during the breath, the elastic recoil forces of the chest decline and so less diaphragmatic activity is needed. However, one singer used a different strategy (B) in which the diaphragm contracts during the high note. The thoracic pressure generated is similar to that in A, but the singer here uses very high abdominal pressure and so contraction of the diaphragm counteracts this to ensure that the thoracic pressure does not rise excessively. This paradoxical use of the diaphragm is not unusual and has been shown in other studies. The dashed traces in B represent the peak of abdominal pressure and the shape of the diaphragm trace from A emphasizes how these differ.

these conditions the diaphragm compresses the contents of the abdomen and forces it to expand outward, increasing the diameter of the base of the rib cage. This may be used to keep the thorax expanded for as long as possible during the singing breath (the pear-shaped up posture), which is encouraged by some teachers (Leanderson, Sundberg, and von Euler 1987). Another possibility is that if the mass of the abdomen was large, small complementary changes in two opposing forces might allow greater control over its movement up into the chest cavity.

By contrast, in other situations all of the singers used the diaphragm in the same way. The group was asked to perform a Renaissance trillo, in which the same note is rapidly repeated interspersed with very brief silences. (The ornament heard, for example, in the Monteverdi Vespers is sometimes unflatteringly described as the goat's trill!) In this rather extreme vocal task, the diaphragm was always activated phasically to create the silences between the notes. The strategy used for singing coloratura passages was also consistent. Surprisingly, perhaps, there was little or no contribution of the diaphragm here to the rapid fluctuations in subglottal pressure that accompany the transitions between each note, which are presumably mainly derived from activity of the muscles of the abdominal wall.

Given the lack of sensory feedback available from the diaphragm, the question of whether it can be brought under conscious control at all is an important one. It has been shown that if diaphragmatic pressure is recorded electronically and presented to singers on a computer screen, they can quickly learn to activate it at will (Leanderson, Sundberg, and von Euler 1987). This generally has the effect of giving the voice a "darker" or more "covered" quality, due to the suppression of the higher harmonic partials of the note that apparently occurs as a result of a shift toward flow-phonation from a more pressed state of the vocal folds (see chapter 5). However, it is also possible with practice to return to a "bright" sound even with the diaphragm active. This implies that the change in tone is a secondary effect of diaphragmatic action, perhaps due to greater tension on the vocal tract or to a change in posture. The experiment also revealed that when the diaphragm is active, there is a reduction in the variability of the formant frequencies of the notes produced. The reasons for this are currently unclear, but it may be the result of a more stable positioning of the larynx.

One distinctive feature of the voice of most modern classical singers is vibrato. Though there is some variation in its nature between individuals, it is typically a fluctuation in the fundamental frequency of the note of about 50 cents at 6–8 hertz (6–8 cycles per second). It appears to be associated with laryngeal muscle activity (see chapter 5), particularly that of the cricothyroid muscles, which stretch the vocal folds, increasing the pitch of the note. There also seems to be some involvement of the vocalis muscles (which tense the vocal folds) and the lateral cricoarytenoid muscles that bring them together, closing the glottis and lowering pitch (Sundberg 1999). Oscillations in phase with the vibrato may also be present in the muscles of the pharynx and tongue, though it is not likely that these would make a significant contribution to the sound. During the vibrato, fluctuations in subglottic pressure and airflow can usually be measured, but their origin is unclear. Though these could be a secondary effect of the oscillations in the vocal folds themselves, they could also result either from rhythmic activity in the diaphragm (at high lung capacities) or in the muscles of the abdomen. As will be seen below, all three of these elements may contribute to the production of vibrato in the flute.

Breathing and Voice Projection

The audibility of a singer's voice against the background of an orchestra is dependent on what is known as the "singer's formant" or "ring" (chapter 5). Though this is largely due to a manipulation of the intrinsic resonances of the vocal tract, it may partly be a consequence of the respiratory element of support. In a study of the supported voice in four male and four female singers (Griffin et al. 1995), it was concluded that in the males this was associated with an increase in subglottal pressure and peak airflow rate, accompanied by a lowering of the larynx. However, the supported voice in females (and particularly sopranos) was reported to employ a different strategy, being linked to tighter closure of the vocal folds (i.e., leading to more pressed phonation) in the upper range, while at lower pitches it actually involved a lower subglottal pressure. Thorpe and colleagues also examined the relationship between respiratory activity and vocal projection; their results partially supported the findings of Griffin et al. (1995). The five singers who took part in the study had all been taught a strategy for voice projection by the same teacher (Thorpe et al. 2001), which stressed the synchronized activation of the lateral abdominal muscles (internal and external obliques, transversus abdominus) during phonation and their complete relaxation at the onset of inspiration. The initial lung volumes used by the singers for each phrase (expressed as a percentage of vital capacity) were the same for projected and unprojected phrases despite the fact that sound intensity increased, though they were of course smaller for much quieter singing. This finding probably reflected the fact that because of their training, the singers had already optimized their respiratory strategies and the initial lung volume was close to capacity. The lateral dimension of the thorax was increased during projected singing while that of the abdomen was reduced. Both of these changes are consistent with increased activity in the lateral abdominal muscles and therefore suggest that the theory behind the strategy was being put into effect. Finally, there was a reduction in the rate of airflow through the vocal tract in the projected voice, which again suggests that this state is brought about by changes in the positioning and vibratory patterns of the vocal folds so that they increase the resistance to the airflow.

While it is understandable that both studies were able to recruit only small numbers of singers, this raises some problems for their interpretation. For example, both involved three or four different types of voice (bass, tenor, mezzo-soprano, and soprano) and, as we have already seen, these may not use the same mechanism for voice projection. Furthermore, while all of the singers in the second study had been pupils of one teacher, this was apparently not true of the first. Consequently it is the similarities rather than the differences between the studies that are likely to be most significant. As the subjects were all classically trained professional singers, it is likely that they were already using breathing strategies optimized for projection even in their unsupported singing. This may make the critical mechanisms underlying each style of singing harder to determine. From the viewpoint of young singers in training, an examination of the evolution of respiratory patterns as technical facility is acquired would be useful for guiding their development, but long-term studies of this nature have not so far been carried out.

Wind Playing

Many of the most detailed published studies on respiratory patterns of wind players also suffer from the very small numbers of subjects involved. This may in part be related to the invasive nature of some of the measuring techniques used. Not many players will relish performing with pressure balloons inserted via the nose down into the stomach and esophagus. We cannot therefore be certain that the results so far obtained will prove typical of the majority of elite performers. However, as more information is accumulated clearer trends should emerge, and even players of a professional standard may find it beneficial at least to experiment with different respiratory strategies. Some studies have revealed considerable similarities between players at very different levels of technical development in certain aspects of respiration, for example, in the duration of breaths used for a given piece (Bouhuys 1964), though these may not turn out to be the most significant parameters for performance. Other studies have emphasized differences in the measurements obtained of the same parameter in a single player when practicing regularly compared to those obtained after

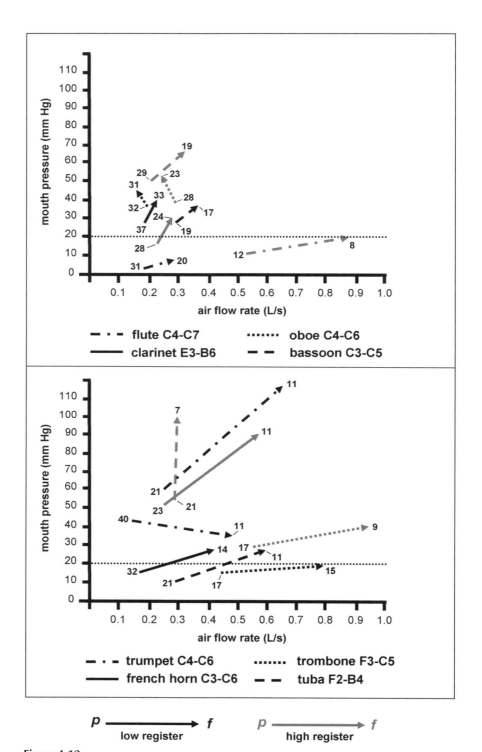

Figure 4-12

a prolonged period without playing the instrument (Roos 1936). As with singers, it is likely that differences in body structure will ultimately prove highly significant for respiratory patterns.

The relationship between respiratory parameters and the type of sound produced has not so far been examined objectively in wind players; for example, the studies generally show no spectral analysis of the sound produced under different breathing regimes or embouchure configurations. Clearly the type of sound that is deemed desirable or which is actually attained will be affected by many factors, such as the personal taste and characteristics (e.g., embouchure configuration) of the individual performer, the prevailing culture of players belonging to different schools of performance (here the age of some studies may be a significant factor), and the characteristics of the mouthpiece or the instrument. Some discrepancies between published studies have been attributed to such factors (see Cossette, Sliwinski, and Macklem 2000). Because a number of these reports are now quite old, differences in the lifestyle of the players may also be significant. For example, the author of one of the few available large-scale surveys of lung volume and breathing patterns in wind players reports that many of the players were heavy smokers (Bouhuys 1964). That smoking has a dramatic effect on lung function is now widely known and so it is unlikely to be as prevalent among today's players, who live in a more competitive and health-conscious society than did those in the 1960s. The respiratory requirements demanded of wind players vary considerably depending on the instrument. The most detailed studies performed to date of the respiratory mechanisms of wind players have been carried out on flutists.

Respiratory Patterns in Flute Playing

Because the flute is played with an unstopped embouchure (i.e., with the mouth open), its respiratory demands are more similar to those of singers than of players of reed and brass wind instruments. In particular, it is only in the flute that respiratory braking is likely to be a significant factor, as in other instruments there is significant resistance to airflow at the mouthpiece or reed (fig. 4-12). Flutists use 70–85 percent of their total vital capacity in playing and typically start a playing breath from 85 to 98 percent of total capacity, though this will obviously depend on phrasing. On a theoretical basis, we described three distinct patterns of expiration in the Konno-Mead diagrams of fig. 4-7: 1) the rib cage may be allowed to descend before the abdominal muscles are en-

Figure 4-12.   Breath pressure and airflow in wind playing. This diagram illustrates the demands made on the respiratory system by woodwind and brass instruments and has been produced from numerical data published by Pawlowski and Zoltowski (1987). Each instrument is represented by a different type of line. The black lines represent a note near the bottom of the register and the gray lines, a note near the top. The beginning of each line represents the note played piano and the end with the arrow, the note played forte. The horizontal dotted line marks the approximate value for the elastic recoil pressure of the thorax at 100 percent vital capacity. The numbers indicate the mean breath duration for each note (usually from four players). Note that some notes in the upper register of the clarinet require less breath pressure than those in the lower register. Among the woodwinds, the oboe requires high pressure but low flow rates, while the flute requires only low pressure but high flow rates in the upper register. For brass instruments, both pressure and flow rate are high in the upper registers.

gaged; 2) abdominal contraction may precede the descent of the ribs; or 3) contraction of the abdominal muscles and descent of the rib cage may occur simultaneously. One study of three professional flutists demonstrated that each employed a different strategy, with no obvious differences in facility or musical outcome (Cossette, Sliwinski, and Macklem 2000). There is therefore no clear evidence at present that any one of these approaches provides a clear advantage over the others, though it must be borne in mind that the investigation of the respiratory dynamics in wind instrumentalists is still at the stage of baseline data collection, and the issue of how changing respiratory patterns might affect different aspects of performance has not yet been addressed. Players who are the subjects of these studies are generally described as being of professional status, but this does not mean that they all make a similar sound. We also have no knowledge of their basic lung function parameters or somatotypes, both of which are significant omissions.

During playing, the flutist must regulate both the flow rate (the volume exhaled per second) and velocity of the air passing through the embouchure. When playing at the bottom of the register, flow rate and air pressure at the embouchure are both low. As a consequence, in the first stages of an expiration, when the lungs are full and the elastic recoil forces of the thorax are high, considerable respiratory braking by the paradoxical activity of inspiratory muscles (particularly the intercostals) is needed for breath conservation. As the lungs empty and the recoil forces decline, the active expiratory muscles of the abdomen become increasingly important to maintain sufficient airflow to support the note. With rising pitch, air pressure at the embouchure must be increased, typically by a factor of 3.5–5 over the three octaves. This is accompanied by a forward projection of the lips to decrease the length of the air jet (Fletcher 1975). The velocity of the airstream increases by a factor of about three over the same pitch range; however, because the area of the embouchure opening is correspondingly reduced (by a factor of 2–3), the flow rate (i.e., the amount of air used per second) remains almost static between D4 and G6, though this rises sharply by C7. Increasing sound volume is supported by rising flow rate and greater embouchure area, accompanied by smaller changes in velocity. The velocity increase with volume declines with rising pitch, particularly in the third octave, where high velocities are required even for relatively low sound intensities.

Vibrato

An important element of the sound that must also be controlled by the respiratory system is vibrato. This is a rapid fluctuation in air pressure leading to an oscillation mainly in intensity, though also to some extent also in pitch. The intensity fluctuations are more pronounced in the upper partials, producing a fluctuation in timbre (Fletcher 1975). Vibrato is particularly important for the flute, as it generates fewer overtones than other woodwind instruments (Bonard 2001) and in the absence of vibrato can sound harsh and lacking in color. In the following account it is important to bear in mind that even a cursory comparison of performances by well-known soloists will reveal very different patterns of vibrato, a factor that is not generally taken into consideration in studies of wind players or singers. Instructions to flutists on how to produce vibrato often refer to the use of the diaphragm. In some players at least, short repeated contractions of the diaphragm do indeed contribute to the production of vibrato through an oscillation in respiratory braking. In the above-mentioned study of three flutists (Cossette, Sliwinski, and Macklem 2000), each was asked to hold a sustained note with vibrato for a period of ten seconds. One of the flutists used the diaphragm rhythmically for the first half of the breath, but its activity then rapidly declined (presumably as the thoracic recoil forces faded), to be replaced with a rapid oscillation of the abdominal expiratory muscles superimposed on their tonic level of activity. The other two flutists appeared to use neither the diaphragm nor the abdominal muscles and it was inferred that the vibrato was produced by oscillatory movements of the muscles of the larynx, which would cause rapid fluctuations in the width of the opening between the vocal cords. This contradicts the belief of many flutists that the larynx is not involved in the production of vibrato; however, direct observation of the glottis (the aperture between the vocal cords) reveals that movements of the vocal folds are probably an almost universal feature of flute vibrato technique (King, Ashby, and Nelson 1988). Even some of the players in this study had previously considered that the diaphragm was the main source of their vibrato. This has been confirmed by several other investigators. The confusion concerning the source of vibrato is perhaps not surprising given the paucity of sensation from the diaphragm and the uncertainty about the sensory supply to the muscles of the larynx. Other players and teachers are more aware of the origin of vibrato, however, and their descriptions of how it should be produced refer to the glottis, throat, or larynx as well as the muscles of the abdominal wall. The frequency of vibrato is generally around 5 hertz; the constancy of this figure between players has led to the suggestion that it represents a resonance phenomenon related either to the mechanical properties of structures that produce it or their control by the nervous system. Though there is as yet no direct evidence for this proposition, the fact that the frequency of vibrato is typically very similar between singers provides some support for it (Sundberg 1999).

One situation in which the action of the diaphragm is both unequivocal and consistent between performers is in the playing of a series of untongued staccato notes (Cossette, Sliwinski, and Macklem 2000). Here each note is initiated by abdominal contraction and terminated by a burst of intense activity in the diaphragm, which rapidly reduces air pressure. This is therefore similar to the situation seen in singers performing the Renaissance-style trillo described previously, though the frequency of the notes generated in the flute study was much slower. However, this is not a task that is usually demanded of players.

Reed and Brass Instruments

Brass and other woodwind instruments have a relatively high pressure threshold for initiation of the vibration of the reed or the lips (figs. 4-12, 4-13). Even at the bottom of their range, the threshold pressure required is above that generated passively by the elastic recoil of the respiratory system at total lung capacity (Bouhuys 1964; Rahn et al. 1946), meaning that respiratory braking is not normally an issue. A possible exception is found in large-bore brass instruments such as the tuba, which appear to make exceptional demands on the respiratory system in terms of the range of respiratory pressures required and the percentage of vital capacity used (figs. 4-12, 4-13).

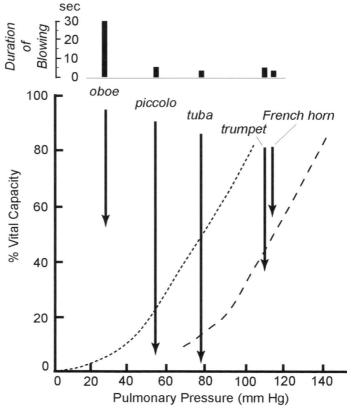

Figure 4-13. Wind instrument breath pressure requirements. This diagram demonstrates the pulmonary pressure generated and the percentage of vital capacity used by wind players when maintaining a note for the longest time possible. The thin dotted line indicates the average pressure generated relative to the percentage of vital capacity and is derived from a study of respiration that used nonwind players as subjects. The dashed line that lies to the right indicates the performance achievable only by the top 5 percent in this study. Oboe players can maintain a single breath for very long durations because their instrument requires only low pressures and small airflow rates. The main limitation to the length of the note is the buildup of carbon dioxide in the lungs. The piccolo and tuba players use up their vital capacity rapidly because the mouth is unstopped in the former case, and the bore of the instrument is very large in the latter. The diagram demonstrates that brass players must develop a level of respiratory performance that is considerably above the average found in the general population. In fact, the pressures needed for playing loudly in the upper registers may approach the limit of what is physiologically possible. Reproduced with permission from Bouhuys (1964). N.B. The pitch and volume of the notes played were not indicated in the original study.

Table 4-1. Mean Intrapharyngeal Pressure for Generating Notes with Different Brass Instruments

	64 Hz *(C2)*	*128 Hz* *(C3)*	*256 Hz* *(C4)*	*512 Hz* *(C5)*	*1024 Hz* *(C6)*
Trumpet	n.a.	n.a.	20	40	120
French horn	35	40	50	110	>150
Trombone	10	15	16	22	70
Tuba	6	8	15	22	n.a.

Pressure units = cm H_2O
n.a. = not applicable, that is, outside the range of the instrument
Reproduced with permission from Stasney, Beaver, and Rodriguez 2003.

The pressure needed to initiate a note increases with frequency for most of these instruments, though in the clarinet it actually decreases in the upper register (Fuks and Sundberg 1999). While increasing the air pressure at the embouchure generally results in a note at a given pitch becoming louder, this tends to follow an asymptotic curve so that it ultimately reaches a limit above which large increases in pressure produce little effect in volume (Fletcher and Tarnopolsky 1999). The highest pressures required among orchestral wind players are found in the upper registers of the trumpet, French horn, and oboe. Professional players can generate pressures considerably in excess of diastolic blood pressure (the peak pressure generated by the heart during a beat). For example, while diastolic pressure in a healthy individual is typically around 19 kilopascals, trumpeters playing loudly at the top of their range can generate intrathoracic pressures of up to 25 kilopascals.

It has been suggested by some brass teachers that the pressure within the airway needed to generate a given pitch is approximately the same regardless of the instrument used. Only one study has investigated this hypothesis directly (Stasney, Beaver, and Rodriguez 2003), and its results are shown in table 4-1. Unfortunately, only one player of each instrument was assessed in each case, but three were section leaders in a major professional orchestra and one, a master's-level student. The results clearly point to considerable differences in the pressures needed to produce the same pitch across the brass family, with the highest pressures being required by the French horn, and successively lower pressures in trumpet, trombone, and tuba. Presumably this relates to the size of the mouthpiece and the depth and tension of the region of the lip that is vibrating, but the precise details await further investigation. It was also found that playing with poor technique increased the pharyngeal pressure required for a given note by about 20 percent. Though it was not made clear what instructions were given to the players to simulate poor technique, direct visualization of the pharynx using a laryngoscope revealed that this involved a retraction of the tongue and an increase in tension in the muscles in and around the larynx. Clearly these important issues merit further study.

Wind instruments also vary considerably in the amount of air expended during playing (Bouhuys 1964). Among the woodwinds, the airflow rates are lowest for the oboe and cor anglais, which allow passages to be sustained for prolonged periods under a single breath (fig. 4-13) even without resorting to special techniques such as circular breathing. The limitation to the duration of the breath in this situation is the buildup of carbon dioxide in the bloodstream, which increases the drive to inhale. Low flow rates are not a feature of all double-reed instruments, as in bassoon players they exceed levels seen in single-reed instruments. The flow rates required by brass instruments when playing at high volume in the upper register are also very high, increasing with the bore of the instrument, and so are greatest in the bass tuba.

Long-Term Effects of High Pressure on Lung Function

The question of whether the high lung pressures needed to play many wind instruments have long-term consequences for lung function has long been a contentious one, and the increasing ease with which it is possible to gather sophisticated information on respirometry has done little to resolve the matter. This may indicate that there are numerous factors related to lifestyle, body morphology, and clinical history that dominate the results and obscure any effect of playing on the data. For example, the increasingly sedentary lifestyles and the rising incidence of asthma in Western society are likely to prove highly significant. A study of one group of young adult brass players (mean age twenty years, with an average of nine years' playing experience) showed a 15 percent greater vital capacity than age-matched controls, mostly due to a large increase in expiratory reserve volume (Tucker, Faulkner, and Horvath 1971). Earlier work by Bouhuys (1964) also suggested an increase in vital capacity in wind players. Recent studies have concentrated on more dynamic parameters of respiration that are now used in the diagnosis of obstructive and restrictive airway disease. Obstructive conditions include asthma, in which the airways of the lungs become constricted, while restrictive diseases lead to a reduction in total lung capacity. In individuals who are not suffering from some overt lung disease, obesity can be a significant cause of restrictive lung function (Spiegel et al. 1988). The lung function in a group of male nonsmoking Turkish naval band members of a similar age and level of experience to those in the study by Tucker et al. was compared with a group of naval nonmusicians (Deniz et al. 2006). This suggested that the bandsmen exhibited a highly significant reduction in many respiratory parameters such as peak expiratory flow rate (PEF) and forced expiratory flow rate (FEF) at various points during the exhalation, and the forced expiratory volume in the first second (FEV1). An observed reduction in forced vital capacity (FVC) appeared to be correlated with the number of years of playing. There was no significant difference between the woodwind and brass players. All of the results were expressed as a percentage of the values expected when corrected for age, sex, and height, helping to eliminate a range of confounding factors. The authors considered the possibility that high-pressure trauma to alveoli and small bronchioles might provide an explanation for the reduction in respiratory parameters. However, in the absence of corroborating evidence from clinical follow-up, they instead suggested that asthma, perhaps aggravated by the inhalation of lung irritants during the deep breathing required for wind playing, might provide a more likely explanation. Though the results of this study are striking, they are in marked contrast to those of a comparison of professional North American wind players, string players, and singers (male and female; average ages forty-one to forty-seven years) that used similar methods (Schorr-Lesnick et al. 1985). This study revealed no difference between the wind players and the other two groups. For most parameters, the percentage values were close to those predicted on the basis of age, height, and gender. One occupational group that shares the necessity to generate high lung pressures with wind players are glassblowers. Though now a relatively uncommon profession, several studies of lung function involving this group have been carried out. In one that managed to track down eighty-five such individuals, forced vital capacity and FEV1 were both significantly higher in the glassblowers compared to controls (Munn, Thomas, and DeMesquita 1990), though some other studies have found no difference. The question of whether a vocational requirement to generate high respiratory pressures has an effect on lung function therefore remains unresolved. Though certain forms of emphysema are associated with high pressure in the lungs and occupations requiring prolonged respiratory effort, there is so far no evidence that this condition is unusually prevalent in the players of high-pressure wind instruments (Gilbert 1998; Harman 1998). The effects of the high pressures generated by wind players on other tissues will be considered in chapter 6.

Role of the Larynx in Playing Woodwind and Brass Instruments

In reed instruments, the contribution of the larynx to the generation of vibrato is much less consistent than in the flute and appears to be more a matter of individual technique than of necessity (King, Ashby, and Nelson 1988). As with brass instruments (Ridgeon 1986), the flow of air is controlled by the size of the gap between the vocal folds (the glottis) together with the degree of arching of the tongue, which alters the area of the opening at the back of the mouth. The partial closure of the glottis during the production of the note can be clearly seen using endoscopy (Weikert and Schlomicher-Thier 1999). When players are encouraged to "relax the larynx," what is actually being encouraged is probably a relaxation of the muscles of the pharynx, which lies above it, as this can also be observed when the area of the glottis is reduced during playing. The vocal folds may also be brought forcibly together to support heavy tonguing and for loud notes. The movements of the vocal folds are greatest in saxophone players. Classical saxophonists generally use the larynx only to regulate airflow (King, Ashby, and Nelson 1988), and neither this nor the diaphragm makes a consistent contribution to the production of vibrato (Weikert and Schlomicher-Thier 1999). However, the vocal folds are used extensively by jazz players to modify the sounds produced. In the "growl" technique, their movements may be forceful and as a result of this style of playing, damage to the surface of the folds can induce hoarseness of the voice.

In some players of brass and woodwind instruments, the larynx may close inappropriately when high pressure is generated in the airway and interfere both with airflow and with articulation (Steenstrup 2004). This can lead to audible noises in the throat as the air is forced through the closed glottis. The tight closure of the vocal folds under these circumstances is called the valsalva maneuver and is seen in weight lifters who, when making a lift, fill their lungs and close off the airway while forcefully contracting the abdominal muscles. This helps to make the trunk rigid to support the weight. Indeed, we may find ourselves doing this when lifting a heavy object. It also frequently occurs in the rather more mundane process of defecation because it is by this means that we raise abdominal pressure to expel feces. This is like squeezing toothpaste from a tube. Unfortunately for some wind players, the valsalva maneuver can become engaged when high pressure is required to support the playing of a note. This is, of course, counterproductive because it reduces the airflow into the instrument, but it may have become a conditioned reflex because the individual has learned to do this in other situations where it is appropriate. In such circumstances, a conscious effort is required to avoid closing the vocal folds during playing until this becomes second nature. Similarly, the rise in airway pressure caused by blocking the airflow with the tongue during articulation may also trigger the valsalva maneuver, which can delay the onset of the attack. The player may not be aware of the true origin of the problem but attribute it to poor control of the tongue.

The level at which the larynx is held is also characteristic for different woodwind instruments. Though the tone quality is mainly a product of embouchure, breath support, and the quality of the reed, resonances in the pharynx and larynx may also contribute and help to give the sound made by different players its individuality (King, Ashby, and Nelson 1988). This is discussed further in chapter 6. The contribution of the larynx to the sound is probably least in flute playing, in which it remains fixed in a neutral position. In single-reed instruments the larynx tends to rise with the pitch of the note, though the degree of movement depends considerably on the individual player. In double-reed instruments the larynx is held low and this may favor the generation of characteristic overtones in these instruments.

Circular Breathing

One of the characteristics of wind playing is the necessity to break the flow of the music into phrases in order to take a breath. While this sometimes is used as a form of punctuation that contributes to musical expression, in many instances it is driven

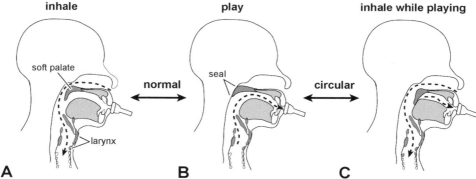

Figure 4-14. Normal and circular breathing in wind instruments. A. During normal inhalation, air is drawn in through both the mouth and nose. The muscles of the soft palate are relaxed to allow free airflow by both routes. B. During playing, the soft palate is raised and held in contact with the back of the throat. This forms a seal, allowing the pressure in the airway to rise sufficiently to generate the sound. C. During inhalation for circular breathing, the soft palate is pulled firmly down against the raised back of the tongue, sealing the mouth chamber. The small volume of air in the mouth is then compressed by the muscles of the cheek to maintain the sound, while air is drawn rapidly into the lungs through the nose.

purely by necessity. One way around this restriction is to use the technique of circular breathing, which allows a continuous flow of air to be maintained from the embouchure. It is regarded as a specialized technique by most classical and jazz musicians, and even those who have developed this skill are likely to use it relatively sparingly. In some instruments, however, most notably the didgeridoo, it is an integral part of standard playing technique. The mechanism of circular breathing is shown in figure 4-14. Prior to starting to play, air is normally taken in through both the nose and mouth. The soft palate is allowed to hang free (fig. 4-14A), neither in contact with the back of the throat nor the tongue, allowing the passage of air into the throat by both routes. When playing, the soft palate is pulled up against the back of the throat, creating a seal that allows the pressure in the airway to rise sufficiently to drive the vibration of the lips or reed (fig. 4-14B). If players suffer loss of seal (see chapter 6), this is due to weakness of the muscles of the soft palate, which hold it in this position. In circular breathing, as the lungs empty during the breath, the cheeks are allowed to puff out like a pair of bellows to form a small air reservoir. During the switch to the following inhalation, the soft palate is pulled downward against the tongue to block off the back of the mouth (fig. 4-14C). While air is taken in through the nose, the cheek muscles (the buccinators) contract to compress the air in the mouth, raising the pressure sufficiently to maintain the sound. As the mouth reservoir is small, the intake of breath must be rapid. This feat of coordination takes considerable practice. One of the most difficult aspects is maintaining a consistent pressure when switching between the lung and the mouth phases of the breath so that the transition is not marked by a dip in sound intensity or pitch. Circular breathing is best suited for instruments that require high pressures and low airflow rates, such as the double-reed instruments, the French horn, and the trumpet. The next easiest are the other brass instruments and the single-reed woodwinds, though it becomes progressively more difficult as the bore becomes larger. The greatest difficulty is found in the flute, in which the mouth is unstopped, but even with this instrument circular breathing is possible.

Wind Playing and Asthma

There is considerable anecdotal evidence for the beneficial effects of playing wind instruments on childhood asthma, both in the scientific literature (Marks 1974; Gilbert 1998; Lucia 1994) and in the personal accounts of individual musicians, some of whom have subsequently become prominent professional players. Though it does not cure the condition, playing appears to reduce the symptoms and improve its management. Asthma episodes can be triggered by stress and exertion, so it may seem paradoxical that wind playing can have a positive effect; however, though playing requires breath control, it does not increase the heart rate to the levels typical of even moderate exercise (Tucker, Faulkner, and Horvath 1971). A common breathing exercise recommended for asthma sufferers is a forced expiration through pursed lips that in many ways resembles the action required to play a wind instrument. While individuals with asthma may have difficulty in finding the motivation to carry out such exercises conscientiously, they are a natural consequence of wind playing, and there is a strong inducement to improve breath control and the duration of expiration for musical ends. Children who are initially unable to hold a sustained note for more than a few seconds may be able to extend this to forty seconds or more over a period of months. Of course, in the event of a severe asthma attack it is important to wait until it is completely over before playing again, but audibly wheezing players who are not otherwise in distress may continue (Marks 1974). Though there is no psychological element in the origin of asthma as a disease, stress and panic may contribute to the onset and progress of an attack. For young wind players, increased confidence in being able to control their respiration and manage their symptoms may be a significant factor in their improvement (Lucia 1994). There is also circumstantial evidence that, over a period of years, increased ventilation of the lungs contributes to the correction of barrel- or pigeon-chest deformities in young asthmatic wind players who are still at an age where the skeleton of the chest is capable of remodeling.

REFERENCES

Bonard, J. M. 2001. The physicist's guide to the orchestra. *Eur J Phys* 22:89–101.

Bouhuys, A. 1964. Lung volumes and breathing patterns in wind-instrument players. *J Appl Physiol* 19:967–75.

Campbell, E. J. M. 1970. Accessory muscles. In *The respiratory muscles: Mechanics and neural control*, ed. E. J. M. Campbell, E. Agostoni, and J. Newsom Davis. London: Lloyd-Luke.

Cossette, I., P. Sliwinski, and P. T. Macklem. 2000. Respiratory parameters during professional flute playing. *Respir Physiol* 121 (1):33–44.

Deniz, O., S. Savci, E. Tozkoparan, D. I. Ince, M. Ucar, and F. Ciftci. 2006. Reduced pulmonary function in wind instrument players. *Arch Med Res* 37 (4):506–10.

Fletcher, N. H. 1975. Acoustical correlates of flute performance technique. *J Acoust Soc Am* 57 (1):233–37.

Fletcher, N. H., and A. Tarnopolsky. 1999. Blowing pressure, power, and spectrum in trumpet playing. *J Acoust Soc Am* 105 (2 Pt 1):874–81.

Fuks, L., and J. Sundberg. 1999. Blowing pressures in bassoon, clarinet, oboe and saxophone. *Acustica* 85:267–77.

Gilbert, T. B. 1998. Breathing difficulties in wind instrument players. *Md Med J* 47 (1):23–27.

Griffin, B., P. Woo, R. Colton, J. Casper, and D. Brewer. 1995. Physiological characteristics of the supported singing voice. A preliminary study. *J Voice* 9 (1):45–56.

Harman, S. E. 1998. The evolution of performing arts medicine. In *Performing arts medicine*, ed. R. T. Sataloff, A. G. Brandfonbrener, and R. J. Lederman. San Diego: Singular Publishing Group.

Hoit, J. D., and T. J. Hixon. 1986. Body type and speech breathing. *J Speech Hear Res* 29 (3):313–24.

King, A. I., J. Ashby, and C. Nelson. 1988. Laryngeal function in wind instrumentalists: The woodwinds. *J Voice* 1:365–67.

Konno, K., and J. Mead. 1967. Measurement of the separate volume changes of rib cage and abdomen during breathing. *J Appl Physiol* 22 (3):407–22.

Lagefoded, P. 1967. *Three areas of experimental phonetics*. London: Oxford University Press.

Leanderson, R., J. Sundberg, and C. von Euler. 1987. Role of diaphragmatic activity during singing: A study of transdiaphragmatic pressures. *J Appl Physiol* 62 (1):259–70.

Lucia, R. 1994. Effects of playing a musical wind instrument in asthmatic teenagers. *J Asthma* 31 (5):375–85.

Marks, M. B. 1974. The 1974 Bela Schick Memorial Lecture. Musical wind instruments in rehabilitation of asthmatic children. *Ann Allergy* 33 (6):313–19.

Miller, R. 1997. *National schools of singing: English, French, German, and Italian techniques of singing revisited.* Lanham, Md.: Scarecrow Press.

Munn, N. J., S. W. Thomas, and S. DeMesquita. 1990. Pulmonary function in commercial glass blowers. *Chest* 98 (4):871–74.

Orozco-Levi, M., J. Gea, J. Monells, X. Aran, M. C. Aguar, and J. M. Broquetas. 1995. Activity of latissimus dorsi muscle during inspiratory threshold loads. *Eur Respir J* 8 (3):441–45.

Pawlowski Z., and M. Zoltowski. 1987. A physiological evaluation of the efficiency of playing the wind instruments—an aerodynamic study. *Arch Acoustics (Poland)* 12:291–299.

Pettersen, V., K. Bjorkoy, H. Torp, and R. H. Westgaard. 2005. Neck and shoulder muscle activity and thorax movement in singing and speaking tasks with variation in vocal loudness and pitch. *J Voice* 19 (4):623–34.

Pettersen, V., and R. H. Westgaard. 2002. Muscle activity in the classical singer's shoulder and neck region. *Logoped Phoniatr Vocol* 27 (4):169–78.

———. 2004. The association between upper trapezius activity and thorax movement in classical singing. *J Voice* 18 (4):500–12.

———. 2005. The activity patterns of neck muscles in professional classical singing. *J Voice* 19 (2):238–51.

Rahn, H., A. B. Otis, L. E. Chadwick, and W. O. Fenn. 1946. The pressure volume diagram of the thorax and lung. *Am J Physiol* 146 (6):161–78.

Ridgeon, J. 1986. *The physiology of brass playing.* Manton, UK: Brass Wind Educational Supplies.

Roos, J. 1936. The physiology of playing the flute. *Arch Néerl Phon Expér* 12:1–26.

Sand, S., and J. Sundberg. 2005. Reliability of the term "support" in singing. *Logoped Phoniatr Vocol* 30 (2):51–54.

Schorr-Lesnick, B., A. S. Teirstein, L. K. Brown, and A. Miller. 1985. Pulmonary function in singers and wind-instrument players. *Chest* 88 (2):201–5.

Spiegel, J. R., R. T. Sataloff, J. R. Cohn, and M. Hawkshaw. 1988. Respiratory function in singers: Medical assessment, diagnoses, and treatments. *J Voice* 2 (1):40–50.

Stasney, C. R., M. E. Beaver, and M. Rodriguez. 2003. Hypopharyngeal pressure in brass musicians. *Med Prob Perform Artists* 14:153–55.

Steenstrup, K. 2004. *Teaching brass.* Aarhus, Denmark: Royal Academy of Music.

Sundberg, J. 1999. The perception of singing. In *The psychology of music*, ed. D. Deutsch. San Diego: Academic Press.

Thomasson, M., and J. Sundberg. 2001a. Consistency of inhalatory breathing patterns in professional operatic singers. *J Voice* 15 (3):373–83.

———. 2001b. Lung volume levels in professional classical singing. *Logoped Phoniatr Vocol* 22:61–70.

Thorpe, C. W., S. J. Cala, J. Chapman, and P. J. Davis. 2001. Patterns of breath support in projection of the singing voice. *J Voice* 15 (1):86–104.

Titze, I. R. 2000. *Principles of voice production.* 2nd printing. Iowa City, Iowa: National Center for Voice and Speech.

Tucker, A., M. E. Faulkner, and S. M. Horvath. 1971. Electrocardiography and lung function in brass instrument players. *Arch Environ Health* 23 (5):327–34.

Vilensky, J. A., M. Baltes, L. Weikel, J. D. Fortin, and L. J. Fourie. 2001. Serratus posterior muscles: Anatomy, clinical relevance, and function. *Clin Anat* 14 (4):237–41.

Waersted, M., R. A. Bjorklund, and R. H. Westgaard. 1994. The effect of motivation on shoulder-muscle tension in attention-demanding tasks. *Ergonomics* 37 (2):363–76.

Watson, P. J., and T. J. Hixon. 1985. Respiratory kinematics in classical (opera) singers. *J Speech Hear Res* 28 (1):104–22.

Weikert, M., and J. Schlomicher-Thier. 1999. Laryngeal movements in saxophone playing: Video-endoscopic investigations with saxophone players. A pilot study. *J Voice* 13 (2):265–73.

Widmer, S., A. Conway, S. Cohen, and P. Davies. 1997. Hyperventilation: A correlate and predictor of debilitating performance anxiety in musicians. *Med Prob Perform Artists* 12:97–106.

Wilder, C. N. 1983. Chest wall preparation for phonation in female speakers. In *Vocal fold physiology: Contemporary research and clinical issues*, ed. D. M. Bless and J. H. Abbs. San Diego: College Hill Press.

Winckel, F. 1952. Electroakustiche Untersuchungen an der Menschlichen Stimmen [Electro-acoustic Investigations of the Human Voice]. *Folia Phoniatr (Basel)* 4:93–113.

Chapter Five

The Voice

Management and Problems

The object of this chapter is to describe the origin of the voice. It will concentrate on how the larynx produces sound and how this is modified by the resonant qualities of the throat (the pharynx) and the mouth (oral cavity) during singing.

THE RELATIONSHIP BETWEEN
THE LARYNX, THROAT, AND MOUTH

The trachea and the esophagus pass down the neck together. The trachea is the route by which air passes into the lungs; in order to keep the airway open, its walls are reinforced by horseshoe-shaped rings of cartilage. The esophagus lies immediately behind the trachea. Waves of contraction run down its muscular walls to propel food into the stomach. It is unsupported by cartilage, so when it is empty it is pressed flat between the trachea, which lies in front, and the vertebral column and the muscles attached to it (see chapter 2), which lie behind. The trachea and esophagus both open into the back of the throat (also known as the pharynx), which is the common conduit for both air and food (fig. 5-1). It is vital that food and drink not enter the trachea during breathing, and the larynx evolved primarily as a valve to prevent this from happening. It sits at the top of the trachea and in humans, its upper opening has a flap called the epiglottis, which is pushed downward by the tongue during swallowing to block off the top of the airway (animation 5-1).

The pharynx, like the esophagus, has muscular walls, but these do not collapse because they are continuous with the cavities of the mouth and nose, which are supported by the bones of the skull. The wall of the pharynx has two muscular layers, an inner one whose fibers run longitudinally (vertically) along its length and an outer one whose fibers run circumferentially. Some of the longitudinal muscle fibers are attached to the palate (the roof of the mouth) and others to the base of the skull or to the opening of the eustachian tube, which runs from the back of the throat to the cavity of the middle ear (see chapter 9). When the longitudinal muscle layer contracts, the pharynx becomes shorter and wider. It is also drawn upward during swallowing

139

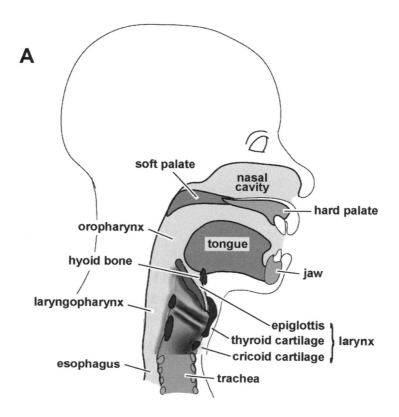

A

soft palate

nasal cavity

hard palate

oropharynx

tongue

hyoid bone

jaw

laryngopharynx

epiglottis
thyroid cartilage } larynx
cricoid cartilage

esophagus

trachea

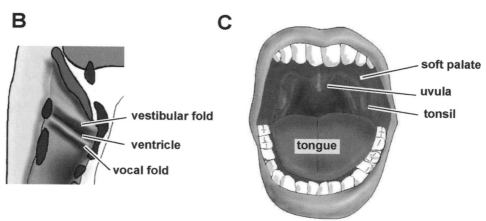

B

vestibular fold

ventricle

vocal fold

C

soft palate

uvula

tonsil

tongue

Figure 5-1. The larynx and pharynx. A. A view of the head and neck showing the different regions of the pharynx and their relationship to the airway. The skeleton of the larynx is composed of the cricoid and thyroid cartilages. The top of the airway is blocked by the epiglottis when it is pushed backward by the tongue during swallowing. B. Enlarged view of the inner surface of the larynx showing the vocal fold (vocal cord) and the vestibular fold with the slitlike cavity of the ventricle lying between them. C. A view into the mouth showing the tonsils. The hard palate forms the bony roof of the mouth. This continues as a muscular shelf known as the soft palate from which hangs a central flap called the uvula.

by a muscle that runs from the base of the skull to the outside wall of the pharynx (stylopharyngeus—fig. 5-2). The outer muscular coat of the pharynx is made up of three sheets of muscle that sit one above the other. When they contract, these muscles make the pharynx narrower and longer and hence are called the superior, middle, and inferior constrictor muscles. The upper constrictor is attached at the front to the muscular wall of the cheek, the middle constrictor to a bone at the root of the tongue called the hyoid (see below), and the inferior constrictor to the cartilages of the larynx (fig. 5-2).

The upper part of the pharynx can be divided into the oropharynx (mouth pharynx), which encompasses the region below the soft palate that opens into the mouth, and the nasopharynx (nose pharynx), which lies above the soft palate and opens into the back of the nose. If you look into your mouth using a mirror, you can recognize the soft palate because of the small, fleshy flap (the uvula) that hangs down from the middle of it (fig. 5-1). Farther forward in the mouth, the soft palate gives way to a horizontal shelf of bone called the hard palate. The oropharynx is a passageway for food and drink as well as for air, while the nasopharynx carries only air and is also the route by which sound emerges in humming or during the production of certain consonants (e.g., *m* and *n*). The soft palate is formed from two pairs of muscles. One pair runs horizontally to meet in the middle, where the muscles are joined together. When these muscles contract the soft palate becomes taut. They are therefore named the tensor palati. The second pair of muscles (the levator palati) raise the soft palate to bring it into contact with the back of the pharynx, sealing off the nasal cavity (animation 5-1, fig. 5-12). If you use the mirror once more to look into your mouth while consciously closing the back of the throat to block off the nose (as you might have done as a child when being given a dose of foul-tasting medicine!), you will see the soft palate, together with the uvula, rise sharply upward to achieve this. The soft palate is held in this position during the playing of wind instruments as these require high oral air pressures to drive the vibration of the reed or lips. Any loss of efficiency of this seal allows air to escape into the nose and has a dramatic effect on the ability to play. It is also possible to close off the back of the mouth from the pharynx by drawing the back of the tongue up against the soft palate. This leaves the airway between the nose and the trachea open. Closing off the mouth in this way to form a small air reservoir is used in circular breathing, a technique used by some woodwind players to extend the duration of the breath (see chapter 4). The passage to the nose and mouth can be closed simultaneously by raising the soft palate and pushing back the tongue. This is the initial phase of the act of swallowing, which serves to drive the food into the lower part of the pharynx, where it is then carried to the stomach by way of the esophagus (animation 5-1).

The pharynx and larynx are lined by a thin sheet of tissue known as an epithelium, which is composed mainly of tall columnar cells. This is kept moist by watery secretions of the mouth (from the salivary glands) and the nose. The epithelium also contains specialized cells (known as goblet cells) that secrete mucus. For this reason it is sometimes called the mucosal epithelium or more simply, the mucosa. In histological terms, it is described as a pseudostratified columnar epithelium with goblet cells. The mucous film has the very important role of trapping dust particles in the airway to prevent them from accumulating in the lungs. The film is moved around by the beating of minute

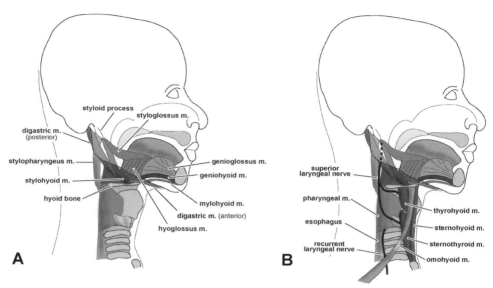

Figure 5-2.   Muscles supporting the larynx and pharynx and hyoid bone. These are active during singing, regulating the level at which the larynx lies, its position relative to the hyoid bone, and the shape of the pharynx. A. This diagram shows the central importance of the hyoid bone, which lies at the root of the tongue. Many of the major muscles of the tongue (glossal muscles) and the floor of the mouth are attached to it. It is suspended from the jaw and from a bony spine on the base of the skull (the styloid process) that is also the origin of a muscle that raises the pharynx (stylopharyngeus). The hyoid bone is attached to the larynx by the tissues of the pharynx and by the thyrohyoid muscles and ligament. B. Muscles controlling the height of the larynx. These are the thyrohyoid above and the sternothyroid below. A longer muscle, the sternohyoid, runs directly from the sternum to the hyoid bone, while the omohyoid passes like a guy rope from the hyoid bone to the top of the shoulder blade. The actions of some of these muscles are shown in animation 5-1. Two nerves innervate the larynx. The superior laryngeal nerve supplies the cricothyroid muscle and carries sensation from the lining of the larynx above the vocal folds, while the recurrent laryngeal nerve supplies all the other muscles and sensation below the vocal folds.

hairlike structures called cilia, which are found on the upper surface of the epithelial cells. From the nose the mucus is propelled downward, while from the trachea and the lungs it is propelled upward. Both streams ultimately reach the esophagus, where the material is swallowed.

CONTROLLING THE HEIGHT OF THE LARYNX

If you were to look beneath the skin that covers the underside of the chin, you would discover that the floor of the mouth is composed of a horizontal sheet of muscle (the mylohyoid muscle) that runs from one side of the jaw to the other. Seen from the inside, most of the floor of the mouth is taken up by the tongue, which plays an important role in the articulation of words and in controlling the onset of the attack in wind instruments. Several sets of muscles contribute to form the tongue. These are usually divided into two groups, the intrinsic and the extrinsic muscles. The intrinsic muscles are those that connect one part of the tongue to another, giving us great control over its shape and the movement of the tip. The extrinsic muscles (fig. 5-2) suspend the tongue between the palate (palatoglossus), the lower jaw (genioglossus), the base of the skull (styloglossus), and the hyoid bone (hyoglossus). It is clear that the common element of each of these names (glossus) refers to the tongue. These muscles allow the tongue to be protruded or drawn back, raised or depressed. The organization of tongue muscles may appear quite complicated at first, but one important point to note is the central role of the small bone called the hyoid, which lies at the root of the tongue and is shaped like a horseshoe with the opening facing backward (fig. 5-2A). It makes no contact with the rest of the skeleton but is linked to many of the structures central to the control of the singing voice. As well as anchoring many of the muscles of the tongue, it is attached to the larynx through the relationship of the tongue to the muscular walls of the pharynx. The hyoid is also directly linked to the larynx by a membrane that forms the wall of the airway at this point (the thyrohyoid membrane) and by a pair of flat, straplike muscles, the thyrohyoid muscles (fig. 5-2B). A second pair of straplike muscles attach the hyoid bone to the breastbone, or sternum (the sternohyoid muscles), while a third pair (omohyoid) runs backward like a guy rope to the shoulder blade. A final pair runs from the larynx to the sternum (the sternothyroid muscles). These strap muscles control the absolute height of the larynx and its position relative to the hyoid bone, and this has an effect on the sound produced during singing (see below). These muscles are also involved in the raising and lowering of the larynx during swallowing. It is this action that enables the backward-moving tongue to make contact with the epiglottis and close off the airway (see animation 5-1). The movements of swallowing must be closely coordinated with the breathing cycle. Just before swallowing, a small breath is taken to draw air into the lungs. This helps to ensure there is a positive pressure in the airway when the larynx is closed by the epiglottis so that any food or fluid that does manage to get into the airway can be blown out. The position of the larynx may also be influenced by activity in the inferior constrictor muscle of the pharynx and by the stylopharyngeus. It is therefore very mobile, something that is amply borne out by studies of how its position changes when singing in different parts of the range (Hurme and Sonninen 1995).

THE VOCAL TRACT

The sounds that we make in speech and singing are not produced by the actions of the larynx alone but involve the entire vocal tract (fig. 5-3). In functional terms this consists of the following:

- **The generator**, which comprises the lungs and the muscles that drive air out of them and control the rate of airflow through the larynx.
- **The vibrator**, which is the larynx itself. The vibrating elements of the larynx are the vocal cords (more correctly called the vocal folds—the term we will use from now on). The pitch of the sound is determined by the degree of tension in the vocal folds,

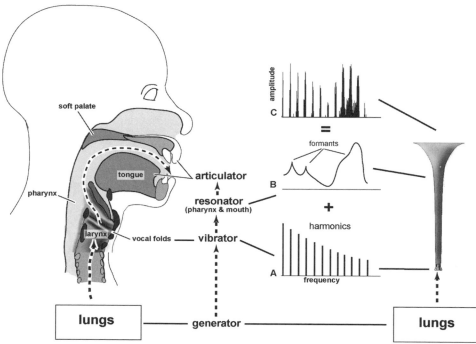

Figure 5-3. The elements of the vocal tract are here compared to a trumpet. The lungs constitute the generator (the source of the airstream), and the vocal folds represent the vibrator or voice source (performing the same task as the lips of a trumpet player). This sets up a complex set of vibrations (A) that are amplified by the resonator. For the voice this resonator is the pharynx and mouth, the equivalent of the tube and bell of the trumpet. This has a set of resonant frequencies called formants (B). In the trumpet these can be altered by changing the length of the tube through the use of the valves, while for the voice, a limited degree of adjustment can be made to both the width and length of the pharynx. The articulator of the voice is formed by the lips, tongue, palate, and cheeks. There is no equivalent for the trumpet; however, placing the hand or a mute across or into the bell and moving it in and out can be used to produce a voicelike modulation of the sound. The sound that emerges is a product of the voice source spectrum modified by the vocal tract resonances. This is shown in C, which comes from a recording of a voice.

which is in turn controlled by the muscles inside the larynx; the greater the tension, the higher the pitch of the voice. The sound made is little more than a buzzing, similar to that produced by a vibrating reed or the mouthpiece of a brass instrument. This is called the voice source. The pattern of vibration is complex and made up of a characteristic pattern of harmonics overlying the fundamental frequency of the vibration. This makes a significant contribution to the timbre and hence the individuality of the voice between singers and in different vocal registers of the same singer.

• **The resonator**, which gives the sound its richness. This is formed by the pharynx and the cavity of the mouth. In terms of the effect it has on the sound, it is equivalent to the tube and bell of a wind instrument.

• **The articulator**, which shapes the sound to produce the vowels and consonants that are combined to form words. The articulator is composed of the soft palate, tongue, cheeks, teeth, and the opening of the mouth. If you think of the way in which the sound of a trumpet can be manipulated by bringing the hand or a mute down over the bell and then up again, it will be clear how even very simple manipulations of the articulator can influence the quality of the sound. The articulator of the human voice is much more complex than this and can be minutely adjusted by the muscles of the palate, tongue, and face to produce the articulations that are characteristic of different languages and of different individuals.

The properties of the generator are dealt with in chapter 4. In this chapter we will examine in turn the nature of the vibrator, the resonator, and the articulator. Though these will be considered primarily from the viewpoint of speech and singing, the elements of the vocal tract also play an important role in the playing of wind instruments. This is discussed in chapter 6.

The Vibrator (Larynx)

The soft tissues of the larynx (which include the vocal folds) are supported by a skeleton formed not of bone, but of cartilage (figs. 5-4, 5-5). The main body of the larynx is formed from two pieces of cartilage. One of these, the cricoid cartilage, is shaped like a signet ring with the larger surface facing backward. Above the cricoid lies the thyroid cartilage, a folded shieldlike structure that is open at the back (fig. 5-5F). The thyroid cartilage looks a little like the prow of a boat except that along the midline fold, the upper surface descends sharply into what is called the thyroid notch (fig. 5-4A). The thyroid cartilage has a hingelike connection with the cricoid that allows it to rotate downward like the visor of a helmet. The thyroid cartilage is more prominent in men, in whom it is also known as the Adam's apple. As already mentioned, when we swallow, access to the trachea must be blocked to prevent food or saliva from entering it. While the epiglottis is mainly responsible for this in mammals, it is a late adaptation of the larynx, and the constriction in the airway created by the vocal folds was the original structure for this purpose. The use of the folds as a means of producing sound for communication evolved only later.

It is possible to look down into the larynx from above using an instrument called a laryngoscope. When we do this we see the narrow opening through which the air flows, bounded on each side by the vocal folds (video 5-1, fig. 5-13A). This opening is known as the rima glottis. Among musicians this is often abbreviated to "glottis" in descriptions of the mechanisms underlying singing and wind playing, though strictly speaking the term applies to the vocal apparatus of the larynx as a whole. The glottis controls the flow of air that is used either to drive the voice or the vibrations of the reed or mouthpiece of an instrument. Immediately above the vocal folds is a horizontal slitlike space called the ventricle of the larynx (fig. 5-4B), above which are two smoothly rounded ridges, the vestibular folds. These are sometimes called the false vocal cords but they make little contribution to the voice except in some extreme forms of vocalization.

Much of the inner lining of the larynx is composed of a sheet of mucosal epithelium similar to that of the pharynx and nose, though its secretions are augmented by pockets

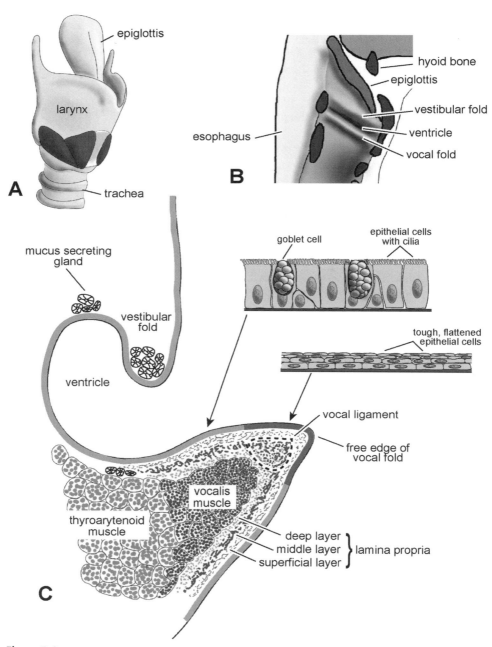

Figure 5-4

Figure 5-4. A. A view of the intact larynx seen from the front. **B.** The inside of the larynx. **C.** A section through the side wall of the larynx at right angles to B, showing the internal structure of a vocal fold. The epithelium that covers the inside of the throat and airway contains tall cells with cilia that move fluid over the surface and goblet cells that produce mucus. Secretions are also produced by glands that lie beneath the epithelium. At the edge of the vocal folds this epithelium is modified to form a layer of tough, flattened cells that are capable of withstanding the impact when the two folds strike each other during vocalization. The epithelium is separated from the muscular core of the fold by a support tissue called the lamina propria, which has three layers. The outer layer is elastic and mobile and together with the epithelium forms what is called the cover of the fold. The inner two layers are composed of fibers that run along the length of the fold, forming the vocal ligament at the fold's free edge. The core of the vocal fold is the thyro-arytenoid muscle. The muscle fibers nearest the edge are sometimes described separately as the vocalis muscle, however, some authors use the terms vocalis muscle and thyroarytenoid muscle interchangeably.

of glandular tissue within the larynx. In places where the surfaces of the two vocal folds come into forceful contact with each other during phonation, the tall columnar cells of the epithelium are replaced by several layers of tough, flattened cells that are more resistant to abrasion. Histologically this is described as a stratified squamous epithelium. Even with this added protection, the forces involved in vocalization may cause physical damage to the surface of the folds, particularly in singers whose technique is imperfect. Just prior to the beginning of phonation, the folds are brought firmly together. How strongly this is done determines the degree of attack at the beginning of the note. One situation in which the vocal folds may be damaged is when the attack is habitually more forceful than is necessary. In addition, the more rapid closure of the vocal folds that is typical of very loud singing also increases the force of impact and risk of damage. The epithelium of the larynx sits on a sheet of supporting tissue called the lamina propria. The properties of the lamina propria of the vocal folds are important for the production of sound. It is usually described as having three layers (fig. 5-4C). The superficial layer is composed of a loosely organized feltwork of randomly oriented stretchy fibers made of a protein called elastin. The intermediate layer is composed primarily of the same type of fibers but is oriented so that they run parallel to the edge of the vocal fold. The deep layer mainly contains similarly oriented collagen fibers that are thicker and much more resistant to stretching, and beneath this lies the muscle that forms the core of the fold. The deep and intermediate layers constitute what is known as the vocal ligament, which is one to two millimeters thick but becomes broader at its ends where it is under greatest mechanical stress during phonation (Titze 2000). The mucosa and the superficial layer of the lamina propria (together known as the cover) have some independence of movement from the underlying tissue; when the two vocal folds strike one another, a ripple runs across these two layers, starting from the free edge of each fold (video 5-1, see below). Unfortunately, there is some ambiguity in how the layers that make up the folds are named, making it difficult to compare accounts of the mechanics of vocal fold vibration in different vocal registers. To help you navigate these treacherous waters, three commonly used schemes are summarized in table 5-1.

We will now consider the structural elements of the larynx and their movements in the context of singing (figure 5-5). The narrow edges of the vocal folds are sup-

Table 5-1. Naming Schemes for Components of the Vocal Folds

Three-Layer Scheme		Five-Layer Scheme		Two-Layer Scheme
mucosa	{	epithelium *superficial layer*	}	cover
vocal ligament	{	*middle layer* *deep layer*	}	body
muscle	{	muscle	}	

Note: Words in italics are components of the lamina propria.
Reproduced with permission from Titze 1994.

ported by the vocal ligaments, which are elastic and lie at the upper opening of a flattened cone-shaped membrane (the conus elasticus) that forms a wall to seal the spaces between the cricoid and thyroid cartilages. The vocal ligaments run from the thyroid cartilage at the front to the small but very important arytenoid cartilages at the back. About a fifth to a quarter of the edge of the vocal folds is composed of a rigid spur (the vocal process) that projects forward from the arytenoid cartilage, so only the region that lies in front of this is supported by the vocal ligament and is able to vibrate during phonation. The space between the vocal folds (the glottis) is opened and closed by muscles acting on the arytenoid cartilages,which therefore provide one of the keys to understanding how the larynx works. Viewed from above, the arytenoid cartilages appear L-shaped, with the two Ls lying back to back (fig. 5-5F, video 5-1). The forward running leg of the L (the vocal process) is attached to the vocal ligaments while the other short leg (called the muscular process) sticks out to the side and is attached to several of the laryngeal muscles. At the junction of the two legs of the L is a vertical projection attached to muscles that prevents the two arytenoid cartilages from being drawn too far apart. The arytenoid cartilages sit on the top of the cricoid cartilage; for the sake of simplicity we will consider that they rotate mainly around a vertical axis. The larynx contains many muscles (fig. 5-5E), but only one pair opens (abducts) the vocal folds. These are called the posterior cricoarytenoid muscles, and the name tells you that the muscles are attached at one end to the back (posterior) of the cricoid cartilage and at the other end to one of the arytenoid cartilages. By pulling on the back of the muscular process of the arytenoid cartilages, these muscles make them rotate in a direction that opens the gap between the vocal folds (see animation 5-2). They are active when we inhale, and if both are paralyzed (a life-threatening situation), air cannot reach the lungs. Two muscles attached to the anterior (front) edge of the muscular processes of the arytenoid cartilages have the opposite action, causing the vocal folds to come together (adduct) to close the glottis. These are the lateral cricoarytenoid muscles (fig. 5-5A, animation 5-2). In this they are aided by the transverse or interarytenoid muscle, which links the two arytenoid cartilages and pulls them together (animation 5-3). Most of the mass of each vocal fold is composed of a muscle running parallel to and in contact with the vocal ligament (fig. 5-5C). This is the thyroarytenoid muscle. As its name suggests, it is attached at one end to the thyroid cartilage, close to the midline, and at the other end, mainly to the muscular processes of the arytenoid cartilages. One part of it forms a thin horizontal shelf in the

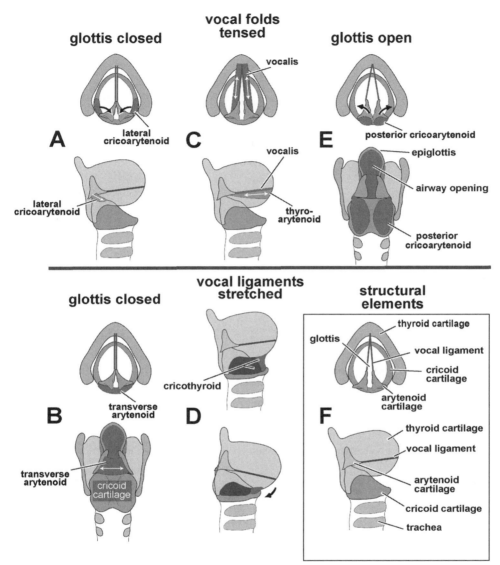

glottis closed

A

lateral
cricoarytenoid

lateral
cricoarytenoid

**vocal folds
tensed**

vocalis

C

vocalis

thyro-
arytenoid

glottis open

E

posterior cricoarytenoid

epiglottis

airway opening

posterior
cricoarytenoid

glottis closed

B

transverse
arytenoid

transverse
arytenoid

cricoid
cartilage

**vocal ligaments
stretched**

cricothyroid

D

**structural
elements**

glottis

thyroid cartilage

vocal ligament

cricoid
cartilage

arytenoid
cartilage

F

thyroid cartilage

vocal ligament

arytenoid
cartilage

cricoid cartilage

trachea

Figure 5-5. A summary of the structure of the larynx and its movements. Each element of the figure shows two views of the larynx, one from above and one either from the side or from behind. The cartilaginous skeleton of the larynx is labeled in F. It is composed of the thyroid cartilage, which looks like the prow of a boat, and the cricoid cartilage, shaped like a signet ring. The two arytenoid cartilages move the vocal ligaments, which form the free edges of the vocal folds, to open and close the glottis. The edges of the vocal folds are formed from both the arytenoid cartilage and the vocal ligament, but only the part supported by the ligament vibrates during phonation. A and B show the actions of two muscles (the lateral cricoarytenoid and transverse arytenoid [interarytenoid] muscles) that bring the vocal ligaments together (adduction). C and D show muscles that tense (thyroarytenoid/vocalis) or stretch (cricothyroid) the vocal folds and E shows the muscles (posterior cricoarytenoids) that open (abduct) the vocal folds. The actions of some of these muscles are shown in animations 5-2, 5-3, and 5-4.

core of the fold, running along side of the vocal ligament; this part is often described as a separate muscle, the vocalis (fig. 5-4C). Unfortunately, there is a tendency for authors to use the terms *thyroarytenoid* and *vocalis* interchangeably, so it is sometimes difficult to know precisely what is being referred to.

Unlike the rest of the thyroarytenoid muscle, the vocalis component is attached to the vocal process of the arytenoid cartilage. There has been some dispute over whether the vocalis can truly be regarded as being functionally distinct from the thyroarytenoid, but studies of distribution of fast and slow contracting muscle fibers appear to support the idea (Sanders, Rai, et al. 1998). The vocalis muscle has been shown to contain a very unusual type of slow-acting muscle fiber that is not seen in other laryngeal muscles (Han et al. 1999). This type of fiber is said to be tonic, which means that it has adapted to remaining in the contracted state for prolonged periods. It has further been suggested that the vocalis component itself has two functionally distinct parts or compartments. The lower compartment is said to be composed of a single large muscle bundle, while the upper part is made up of many small, loosely packed muscle bundles. Standard descriptions of the action of the thyroarytenoid muscle state that it pulls the thyroid cartilage toward the cricoid, slackening the vocal ligament and the cover, while the vocalis is said to slacken the posterior part of the fold and tighten the anterior part. Under these circumstances, the vibration would be confined to the section of the fold overlying the contracted region of the vocalis. This is analogous to shortening the vibrating segment of a string, and therefore increases the frequency of the sound generated. Some mechanism of this kind is needed to explain why the pitch of the voice continues to rise even when the vocal folds can be stretched no farther. This stretching is brought about by the cricothyroid muscle, which opposes the actions of the thyroarytenoid muscle. The cricothyroid muscle runs between the cricoid and thyroid ligaments at the side of the larynx. This rotates the thyroid cartilage toward the cricoid cartilage, stretching the vocal folds (fig. 5-5D, animation 5-4). There is also some disagreement as to whether this is achieved by an upward movement of the cricoid arch or a downward movement of the thyroid cartilage. Though some authors emphasize the movement of the cricoid, this is to some degree restricted by its attachment to the first ring of tracheal cartilage. Furthermore, during phonation, the lamina of the cricoid cartilage (the large, flat, backward-facing surface of the "signet ring") is said to be pressed firmly against the vertebral column, limiting its ability to rotate upward (Gray and Williams 1989). On the other hand, though the laryngeal cartilage should be more free to move, it is attached to the strap muscles at the front, and depending on their state of contraction, these may aid or inhibit its forward and downward movement. It therefore seems most likely that some degree of movement of both the thyroid and cricoid cartilages may occur through the action of the cricothyroid muscle, but that which moves most may depend on the state of other muscles.

The length of the vibrating part of the vocal folds (i.e., the part occupied by the vocal ligaments) is difficult to measure in a living person without using X-rays or other specialized equipment; however, it has recently been discovered that this has a relatively fixed relationship to the distance between the lower border of the cricoid cartilage and the thyroid notch (Williams and Eccles 1990). This external feature of the larynx can easily be measured with simple instruments and can predict the fundamental frequency of the voice. If we call this measure M, the frequency is predicted by the following equations:

Fundamental frequency (hertz) = 190 or (M $\times$ 1.7) for men
Fundamental frequency (hertz) = 260 or (M $\times$ 1.4) for women

The typical average fundamental frequency as revealed by a reading task is about 112 hertz (Hz) for males and 206 Hz for females. Though there is a significant overlap in laryngeal size between males and females, studies involving large numbers of subjects have revealed little or no overlap in fundamental frequencies between the sexes. Consequently, other factors must contribute to the differences in fundamental frequency between the sexes. The most likely explanation is that in the male, the vocal folds have a greater mass per unit length (Williams and Eccles 1990).

The muscles of the larynx are supplied by two pairs of nerves (one pair on each side). The cricothyroid muscle is controlled by the superior laryngeal nerve, which runs down the side of the larynx, while all the other muscles are controlled by the recurrent laryngeal nerve, which enters the larynx from below (fig. 5-2B). Unlike most of the other muscles in the body, we do not have any conscious sensation of the activity of the laryngeal muscles, so we are not aware when they are contracting. Any sensation of tightness that is felt in the throat probably comes from the pharynx. The lining of the larynx is very sensitive to touch, however; something brought to our attention only too clearly when a fragment of food "goes down the wrong way." The region of the mucosa above the vocal folds is supplied by the superior laryngeal nerve and the region below by the recurrent laryngeal nerve. The nerves supplying the larynx are potentially vulnerable during surgery to the front of the neck (e.g., involving the thyroid gland). Damage to one of the recurrent laryngeal nerves can result in paralysis of almost all of the muscles on that side of the larynx. The inability to move the vocal folds results in a husky voice due to paralysis of the posterior cricoarytenoid muscle, which cannot therefore open the fold on the affected side. The nerve branches may be able to regain contact with the muscles as long as they can find a way back to their appropriate targets, but this takes several weeks, as they grow at a rate of around one millimeter per day, at best.

Movements of Vocal Folds

The classical description of the movement of the vocal folds during singing is as follows. At the beginning of phonation, just before the air is driven from the lungs through the larynx, the vocal folds are brought together (i.e., the glottis is closed). As the air is then driven from the lungs against the closed folds, the subglottic pressure (the pressure in the region below the glottis) rises until it is capable of pushing the vocal folds apart. The edges of the vocal folds are elastic; as the airstream begins to flow between them, they become progressively more stretched. The farther apart they become, the greater are the elastic forces trying to close them again. Finally, this exceeds the subglottic pressure, and the folds snap shut and the cycle repeats itself (fig. 5-6, animations 5-5 and 5-6, video 5-1). Other factors also help to close the glottis.

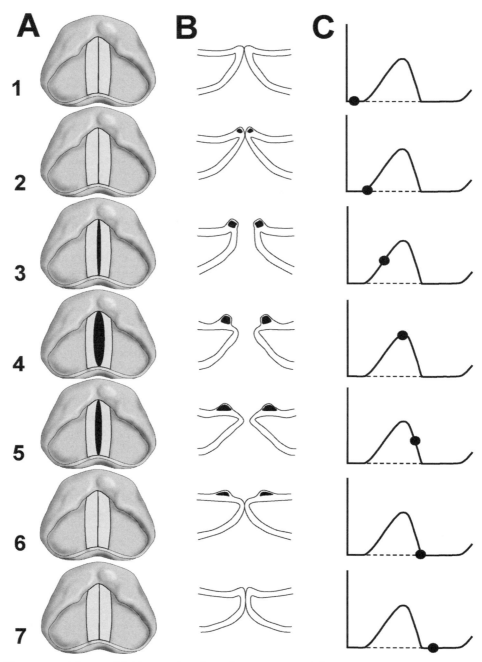

Figure 5-6. The vocal folds. A and B show the movement of the vocal folds through one complete vibratory cycle. The column in A shows a series of views of the vocal folds as seen from above. B shows a series of transverse sections through the folds corresponding to each stage in the cycle. In B the black patch indicates a ripple on the surface of the vocal fold that moves across it during the cycle. In C, the black dot indicates the position on a flow glottogram (see fig. 5-8) represented by each image in A. The movements of the folds can also be seen in animations 5-5 and 5-6 and video 5-1.

The faster the air rushes through the gap between the folds, the lower the pressure between them, a physical phenomenon known as the Bernoulli effect. This sucks the vocal folds together and aids the elastic forces that are trying to close the glottal opening. This description of the mechanism underlying the oscillation of the vocal folds does not offer a complete explanation of the events that take place. In particular, it would not explain how vocal fold oscillation can be maintained in a situation in which the glottis does not close completely, for example, during breathy phonation (see animation 5-3). An important element of the mechanism that ensures the sustainability of the oscillation is a process known as inertive reactance (Titze 2008). When the subglottal pressure first drives the folds to open, the air passing between them encounters a mass of stationary air in the space immediately above. It takes some time for this air mass to accelerate to a steady velocity, and during this period, the barrier it presents causes the pressure of the air being driven from below to rise. This helps to force the folds open farther. Later, as the elasticity of the vocal folds acts to close again, the inertia of this air mass means that it takes some time to decelerate. This leads to the formation of a region of low pressure immediately above the folds that helps to suck them closed again. Inertive reactance serves to give the oscillation a periodic kick, analogous to pushing a swing in phase with its movement, which helps maintain the oscillation. Readers with a mathematical bent will find a full description of this and other processes that support vocal fold oscillations in Titze (2000).

The frequency of the opening and closing of the glottis determines the pitch of the note, so if this happens 440 times a second (i.e., at 440 Hz), the pitch of the fundamental note produced will be A4. When the vocal folds come together to produce a note of low frequency, they first make contact deep in the glottal opening. As a result of the impact, a long ripple is generated on the upper surface of the vocal folds that runs away from the opening, parallel to the free edge (fig. 5-6B, animations 5-5 and 5-6, video 5-1). This is called the mucosal wave and represents a displacement of the cover (see table 5-1), which indicates that it is not under significant tension and is only loosely attached to the underlying vocal ligament and muscle. The ripple plays a significant role in making the vocal fold oscillation self-sustaining. If the wave is absent for some reason, considerably greater subglottal pressure is required to maintain vocal fold vibration, particularly in the upper registers (Titze 2000). Current wisdom is that the folds must be adequately hydrated to maintain the mobility of the cover and consequently that the singer must take in a sufficient quantity of fluid on a daily basis to ensure that this is the case.

At high frequencies (e.g., in the falsetto register), the tension of the vocal folds is carried mainly by the vocal ligament and cover, with the result that no ripple is generated. It has been proposed by some that the mobile cover part of the vocal folds may contain the upper compartment of the vocalis muscle and that this is controlled separately from the lower compartment (Sanders, Rai, et al. 1998). If this is true, it implies that the upper compartment plays an active role in controlling the shape and tension of the edge of the vocal fold, which in turn contributes to the control of pitch, particularly in the falsetto register (see animation 5-4).

One way of displaying the airflow through the glottis during vocal fold vibration is what is known as a flow glottogram (figs. 5-6C, 5-7, animations 5-5, 5-6). The velocity of the airflow fluctuates in time with each cycle of opening and closure of the vocal folds. The louder we sing, the greater the peak flow rate during the open phase and the more abruptly the flow is cut off as the vocal folds snap shut. There is a linear relationship between the intensity of sound produced and flow rate—a doubling of flow rate produces about a 9 decibel (dB) increase in volume (Bouhuys, Proctor, and Mead 1966). However, as the flow rate increases, the intensity of the upper harmonics rises to a greater extent than that of the lower harmonics. For example, an increase that produces a rise in intensity of 10 dB at a fundamental frequency of 600 Hz, sung by a baritone, generates a 16 dB increase in harmonics close to the singer's formant at 3 kilohertz (kHz) (Sjolander and Sundberg 2004), which alters the timbre of the sound. Increasing subglottal pressure and flow rate also causes a rise in the pitch of the note, so to stay in tune during changes in volume, the singer must adjust the strength of contraction in the muscles that close and tense the vocal folds. Because the degree of opening of the folds is also related to their length, singers with longer vocal folds (i.e., those with low voices) have stronger fundamentals in the notes they produce than do singers with short vocal folds.

The quality of the sound generated by air passing through the glottis varies depending on the precise action of the vocal folds. If the vocal folds are held strongly

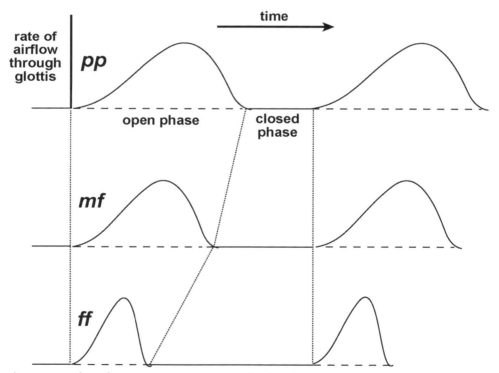

Figure 5-7.   Flow glottograms are a measure of airflow through the glottis (the space between the vocal folds). As the folds open and close at the fundamental frequency of the note sung, flow glottograms show the rapid fluctuations in airflow. These idealized glottograms show that as the singing gets louder, the folds closer ever faster and the open phase becomes shorter.

together, this results in what is known as "pressed phonation" (see animation 5-3). In this mode, the fundamental frequency of the note generated is weak, giving the voice a harsh sound due to the greater prominence of the upper harmonics. This is a result of increasing the stiffness of a vibrating surface, which leaves it more prone to damping the lower frequencies and better able to sustain higher frequencies. When the vocal folds are not so strongly pressed together, the result is "flow phonation," in which the fundamental frequency is strong (up to 15 dB greater in intensity than in pressed phonation). However, if the vocal folds are so weakly brought together that the opening is not closed completely (animation 5-3), the fundamental is again weak and the voice is described as "breathy." Many young singers exhibit a degree of breathiness in their phonation. This is normal and may be particularly associated with weakness in the interarytenoid muscle, with the result that a triangular gap or "chink" is left between the arytenoid cartilages during phonation. As the laryngeal muscles mature and strengthen, the breathiness generally disappears. Most Western classical singers base their singing voice on flow phonation, though the other types of phonation may also be used for expression and in particular contexts. In speech, flow phonation is characteristic of low pitch and quiet vocalizations, and pressed phonation with higher and louder vocalizations such as shouting.

In whispering, the vocal folds do not vibrate and are kept partly open because the posterior cricoarytenoid may be partly active and the interarytenoid muscle relaxed (animation 5-3). The edges of the folds are either held straight for their entire length like an inverted V or are first straight then angled outward toward the ends, which attach to the arytenoid cartilages like an inverted Y whose stem is either closed completely, or itself a narrow V (Solomon et al. 1989). As a result, most of the air bypasses the vocal folds, and the sound is generated as a result of turbulence in the airflow. The false vocal folds are often displaced downward in whispering and may even be brought into contact with the true vocal folds, limiting their ability to vibrate (Tsunoda et al. 1997).

Vocal Registers

Any account of how the larynx is used in singing must explain not only how the pitch of a note is regulated, but also why the quality of the sound changes in different vocal registers. A vocal register is a pitch range over which the timbre (harmonic richness) of the sound remains relatively constant. The vocal range of a singer generally has two or more registers; for example, in a male voice there is typically a modal register (also known as the chest or normal register) and a falsetto register. In some musical cultures (e.g., in Russia and Eastern Europe) a very low *Strohbass* (or pulse) register is also used by the lowest male voices. For the female voice, a chest and a head register are generally distinguished. The situation is made confusing by the presence of several naming schemes. Table 5-2 summarizes the features of the main registers and lists some of their more common synonyms.

The timbre depends on what elements of the vocal folds are vibrating; this is shown schematically in animation 5-7. When most of the mass of the fold is in motion (the muscle plus the overlying tissue), the timbre is rich in strong lower harmonics. This is typical of the modal register. If the muscular core of the fold is allowed to relax so

Table 5-2. Main Register Features

Register	Muscles Active	Vibrating Region of Fold	Voice Quality	Pitch
Pulse (*Strohbass*)	TA only	Most of the thickness of the fold	Pulsating; vocal fry	Lowest; below normal singing
Chest (modal)	Mostly TA, some CT	Most of the fold, both cover and body	Heavier, richer tone; vibration felt behind breastbone	Lower part of singing range
Head (middle or mixed)	Mostly CT, some TA	Cover only tone; vibration	Lighter, thinner, felt in head	Upper part of singing range
Falsetto	CT only	Only outer cover layers	Lightest possible	Highest sung pitches; above normal range

TA = thyroarytenoid; CT = cricothyroid
Reproduced with permission from Titze 1994.

that most of the tension is carried by the vocal ligament, then the harmonic structure of the sound is depleted. This is typical of the falsetto register, in which the vocal folds are also more stretched, less flexible, and thinner than in the modal register and the glottis is rarely completely closed. The characteristics of the pulse register have a different origin. When the folds are vibrating very slowly, the resonances set up by each opening and closing event may die out before the next one occurs. The result is that the sound is heard as a series of separate pulses said to be like the crackling of breaking straw when it is walked upon (hence *Strohbass*) or like the sound of frying fat (vocal fry). This is generally heard only at pitches below 70 Hz (about C2) and can take a number of forms (Scherer 2006). At very low pitch (e.g., around 30 Hz), the vocal fry may represent each single cycle of vocal fold opening and closing. A roughness at higher frequencies may be the result of alternate cycles of different amplitudes, producing an audible pulsation at half the frequency of the note; this is the most typical form. More complex patterns can be produced in which the flow rate through the glottis waxes and wanes at regular intervals through succeeding cycles. An example shown by Scherer shows a low-amplitude pulse at 93 Hz superimposed on a larger one at 7.5 Hz.

When crossing from one register to another, the voice of an inexperienced singer may show a break, that is, an abrupt change in timbre, something that vocal training aims to eliminate. One of the complicating aspects of registers is that because their ranges overlap, a singer will often be able to produce a note of a particular pitch in two or even three registers (Hirano, Vennard, and Ohala 1970; Hollien and Moore 1960). One can liken this to playing the same note on two guitar strings, one of which is a thin nylon monofilament string and the other a string overwound with metal wire to increase its mass. The heavier string can match the pitch of a note played on the thinner one by being shorter or under greater tension; however, the quality of the note is not the same because they have different harmonic structures.

Laryngeal Muscle Activity during Singing

The precise way in which the muscles act during singing is controversial. Observing the activity of muscles in the larynx, which are small and delicate, is difficult and involves the placing of fine-wire hook electrodes into them. This is both uncomfortable and potentially risky for singers and as a consequence there have been few investigations of this nature. Unfortunately the results of those that have been carried out are not in complete agreement (Shipp, Doherty, and Morrissey 1979; Hirano, Vennard, and Ohala 1970; Hillel 2001). For this reason we will start by considering the principles underlying the control of pitch and register and then consider the experimental evidence to support them.

During phonation, the vocal folds are brought together (adducted) by the lateral cricoarytenoid muscles, which rotate the arytenoid cartilages toward each other. At the same time, the interarytenoid muscle draws the arytenoid cartilages closer together (animation 5-3) and the thyroarytenoid muscle contracts to bring the vocal folds under tension. Electrical recordings show that these three sets of muscles are activated simultaneously immediately prior to vocalization, but that once this has started, activity in the interarytenoid muscle dominates (Hillel 2001). In singing, the cricothyroid and

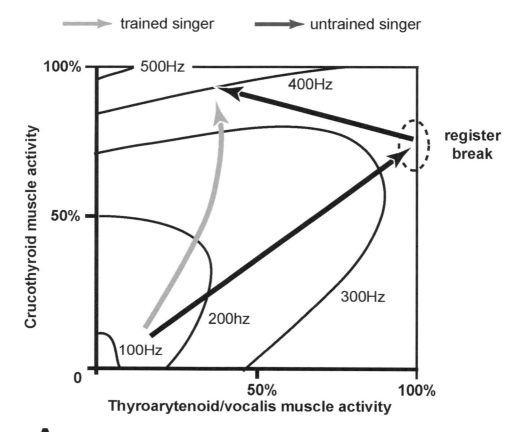

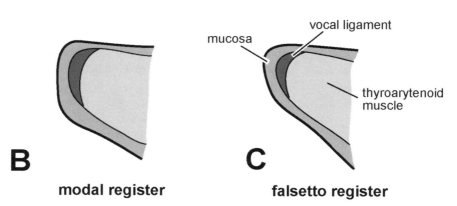

Figure 5-8

Figure 5-8.   A. The relationship between activity in the thyroarytenoid and cricothyroid muscles and the vocal pitch. This graph demonstrates how pitch can be increased by activity in either the thyroarytenoid or cricothyroid muscles alone or by the two acting in concert. The degree of muscular effort required to produce the note also depends on the air pressure generated by the respiratory system. The lines represent the generation of sound at 200, 300, 400, and 500 Hz. Increasing subglottal pressure raises the frequency of the sound, so at higher pressures, less muscular effort (less tension in the folds) is needed to generate a note of a given pitch. The quality (timbre) of the sound will depend on how the note is achieved. If the tension in the folds is increased mainly by the thyroarytenoid muscle, a point is ultimately reached when the muscle can contract no more. To raise the pitch further, the thyroarytenoid must be relaxed and the cricothyroid brought into play (black arrows). This will lead to an abrupt change in timbre (i.e., a register break) between the modal to falsetto registers. The trained singer (gray arrow) learns to avoid this by continuously adjusting the activity of both muscles. The result is a gradual change in timbre. B, C. Cross-sections through the vocal fold when singing in the modal or falsetto registers. In the modal register, the thyroarytenoid muscle is contracted, which makes the edge of the fold blunter in cross-section and increases the contact area between the two folds. The entire thickness of the vocal fold vibrates and the sound is rich in low harmonics. In the falsetto register, the thyroarytenoid relaxes and the cricothyroid contracts, the edge of the fold becomes thinner as the tension is transferred to the vocal ligament, and the vibration is mainly in this and the mucosa, leaving the sound with weak lower harmonics and hence brighter. Reproduced with permission from Titze (2000).

thyroarytenoid muscles act to some extent antagonistically. The cricothyroid rotates the thyroid cartilage downward and in so doing stretches the vocal folds. However, as we have seen, these are made up of several components, including the thyroarytenoid and vocalis muscles, the vocal ligament, and the mucosa. If the thyroarytenoid muscle is relaxed when the folds are stretched, their edges become thinner and most of the tension is carried by the thin vocal ligament (fig. 5-8A, B, animation 5-7). This can vibrate at high frequency, and the timbre is light and typical of the falsetto register. The thyroarytenoid muscle shortens the vocal folds and resists the action of the cricothyroid. When both muscles are active, most of the tension and vibration in the vocal folds is transferred to the much more massive thyroarytenoid muscle (animation 5-7). This favors lower fundamental frequencies and the rich timbre typical of the modal or chest register (table 5-2, fig. 5-8A). The contraction of the thyroarytenoid also thickens the edge of the vocal folds, increasing the contact area when the glottis is closed (fig. 5-8C). Figure 5-8 illustrates a theoretical explanation for the abrupt register transition seen in untrained singers (Titze 2000). Both the cricothyroid and thyroarytenoid muscles are active in the modal and falsetto registers, and to achieve a particular timbre what is important is not the absolute level of activity in each muscle but the relative activity in the two muscles. Thus the same pitch can be achieved in a variety of ways, but the timbre will depend on which muscle is dominant. It is hypothesized that in the untrained singer, activity in the thyroarytenoid dominates in the modal register. This produces a rich timbre but when the muscle is fully active, the pitch can increase no further in this register. To raise the pitch, the thyroarytenoid must be relaxed abruptly to allow the cricothyroid to increase the tension in the vocal fold further. Over a very small frequency interval, the tension in the vocal fold is switched from the muscle to the vocal ligament, leading to a noticeable change in timbre characteristic of a register break (black arrows). It is envisaged that with training, the singer learns to modulate the pitch by a more gradual change in the pattern of activity in the two muscles, which leads to a smooth and continuous change in timbre throughout the vocal range (gray arrow).

Experiments that directly monitor the activity of laryngeal muscles through implanted electrodes (Hillel 2001; Hirano, Vennard, and Ohala 1970) confirm that cricothyroid activity increases as pitch rises within a given register. Noninvasive ultrasound measurements of changes in the dimensions of the space between the cricoid and thyroid cartilages are consistent with this observation (Laukkanen et al. 2002). This confirmation is important, as the risk that direct recordings from the muscles may alter the way they are used is a significant one. However, the downside of ultrasound studies is that the evidence of muscle activity is rather indirect, so it is important that the two approaches be used in concert. Hirano concluded that activity in the lateral cricoarytenoid (which closes the gap between the vocal folds) also increases with pitch and that this appears to be matched by activity in the interarytenoid muscle, which draws the two arytenoid cartilages together. Both therefore act to keep the glottis closed and will also help to prevent the arytenoid cartilages from being pulled forward by the action of the cricothyroid and thyroarytenoid muscles. We previously simplified our consideration of the movement of the arytenoid cartilages by describing only rotation around a vertical axis, but the shape of the surfaces of their joints with the cricoid cartilage also allows them to slide forward.

Hirano et al. reported that when the limit of the register is reached and the voice switches to a higher register, activity of both the cricothyroid and the vocalis muscle declines sharply. It is probable however, that what they meant by the term *vocalis* was the thyroarytenoid muscle, as it is almost inconceivable that the recording techniques used could access the vocalis selectively, and no mention is otherwise made of the thyroarytenoid. Relaxation of the thyroarytenoid would reduce the resistance of the vocal folds to stretching under the action of the cricothyroid muscle and allow the vocal fold to become thinner. As a result, tensioning the fold to a given pitch would require less effort by the cricothyroid and might explain the reduction in its activity. Though this is not predicted by figure 5-8A, which is intended as a simple diagram to illustrate a theory of register change, it is not inconsistent with the ideas on which it is based.

The ultrasound studies of Laukkanen (2002) found that the pitch can still rise after the vocal folds have reached their maximum level of stretch. This must therefore be achieved by other mechanisms. One would be to increase the airflow through the glottis, which, as we have already seen, increases pitch. Another is the one previously mentioned, that in the upper falsetto register, the posterior parts of the vocal folds are held together and only the anterior parts are allowed to vibrate, that is, as the vibrating surfaces effectively become shorter the frequency would rise. For this to be possible, different parts of the vocalis muscle would have to be under separate control (Sanders, Rai, et al. 1998), for which there is as yet no direct evidence.

Though the description of the activity patterns in the laryngeal muscles by Hirano et al. appears quite rational, a second study of laryngeal muscle activity failed to show similar patterns during register changes (Shipp, Doherty, and Morrissey 1979). This might indicate that there are several ways of achieving the same vocal goals (Sundberg 1987) and that these might, for example, be influenced by the specific laryngeal architecture of individual singers (Shipp, Doherty, and Morrissey 1979). Unfortunately, Shipp et al. do not discuss why their data differ from those of Hirano. Closer examination of these two studies reveals a number of factors that make it difficult to compare them in a satisfactory way. These reflect problems that are typical of the current state of the published literature on the physiological basis of singing. Both used only four singers and the data obtained are presented in different ways. In the study by Hirano, the singers were two sopranos, a tenor, and a bass who were all trained professionals. The study by Shipp used only four males whose vocal range and proficiency is not reported, though the pitches sung cover the bass to tenor ranges. The data presented also appear to show that even these four may not all have been using the same strategy for vocalization. They were also given a number of drugs to reduce the undeniable discomfort and stress of implanting the electrodes into the laryngeal muscles, including topical anesthetic to the vocal tract, which has a fundamental effect on singing performance (see below). Hirano does not describe how his singers were treated to control discomfort, though this was most probably done. Finally, it was not clear how the correct placement of the electrodes into the target muscles was ensured. While these are very difficult experiments to do on human subjects, it is likely that such approaches will ultimately give considerable insight into singing strategies. It is therefore a pity that so few have been carried out and that for the time being, the results of existing studies must be treated with some circumspection.

Nervous Control of the Laryngeal Muscles

In considering the nervous control of the larynx, it is important to remember that in addition to its role in phonation, the larynx also provides a line of defense for preventing food material or fluids from entering the trachea. The lining of the larynx has an extremely abundant sensory innervation, and the purpose of many of the nerve endings on its inner surfaces is to detect the presence of foreign bodies (Andreatta et al. 2002; Yoshida et al. 2000). Some of these produce the sensations of pain or discomfort with which we are all familiar. In addition, however, there are many receptors that gather information needed by the brain to control the laryngeal muscles during phonation. This includes feedback from the muscles, joints, and mucosal epithelium within the larynx as well as from muscles attached to the outside, which adjust its height.

Current theories about how the laryngeal muscles are controlled depend largely on ideas put forward by Wyke and colleagues, based on a series of studies carried out in the 1960s and 1970s (Wyke 1974). Only some of the key papers on which these results are based show raw experimental data, so it is often not possible to assess the quality of the evidence. Though most of the ideas appear quite reasonable, there have been few new studies performed in intervening decades using the superior techniques that are now available. According to the hypotheses presented by Wyke, just before the onset of vocalization and the accompanying rise in subglottic pressure, there is a brief burst of activity in the muscles that close the glottis. This would indicate that the tension, length, position, and shape of the vocal folds is preset prior to any sound being produced. Most people can quite accurately sing the pitch of a note played on the piano; however, it has been demonstrated that trained singers generate sounds of the correct frequency within a few cycles of onset of vocal fold vibration (i.e., within a very small fraction of a second). As anyone can demonstrate for themselves, this is under conscious control, but it is too rapid to be a response to hearing the initial pitch of the sound produced by the voice and then adjusting it to the correct value. Once the sound is initiated, a considerable amount of sensory information about the vibration and stretching of the vocal folds and the pressure in the region of the glottis will be generated as it rapidly opens and closes under the influence of the airstream (Shiba et al. 1999). Vocal training improves laryngeal control, for example, the ability of a singer to match a sound whose pitch changes continuously. It is not clear, however, whether this is primarily a result of an enhanced auditory ability to discriminate pitch or of a more precise control of the laryngeal muscles in response to sensory feedback. We are not, in general, conscious of this sensory feedback, though we may feel vibrations from other parts of the vocal tract or the tissues in the throat surrounding it. Wyke's theory proposes three mechanisms that underlie the control of vocalization and allow us to match the sound from our own voice to the one we seek to produce.

The first mechanism is a myotactic reflex that causes contraction of the muscles that close or tense the vocal folds. It is said to be driven by sensory signals from the laryngeal muscles themselves, generated by the stretching of the vocal folds as they open and close. The actions of most muscles in the body are monitored by sensory structures called muscle spindles. In a major review of the control of the larynx written by Wyke more than thirty years ago (Wyke and Kirchner 1976) it was stated that there was considerable controversy concerning whether muscle spindles are present in human laryngeal muscles. Despite more sophisticated methods of investigation available today, this controversy remains unresolved (Brandon et al. 2003; Sanders, Han, et al. 1998; Hirayama et al. 1987; Keene 1961). The one muscle that remains above this controversy is the interarytenoid muscle that runs between the two arytenoid cartilages. It clearly does contain muscle spindles (Tellis et al. 2004; Hirayama et al. 1987), suggesting that it may play a key role in the positioning of the vocal folds and stabilization of the joints between the cricoid and arytenoid cartilages. As we have seen, these are not simple pivot or ball joints, but allow the arytenoid cartilages to glide forward as well. Given the degree of freedom this allows, precise control of the position of the arytenoid cartilages is likely to be central to laryngeal function.

In the absence of muscle spindles, the action of the other intrinsic muscles of the larynx may therefore be monitored by other types of sensory endings. Amongst these are so-called spiral endings within the muscle and Golgi tendon organs associated with the attachment sites of the muscles to the cartilages of the larynx (Wyke and Kirchner 1976; Nagai 1987). Some physiological studies have found sensory nerve cells with properties matching what would be expected from such receptors (Shiba et al. 1999; Sampson and Eyzaguirre 1964), though their presence has not been identified unequivocally. However, one animal study found that in the thyroarytenoid muscle, the myotactic reflex is lost following the rather extreme measure of removing the mucosa. The authors interpreted this as implying that there was no sensory contribution from the muscles themselves (Andreatta et al. 2002); however, it is also possible that the nerves carrying information from the muscles were damaged by the considerable disruption that was caused when the mucosa was removed.

The second mechanism proposed by Wyke involves receptors in the mucosa of the larynx that are said to provide sensory feedback that influences muscle activity during vocalization. There is a particularly high density of these receptors in the region of the arytenoid cartilages (Davis and Nail 1987; Sanders and Mu 1998). Their physiological properties have been quite well studied (Shiba et al. 1999; Shiba, Yoshida, and Miura 1995; Shiba et al. 1997; Andreatta et al. 2002; Davis and Nail 1987), but the precise roles of many of the different types remain unclear (Bradley 2000). Nevertheless, the basic properties of these receptors, which are found both above and below the glottis, appear similar to those proposed by Wyke. Some are said to be responsible for the abrupt rise in the tension in the muscles that close the vocal folds just as the subglottic pressure reaches the level necessary to produce sound (Shiba et al. 1997). With further increases in subglottic pressure, the tension in the muscles rises more slowly. Most of the receptors in the mucosa are sensitive to vibrations and some will follow these accurately up to frequencies of 400 Hz (near G4) (Davis and Nail 1987; Shiba et al. 1997); however, they are generally most sensitive to lower frequencies. Whether this frequency information is important for the control of the laryngeal muscles or whether pitch control is mainly learned through auditory feedback and the memory stored is not clear. Because they lie close to the surface of the mucosa, the receptors are rapidly affected by local anesthetics applied to the inner surfaces of the larynx (Shiba, Yoshida, and Miura 1995). There is some controversy as to the effect this has on humans. The application of local anesthetic to the mucosa below the vocal folds has little effect on normal speech, but it was long believed to make singing almost impossible (Gould and Okamura 1974) because blocking the responses of the subglottal pressure receptors led to a rise in glottal resistance and subglottic pressure (i.e., the vocal folds were held more tightly closed than normal). However, a more recent study (Sundberg, Iwarsson, and Billstrom 1995) reported no consistent effect on subglottal pressure and that singing remains quite possible, though there is a marked deterioration in pitch control.

The third component of the mechanism proposed by Wyke for the control of laryngeal muscles is driven by sensory receptors that monitor the position or movements of the joints between the cartilages of the larynx, particularly those linking the cricoid cartilage with the thyroid and the arytenoid cartilages (Kirchner and Wyke 1964a, 1964b). Some recent findings have been interpreted as suggesting that sensory information from joints may not after all be involved in the reflex control of muscles that close the vocal folds (Andreatta et al. 2002). However, this conclusion is again based on the observation that removing the mucosa abolishes the responses attributed to joint receptors, and even the authors did not completely dismiss a possible role for joint receptors in laryngeal control circuitry.

From the foregoing account it will be appreciated that the way in which the larynx is controlled is still uncertain and that recent studies have complicated rather than clarified our understanding. Most of our knowledge of the control of the larynx is based on studies of animals. The sophistication of their vocal repertoire is much less than that of humans, and though the principles under which they operate are likely to show many common features, we should expect that the systems controlling human vocalization will be considerably more complex and precise.

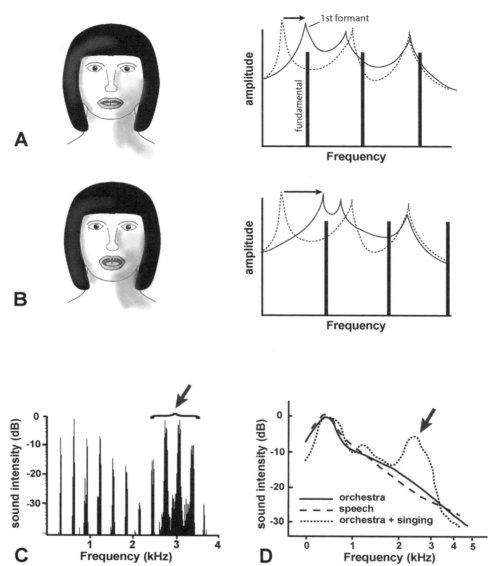

Figure 5-9. The manipulation of formants in voice projection. A, B. Soprano voices. In these diagrams, the harmonics of the nonprojected voice are indicated by the dashed lines. When these do not coincide with the harmonics of the voice source (vocal folds), projection is weak. This can be improved by manipulating the throat and mouth opening to tune the lowest formant toward the first harmonic of the note (solid line). As the pitch of the note rises (A to B), the lowest formant tracks the first harmonic (e.g., by opening the mouth wider) to maintain vocal projection. C, D. Low voices use a phenomenon called the "singer's formant" in voice projection. A peak in the intensity of the sound spectrum of the sung note is produced at 2.5 and 3.0 kHz by the clustering of several formants. In C, which was recorded from a mezzo-soprano singing a note with a fundamental frequency of around 300 Hz, the increase in the amplitude of the harmonics due to the singer's formant is clearly evident (arrow—see also video 5-2). D. In this frequency range, the average intensity of the sound from the orchestra is on the wane and so the voice can be heard above it. This peak will not generally correspond to the pitch of the note, but to some of its upper harmonics. As will be seen in chapter 9, the brain can nevertheless compute the pitch of the fundamental from its harmonic structure. D is reproduced with permission from Sundberg (1972).

The Resonator

As already mentioned, the pharynx and the mouth represent the resonator for the voice and are largely responsible for the harmonic richness that we hear. As with any wind instrument, the vocal tract resonates best at particular frequencies that depend on its length and its shape. These resonant frequencies are called formants, and efficient projection of the voice depends on matching these formants to the frequencies of the notes being sung (fig. 5-9). A particularly clear discussion of the significance of formants in singing is given by Sundberg (1977). The frequencies of the formants set some limits to the effective singing range of individual performers. Experienced teachers can often predict the likely range of untrained singers by identifying the formant frequencies of sung vowels, even before the full tessitura of the voice (which will depend on the structure and muscles of the larynx) has been fully developed. The pitch of the formants of the vocal tract can, within limits, be manipulated by changing its dimensions. The formants are derived from standing waves that have a peak amplitude at the vocal folds and a minimum near the mouth opening. If the vocal tract were a straight tube with a typical length of 17.5 centimeters, the first four formants would occur at about 500, 1500, 2,500, and 3,500 Hz, which are equivalent to one-quarter, three-quarters, one and one-quarter, and one and three-quarters of a wavelength.

There is an inverse relationship between the formant frequencies and the length of the vocal tract and this is reflected in the characteristics of voices with different ranges, and of voices of the same range but different qualities. For example, the average formant frequencies found in bass singers are about 15 percent lower than those in tenors, which is thought to reflect a corresponding difference in vocal tract length (Titze 2000). In singers with the same range, darker voices may reflect longer vocal tracts than brighter voices. The effective length of the vocal tract in any one individual can be altered by about 10 percent by changing the position of the larynx and by extending or retracting the lips. When the larynx is raised, the pharynx becomes shorter and its walls tend to sag inward. This leads first to the narrowing and then the closing off of a cavity that surrounds the upper end of the laryngeal opening called the piriform recess (Yanagisawa et al. 1991; Benninger et al. 1989). Raising the larynx increases formant frequencies, which will enhance the upper harmonics, perhaps at the expense of the fundamental frequency (Sundberg 1999), making the voice sound brighter or more shrill. When the larynx is lowered, the opposite effect is achieved. The walls of the pharynx become stretched and its diameter increases, particularly at the base. This reduces the frequencies of the formants, which results in the lower harmonics of the voice being more efficiently projected, leading to a darker, more covered quality in the voice. Many teachers encourage singers to try to maintain a laryngeal position that is lower than the rest position seen during normal respiration; however, in many, though not all, trained singers there remains a tendency for the larynx to move upward with rising pitch, particularly at the upper end of the range (Shipp 1987; Sonninen, Hurme, and Laukkanen 1999; Yanagisawa et al. 1991). The shape of the vocal tract is not determined by the position of the larynx alone, however, but by its position relative to other mobile structures in the neck such as the hyoid bone (Hurme and Sonninen 1995). We have seen that the larynx can be lowered by the action of the sternothyroid muscles and raised by the thyrohyoid muscles. However, the actions of the sternohyoid and omohyoid may also indirectly affect its position and its relationship to the hyoid. Direct radiographic observations of singers carrying out different vocal tasks reveal complex and highly variable pitch-dependent changes to the relative position of the larynx and hyoid and to the shape of the pharynx, whose significance is not currently well understood (Sonninen, Hurme, and Laukkanen 1999; Hurme and Sonninen 1995).

The position of the larynx may also be affected indirectly by how the singer breathes. When breathing in, the diaphragm contracts and pulls downward, drawing the base of the lungs with it. It has been suggested that this may put tension on the trachea and draw the larynx downward (Iwarsson and Sundberg 1998), especially if the abdomen is allowed to bulge out (the "pear-shape up" posture—see chapter 4). However, some singers hold the wall of the abdomen in (the "pear-shape down" posture), which should theoretically limit the downward movement of the diaphragm and its pull on the larynx. Studies of what happens in practice with these two breathing strategies reveal a more complicated situation (Iwarsson 2001). When singers prevent the abdomen from bulging outward, they tend to tilt the head forward, rotating the chin down toward the neck, which has the result of allowing the larynx to fall lower in the situation where otherwise it might be predicted to remain high. By contrast, any tendency to tilt the chin up will increase the upward pull on the larynx, making it rise. Consequently, when considering the control of the height of the larynx, it is necessary to take into consideration not only the role of the muscles attached to it, but also posture and breathing technique.

Up until now, we have considered the vocal tract as being analogous to the straightened tube of a trumpet or trombone, but this is too simplistic a notion, as it bends sharply forward at the back of the throat and its width is far from uniform (fig. 5-1). Furthermore, its internal diameter can be varied at a number of levels, for example, by exposing or occluding the piriform recesses (a pair of shallow bowl-shaped spaces lying on either side of the larynx), by contracting the stylopharyngeus muscle (fig. 5-2), by altering the position and shape of the tongue so that the mouth cavity becomes narrowed at different points, or by changing the size and shape of the mouth opening itself. In the male voice, such means can be used to place the first formant anywhere between 250 and 700 Hz, and the second formant between 700 and 2,500 Hz (Sundberg 1977). For example, the frequency of the first formant is raised when the jaw is dropped to widen the mouth opening. The second formant can be altered by moving the body of the tongue and the fourth formant by moving its tip.

Singers with high voices (sopranos) can project the voice adequately when the fundamental frequency of the note being sung lies below that of the first formant, but in the upper part of the range it will generally rise above it. The intensity of the sound then falls progressively as its pitch diverges more and more from the first formant. To correct this situation, the singer alters the shape of the pharynx, for example, by opening the mouth aperture to allow the first formant to track the fundamental frequency of the sung note (fig. 5-9A, B) (Joliveau, Smith, and Wolfe 2004). Constantly moving the formant frequency in this way not only helps to ensure that the notes are all of equal volume, but minimizes the vocal effort required by eliminating the damping effect that the pharynx imposes at pitches where it does not resonate well.

In singers with lower voices, the sung note does not generally exceed the frequency of the first formant, and another mechanism is used for voice projection. When performing with an orchestra, a major problem that singers must overcome is to project the sound of the voice over it. The sound intensity of the orchestra typically peaks at between 400 and 500 Hz, and below 100 Hz in particular will quite readily mask the singer (fig. 5-9C). In classically trained mezzo-sopranos, baritones, and basses, one noticeable feature of sung vowels is that there is a peak in sound intensity between 2.5 and 3.0 kHz, which is not found in speech (fig. 5-9B, video 5-2). This is called the singer's formant (or ring) and is not present to the same extent in sopranos (Sundberg 1999). It appears to be due to a clustering of the third to fifth formants and falls in a frequency range in which the mean sound energy of the orchestra is declining (fig. 5-9D). Of course, this does not represent the fundamental of the note being sung and so does not match its pitch. The perception of pitch is dealt with in detail in chapter 9, but here it suffices to say that under these circumstances the central nervous system may use a series of upper harmonics to compute the actual pitch of the voice even though the fundamental is not clearly audible above the orchestra. There is also another way in which the singer's formant may contribute to the audibility of the voice, that the higher frequencies typical of this range are more efficiently radiated forward (i.e., toward the audience) than frequencies of the lower harmonics of the voice. The singer's formant is achieved by widening the pharynx and lowering the larynx (Sundberg 1987), actions that are typical of many male singers (Shipp and Izdebski 1975). As the pitch of the voice rises, the upper opening of the larynx where it joins the pharynx may increase considerably in diameter. This changes the sound-projecting properties of the vocal tract and may compromise the formation of the singer's formant. To avoid this eventuality, the larynx must be lowered still farther. This is the opposite of what happens in normal speech, where the larynx tends to rise as the pitch of the voice increases, a tendency that the singer must therefore learn to counteract (Sundberg 1987). The lowering of the larynx does not require much muscular effort, so the considerable increase in projection that results is still obtained with little extra expenditure of energy. The importance of the singer's formant may depend on the context, however. There appears to be a greater enhancement in this range in solo singing, while in choral singing more power is generated at the fundamental frequency (Rossing, Sundberg, and Ternstrom 1986). Boosting power at the fundamental frequency is thought to be achieved by modification of the voice source, that is, by manipulating the larynx. This would help to enhance the audibility of the bass parts in choral singing.

The disadvantage of adjusting formant frequency to increase projection of the soprano voice is that it alters the characteristic of the vowels, and both intelligibility and some of the expressiveness and inflection present in everyday speech must be sacrificed in the interest of singing efficiency. However, in lower voices, production of the singer's formant has little effect on vowel sounds. To understand the reason for this effect, it is necessary to consider what gives different vowels their particular characteristics. This depends on how the properties of the sound source (the harmonic series generated by the larynx) are modified by the acoustical properties of the pharynx (i.e., its formants). In normal speech, the frequencies of the two lowest formants

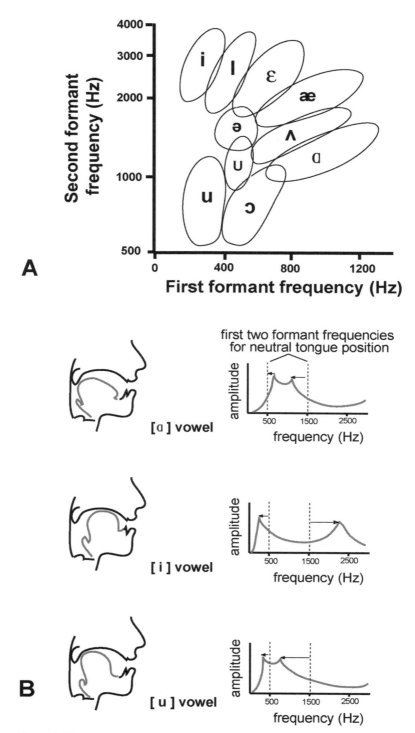

first two formant frequencies
for neutral tongue position

[ɑ] vowel

[i] vowel

[u] vowel

Figure 5-10

are crucial in enabling us to distinguish between different vowel sounds (Titze 2000). This can clearly be seen in figure 5-10A, which plots the frequency of these two formants against one another (Peterson and Barney 1952). Figure 5-10B demonstrates how changing the shape and position of the tongue is used to control the formant frequencies that distinguish [α] (as in car) from [u] (as in boot) and [i] (as in tree). From this it will be apparent that any manipulation of the vocal tract that alters the position of these formants to improve voice projection may have the additional consequence of transforming one vowel into another. Some rules for this are as follows. Constricting the mouth opening lowers the first formant and raises the second, transforming the sound toward vowels in which the first two formants are relatively far apart, such as [i] (as in tree) and [ε] (as in bet). Opening the mouth or constricting the pharynx at the other end of the vocal tract brings the formants closer together by raising the first and lowering the second, which pushes the sound toward [α] (as in car) and [o] (as in bought). As the soprano alters the shape of the vocal tract to optimize the projected voice as it rises ever higher, the first and second formants of the different vowels converge and so they progressively sound more and more similar (fig. 5-11). Above F4 (698 Hz), all vowels in a classically trained projected voice become essentially identical, though placing the vowel between two consonants does improve matters to some extent (Smith and Scott 1980). This phenomenon is well understood by composers, who do not score words that must be understood in the upper soprano register but in this range use the voice purely as an instrument. Interestingly, the question of vowel intelligibility is rarely raised in the contemporary debates over whether surtitles should be used for opera sung in the language of the audience.

In singing styles, such as folk or pop, where the intelligibility of the words and their expression can be particularly important, a more flexible approach to voice production is needed than can be achieved in classical singing styles. This depends on a technique that is more akin to speech and which would make it difficult to sing at high volume. If the performance takes place in a small venue using acoustic instruments there is little problem, but where the venue is large or the accompaniment is electronically enhanced, it may be necessary to use a microphone to maintain the appropriate balance between the instrumental accompaniment and the voice. The same approach may be taken in musicals. In nineteenth-century operettas, such as those of Gilbert and Sullivan, where intelligibility is at a premium and the option of amplification was not originally available, the more complex soprano arias were scored low in the vocal range, backed by only light orchestration, and many male arias are sung in a speechlike declamatory style. In opera, recitative or even speech may be used to take the story forward.

Figure 5.10.   The formant theory of vowel production. The sounds of different vowels can be characterized by the frequencies of the first and second formants, which are controlled largely by the placement of the tongue. A. The relationship between vowel sounds and the first two formant frequencies. The sounds [i], [α], and [u] are known as the corner vowels because they represent the extremes of the vowel space on the graph and also represent the extreme positions of the tongue. B. The tongue positions for the corner vowels together with the frequencies of the first two formants. The broken lines at 500 and 1500 Hz indicate the position of the formants with the tongue in a neutral position, represented by the vowel [ə]. Reproduced with permission from Titze (2000) and Peterson and Barney (1952).

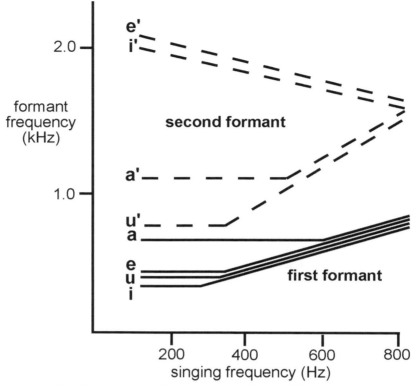

Figure 5-11. Changes in the formant frequencies of different vowels brought about by the tuning of the soprano vocal tract to optimize voice projection. To project the voice efficiently, the singer alters the first formant frequency to track the pitch of the fundamental of the note being sung, for example, by opening the mouth wider. This causes the frequencies of both the first and second formants of different vowels to converge and ultimately become identical, making it impossible to distinguish between them. Reproduced with permission from Sundberg (1972).

The most extreme examples of formant manipulation are encountered among the practitioners of various forms of throat singing (Levin and Edgerton 1999). This is a traditional form of vocalization found in areas of central Asia such as Siberia (e.g., in Tuva), Mongolia, and Tibet. A single drone note, often with *Strohbass* qualities, is sung, sometimes with the involvement of the false vocal folds. The formants of the vocal tract are tuned to a very narrow peak by manipulating the tongue and lips to isolate single harmonics of the drone (typically the sixth and above). By picking these out in a sequence using formant tuning, a melody can be created. Some of the harmonics are out of tune and so must be avoided. By reducing the opening time of the vocal folds during each oscillatory cycle, more energy is transferred to the upper harmonics and sound leakage back into the trachea is reduced, which strengthens the resonance. There are several styles of throat singing, whose qualities vary from the gruff to the ethereal.

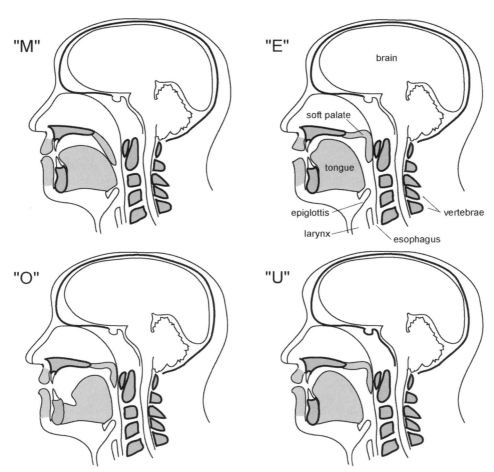

Figure 5-12. Diagrams of the vocal tract during singing the consonant *m* and the vowels *e, o,* and *u*. This shows the different position of the elements of the resonator used in producing these sounds. For *m*, the soft palate is allowed to descend, but for the vowels it seals off the nasal cavity (this is different from speech). Note also the different shape of the tongue and degree of opening of the lips in each case. Adapted from Dana (2000).

The Articulator

We take the role of the tongue and lips in the production of the consonants completely for granted, but with a little experimentation and self-observation, how this is achieved becomes quite obvious. Figure 5-12 shows drawings based on magnetic resonance scans of the head that reveal the different position of the lips, tongue, and soft palate in the generation of different sounds (Dana 2000). The figure shows the soft palate lowered for the consonant *n*, and the same is true for *m*. The sound comes partly or entirely from the nose. For all of the vowels, the soft palate is raised, blocking off the nasopharynx; however, for each the tongue is held in a characteristic way.

This has a dramatic effect on the shape of the oropharynx, and we have already seen its consequences for formant frequency and the sound of individual vowels.

Some languages lend themselves better to the meter and sound-generating requirements of singing; for example, Italian with its many terminal vowels works well while in French, it may be necessary to distort the language, for example, by sounding the letter *e* at the ends of words where it is normally silent in speech. What is more, not all languages have the same repertoire of sounds and inflections; some are completely unique to a particular language or group of languages while others, which at first seem to be similar, may be made in subtly different ways. As a result, learning to speak or sing in another language often requires the learning of new motor patterns for controlling the elements of the articulator. There is, however, a more insidious problem, which is that by the time we reach adulthood, we may have lost the ability to identify or distinguish aurally between certain types of sounds that are not found in our native language. Without this ability, producing the sounds in speech or singing with complete authenticity becomes virtually impossible. This is one reason why someone may be completely fluent in a nonnative language, yet still persist in speaking it with an accent that is strongly foreign to native speakers, reflecting incorrectly produced vowels and consonants.

VOICE PROBLEMS

Singing, particularly if this requires strong projection, makes considerable demands on the physical integrity of the functional elements of the larynx. The vocal folds and their epithelial covering are delicate structures that are vulnerable to hard usage. Direct examination of the folds in a number of studies of singers has revealed a high incidence (60 to 95 percent) of abnormalities, most of which were not at the time associated with voice dysfunction (Lundy et al. 1999; Elias et al. 1997; Heman-Ackah, Dean, and Sataloff 2002). While it is likely that many of these will be a direct consequence of singing itself, others may be a reflection of general health problems that may or may not be obvious to the individual. Stress, poor diet, overindulgence in food or alcohol, and lack of exercise or rest may all contribute to problems with the voice. However, there have so far been no comparisons between matched groups of singers and nonsingers, which might help to clarify these issues.

Environment, Lifestyle, and Medication

Some voice problems arise from environmental conditions. Living or working in an atmosphere that is dry, dusty, or smoky will almost certainly have consequences for the voice. Breathing through the nose, rather than the mouth, ensures that the incoming air is warmed and humidified. The inner walls of the nose carry a set of curved projecting shelves called conchae or turbinate bones, which increase their surface area. These and the other surfaces within the nose are covered with a moist epithelium that humidifies the air passing through it as well as trapping dust particles. The epithelium is well supplied with blood vessels, which also warm the incoming air. In a continental climate, at temperate latitudes, the humidity of the atmosphere can at times be very low, making humidification a much more important issue than it is in more maritime environments. This is particularly acute in winter during prolonged periods of low temperature. Habitually sleeping with the mouth open may contribute to dryness of the vocal tract, and any airborne pollution will also affect the vocal folds. Smoking generates a particularly acute form of irritation due to the high concentrations of smoke particles that are inhaled. This not only irritates the epithelium of the vocal folds; the chemicals in tobacco smoke can also damage the structure and the properties of its cells. This will cause changes to the voice, and may ultimately lead to the appearance of cancerous growths.

Anything that changes the physical properties of the vocal folds will alter the characteristics of the voice. A number of factors can lead to an accumulation of fluid in the tissue of the folds (edema); this may make the voice sound muffled or reduce its vocal range (Sataloff 1995). The fluid often accumulates, particularly within the lamina propria, which lies between the mucosal epithelium and the muscular core of the folds. This region is sometimes known as Reinke's space and, consequently, the fluid retention, Reinke's edema. In extreme cases, the edge of the fold becomes extended and floppy, giving it a characteristic "elephant's ear" appearance (video 5-2). This has a marked effect on voice quality. Paradoxical as it may seem, edema can occur simultaneously with a drying of the surface of the folds.

In women, mild edema may occur for a few days before menses, during pregnancy, or, in a small proportion, as a result of taking oral contraceptives. Common medications such as antihistamines or aspirin may also have effects on the larynx. Antihistamines reduce the secretions from the lining of the nose and throat and may lead to dryness, while one effect of aspirin is to reduce the ability of blood to clot, so any hemorrhaging (bleeding) of the vocal folds may be aggravated. Even elements of the diet can cause vocal problems. In some people, for example, milk products or fats cause changes in the mucus secretions of the nose and throat, making them thicker and more troublesome after eating.

Laryngitis

This is one of the most common vocal disorders. It is caused by an inflammation of tissues in the larynx and is most often the result either of an infection or of gastroesophageal reflux (heartburn—see below). Infection of the respiratory tract by bacteria or more commonly by viruses (e.g., during a cold infection) results in a swelling of the lining of the larynx due to fluid retention (edema), which is part of the normal response of the body to infection. This causes hoarseness as the thickening of the vocal folds that results restricts their freedom to vibrate. Normal cold treatments together with resting of the voice are in order, and though corticosteroids are sometimes employed to counter severe swelling, their frequent use is not recommended. In fact, inhaled steroids and anesthetic sprays seldom help and may actually cause harm, particularly if they are used to allow performance to continue before the infection has been resolved. Though steroids may reduce inflammation of the vocal folds, the blood vessels within them remain fragile; singing under these conditions is associated with an increased risk of bleeding, which may have both short- and long-term consequences for the voice (Hanson and Jiang 1998). We have seen that the precise control of the larynx is dependent on feedback from sensory nerves in the vocal folds; anesthetic sprays used to block the pain of a sore throat will equally affect nerves carrying information that is needed to control the pitch of the voice and therefore be avoided if the singer absolutely must perform. During laryngitis, it is important to rest the voice as much as possible (even from talking), particularly at the height of the infection when heavy voice use may result in long-lasting problems (Koufman 1992). Many singers believe that even whispering should be avoided in these circumstances. The major reason for this is that though the vocal folds are held predominantly open, the edges may make periodic contact during whispered speech. Because the tissue is inflamed in laryngitis, it is particularly vulnerable to abrasion. The likelihood of vocal fold contact during whispering appears to be greater in individuals in whom the folds show an outward kinking during this form of speech than in those in whom the vocal folds are held straight, so it may not be an equally risky activity in all singers (Solomon et al. 1989). The air turbulence generated in the larynx during whispering may also tend to dry out the mucosa, which will not be beneficial to recovery.

Gastroesophageal Reflux (Heartburn)

Laryngitis is sometimes the result of damage to the mucosal epithelium caused when the acid contents of the stomach rise up into the esophagus and reach the larynx. The lining of the stomach is resistant to attack by the acid, which is produced by glands in its walls as a normal function of digestion, but the lining of the esophagus and larynx is not so protected. When the acid enters the esophagus, it is perceived as heartburn due to the irritation it causes to the epithelium. Singers with this condition do not always experience heartburn, but symptoms such as occasional hoarseness not associated with infection, a feeling of a lump in the throat, difficulty in swallowing, halitosis, or a bitter taste in the mouth may all be a consequence of acid reflux. The symptoms are often experienced on first waking. Frequent throat clearing to remove excess mucus, which is produced in order to protect the pharynx from the acid, may also be a symptom. Many aspects of professional singers' lifestyles predispose them to gastroesophageal reflux (Sataloff 1987). Singers generally perform with an empty stomach, as a full one makes optimal breathing strategies and support difficult and because the redistribution of blood to the digestive organs induces a feeling of mental and physical lethargy. Consequently, the main meal is frequently eaten late at night after the performance and therefore not long before sleeping. This means that the stomach is active and filled with acidic liquid when the body is lying horizontally in bed, making reflux more likely. Treatments for gastroesophageal reflux include medications that neutralize or reduce the secretion of gastric acid. Simple changes in behavior, such as not lying down until a couple of hours after eating, and raising the head, neck, and upper body with pillows while sleeping, will also help (Hanson and Jiang 1998).

A number of other vocal fold problems may result from gastroesophageal reflux, including the development of growths of various types. Reinke's edema we have already mentioned. Another is the appearance of granulomas, which are swellings filled with white blood cells that are removing damaged cells or infectious agents that have entered the affected area. The first stage of treatment for any such secondary problem is to identify and address the underlying cause, but surgery may occasionally be appropriate for granulomas and for Reinke's edema if persistent in the face of this approach. If this is necessary, great care must be taken to prevent damage to the free edge of the vocal fold, which will produce scarring that will badly affect the voice (Sataloff 1998). However, it must be remembered that the characteristically low pitch and instability of the voice produced by the edema is for some people an integral part of their vocal identity, in which case radical treatment is inappropriate unless it is thought to be related to some serious pathology such as cancer (Sataloff 1998). Small cancerous growths are sometimes seen on the vocal folds, though these are far less common than most of the other lesions described here.

Vocal Fold Polyps

Polyps are swellings that are typically seen on only one vocal fold. They may arise directly from the surface of the fold, or be attached to it by a thin stalk, and are often supplied by a well-developed small blood vessel. Indeed the polyp may first arise as a result of a hemorrhage (bleeding) from such a vessel. Though benign (noncancerous), they may, if allowed to grow, ultimately interfere with the movement of the other vocal fold. In some cases they will disappear spontaneously following rest and mild steroid treatment but often require surgery.

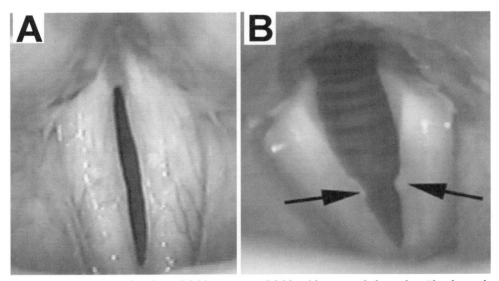

Figure 5-13.   Photographs of vocal folds. A. Normal folds with a smooth free edge. Blood vessels run mainly parallel to the edge. B. Vocal folds with nodules. Note that there is one on each fold and that these lie opposite each other. They resemble calluses and are formed where the folds impact most strongly together. In this photograph the folds are open (abducted) to reveal the rings of the trachea beneath. In both images the back of the larynx is at the top. Reproduced with the permission of Clark Rosen, M.D., University of Pittsburgh Voice Center (voicecenter.upmc.com).

Voice Abuse

This rather dramatic term refers to very loud singing or shouting, overuse of pressed phonation, or forcing the voice beyond its natural range. Problems can also arise as a result of using a very strong glottal attack at the onset of the note. The damage caused to the vocal folds is due to the force with which they are brought together under these conditions. This can cause bleeding, tearing of the mucosal epithelium covering the folds (ulceration), and the development of granulomas (see above) or of vocal nodules (fig. 5-13, video 5-2). Vocal nodules are small calluses (thickenings of the epithelium) that always appear in pairs, opposing each other where the vocal folds impact most strongly (Koufman 1992). Though they do not always affect voice quality, they are, together with other effects of vocal abuse (Elias et al. 1997), often associated with hoarseness (dysphonia). Vocal nodules are more common in rock, jazz, and gospel singers, who frequently employ singing techniques (such as pressed phonation) that have similarities to shouting or screaming (Koufman 1993). The treatment of vocal nodules has excited some debate. As for most medical conditions that are the result of a particular activity, the best approach is to eliminate the cause. If this is not done, then even if the nodules disappear following treatment or are surgically removed, they will return again when the original singing pattern is resumed. Vocal nodules will generally (though not always) reduce spontaneously, either with voice retraining alone or, if appropriate, with treatment for gastroesophageal reflux. This is reflected in an improvement in voice quality (Holmberg et al. 2001). The growth of vocal nodules is often associated with a forward movement of the arytenoid cartilages. As a result, the posterior parts of the vocal folds are hidden when viewed from above, and the posterior part of the glottis may fail to close during phonation (Pontes et al. 2002; Koufman 1993). This symptom can be seen to disappear as retraining progresses. The training may have to continue for several months, but has an almost identical success rate in terms of restoration of voice quality (70 percent) to surgical intervention (Koufman and Blalock 1991), which is popular with some practitioners but carries significant risks. Retraining should therefore always be the treatment of first resort. If this fails, surgery may be indicated and if carried out by a careful and experienced surgeon can be highly successful, but the singer must be fully aware of the risks in order to give informed consent to the operation.

Vocal Misuse

Like vocal abuse, vocal misuse refers to inappropriate use of the voice, which in the long run is unsustainable. It can also arise from singing outside the natural range (tessitura) of the voice or by altering its quality deliberately for the purpose of characterization (Koufman and Blalock 1991). The difference between vocal abuse and vocal misuse is that the effects of the latter are less extreme, but because the causative behavior is sustainable for longer, it may have become more ingrained and therefore is harder to correct. The problems may arise from using higher tensions than are necessary in the laryngeal muscles. High muscle tensions may also be used in an attempt to compensate inappropriately for mild laryngitis when swelling of the laryngeal tissue makes it more difficult to maintain vibrations of the vocal folds. Good vocal technique involves the optimization of all aspects of phonation: breath support, control of laryngeal height and muscle activity, voice projection, and articulation. If one or more of these elements are deficient, a short-term compensation may be possible through overuse of the laryngeal muscles, however, ultimately this will break down, and the only recourse is to perfect all aspects of voice control. Singing, like many other musical activities, requires prolonged, highly controlled, and sometimes forceful muscle activity. Warm-up routines, in which the muscles are gradually prepared for heavy use, are very beneficial in preventing unnecessary tension when the full voice is finally unleashed. Mental preparation is equally a part of this process, as it allows the techniques required for the coordination of each of the various aspects of voice production to be refreshed and rehearsed in a nonstressful way.

In terms of voice care, a singer will naturally concentrate mainly on regulating his or her singing activities, but care of the voice when speaking should not be neglected. The ambient noise at social events can reach very high levels, particularly in restaurants or reception rooms with bare, reverberant walls. Speaking loudly to maintain a conversation in such places may entail using pressed phonation, which can be damaging to the edges of the vocal folds in just the same way as other forms of voice misuse. This can be easily forgotten in the relaxed atmosphere of a postperformance meal or party.

Singers are fortunate to have many sources of practical information on voice care as well as access to significant numbers of clinicians with experience of the singing voice. For example, *Care of the Professional Voice* by Davies and Jahn is a compact source of useful authoritative information (Davies and Jahn 2004). Those who wish to go into this in more detail may find it useful to consult Sataloff's two-volume *Vocal Health and Pedagogy*, now available in paperback (Sataloff 2006a, 2006b).

HOW THE VOICE CHANGES THROUGHOUT LIFE

The Young Voice

The two most important factors in determining the pitch of the voice are the length and the mass of the vocal folds (fig. 5-14A). At birth, the larynx is small, the vocal folds are short, and the mean pitch of the voice is about 500 Hz (around B4). The larynx initially grows rapidly so that by the age of three mean pitch has fallen to around 300 Hz (D4), but from this age until puberty, growth is much slower and mean pitch falls only a further 25–30 Hz. During this period, however, other changes take place. For example, at birth there is no well-defined vocal ligament; this only becomes distinct from the rest of the lamina propria at about the age of eight. At this age the voice typically has a range of up to two and a half octaves. This remains virtually constant until the midteens, and any attempt to increase range during this period is likely to be damaging. Voice training of children should therefore be restricted to improving sound quality and pitch control (Sataloff, Spiegel, and Rosen 1998). The muscles and the mucosal lining of the larynx are delicate in children and easily damaged. Child performers should not be expected to sing as frequently as adults, and in shows with regular performances, child leads should be alternated among several individuals to

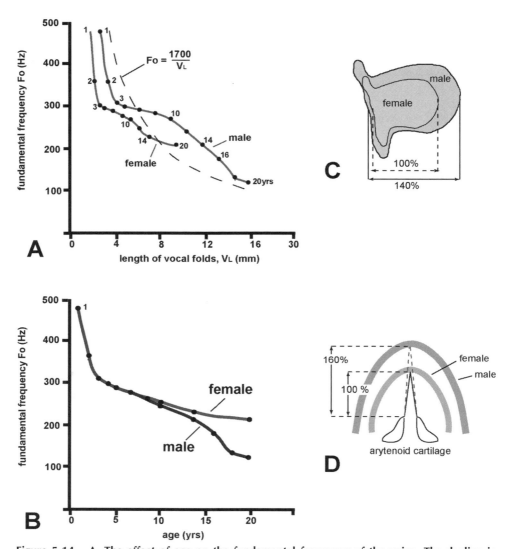

Figure 5-14. A. The effect of age on the fundamental frequency of the voice. The decline in fundamental frequency from childhood to maturity reflects a change in the length of the vibrating segment of the vocal folds (the vocal ligament). This is plotted for males and females. The dashed line indicates the ideal curve that would be produced if vocal fold length was the only factor controlling frequency. The deviations from this are probably due to changes in the structure and physical characteristics of the folds. Because the data are averages, the abrupt change in frequency when the voice breaks in adolescent males is smoothed out. In B, the data has been replotted to show the change in pitch with age. C. The difference in the dimensions of the laryngeal cartilages in adult males and females. This is shown in the horizontal section in D. Because the arytenoid cartilages form proportionately less of the fold in males, the difference in the length of the vocal ligaments is 60 percent while the difference in the depth of the thyroid cartilage is only 40 percent. Reproduced with permission from Titze (2000).

avoid damaging the voice. The signs of vocal abuse (e.g., hemorrhaging of the vocal folds, the development of vocal nodules, edema) are seen in children as well as adults and can arise either as a result of singing or from prolonged habitual screaming (Reilly 1997).

Of course, the most rapid changes in voice quality take place at puberty. This typically begins between the ages of nine and fifteen and lasts around eighteen months, though it can take up to twice as long (fig. 5-14A, C). The greatest changes in voice quality are generally experienced between the ages of twelve and fourteen (Spiegel, Sataloff, and Emerich 1997). In young children, the larynx is the same size in both sexes, but during puberty the male larynx grows more rapidly. By the end of puberty the thyroid cartilage of the larynx is 40 percent greater in the male than it is in the female (fig. 5-14B, D). It sits prominently in the neck as the Adam's apple, which has a sharper prow-shaped front edge than the female larynx. The male vocal folds increase in length by up to 60 percent. The change in pitch that occurs around puberty cannot be accounted for solely by the increased length of the vocal folds (fig. 5-14C). It is also affected by an increase in the mass of the muscular core of the fold and a thickening of its mucosal covering, both of which are affected by rising levels of male sex hormones (androgens) such as testosterone. As a result, the mean vocal pitch falls by about an octave to 130 Hz (C3). In females, the vocal folds exhibit only about half the increase in length seen in males and mean vocal pitch descends by only two to three half-steps to about 220 Hz (A3). The maturation of the muscles of the larynx lags behind the growth of the vocal folds. One consequence of this is a tendency toward breathiness in the voice of adolescent female singers. This may be due in part to a weakness in the interarytenoid muscle, which appears to play a key role not only in holding the vocal folds closed, but also in stabilizing the joint between the arytenoid and cricoid cartilages (Tellis et al. 2004).

The changes in the voice at puberty are not due solely to the development of the larynx. As the body grows, the length and width of the pharynx also increase, changing its resonant properties. In addition, the tonsils are large in children and can block the passage to the back of the nose, making the voice sound nasal. In most children, the tonsils are easily visible at the back of the throat but they decrease rapidly in size during the teenage years and in most adults are barely detectable. The respiratory muscles also become stronger and the volume of the chest increases postpubertally. Muscle strength peaks in the early twenties before vocal skills are fully developed, and the young adult singer must resist the temptation to use brute force to increase the volume of the voice in order to compensate for inadequacies in vocal projection techniques, as this can have long-term consequences for vocal health (Spiegel, Sataloff, and Emerich 1997). Empirical evidence suggests that when the voice is changing during puberty, adolescents should be discouraged from heavy voice use and that boy sopranos and altos should not try to maintain these voices for as long as possible in the face of the hormonal onslaught. Sataloff proposes that a light diet of choral singing can be safely continued by allowing the male voices to break naturally during a piece so that each phrase is delivered in the register that is most comfortable (Sataloff et al. 1997). Though some authors have suggested that intensive vocal training can continue and indeed be beneficial during this period (Blatt 1983), such a view is highly contro-versial and is not supported by the majority of vocal teachers.

Psychological factors have the ability to influence the voice at many ages, but emotional turmoil is often particularly acute during adolescence and young adulthood. Insomnia, anorexia, and bulimia are common consequences of this in today's world. Bulimia has a particularly direct effect on the voice, as bringing up food from the stomach exposes the throat and vocal folds to acids that can damage and ultimately scar them. A stressful or frantic lifestyle involving poor eating and drinking habits can also lead to gastroesophageal reflux, with similar consequences (Spiegel, Sataloff, and Emerich 1997; Tepe et al. 2002).

Hormones and the Female Voice

For young women, the onset of puberty heralds the appearance of the cyclical hor-monal fluctuations of the menstrual cycle and for some (though not all) this can have significant consequences for vocal performance. In order to understand how this comes about, it is first necessary to describe the sequence of events that underlie the cycle. The menstrual cycle is ultimately controlled by signals that originate in the brain, which cause the release into the bloodstream of follicle-stimulating hormone and leutinizing hormone from the pituitary gland. The effects on the body are brought about by fluctuations in the levels of sex hormones that as a result are released into the bloodstream. These come mainly from the ovaries, and the most important are estro-gen and progesterone. As its name suggests (*menses* is the Latin word for "month"), the cycle lasts approximately twenty-eight days (though there is some variation be-tween individuals), and it can be divided into a number of distinct phases (fig. 5-15). Because menstruation is the most obvious manifestation of the cycle, the day on which this commences is designated day 1. Menstruation lasts about seven days, during which time the inner lining (endometrium) of the uterus (womb) is shed. The ovaries contain a large number of egg cells (ova), each of which lies within a structure known as a follicle, which is responsible for hormone production. From the end of menses, the amount of estrogen released by the follicles starts to rise rapidly, stimulating the regeneration of the endometrial lining of the uterus in preparation for the possible im-plantation of an egg. The uterine lining must acquire a structure capable of supporting a fetus. In order to do this, it becomes thicker and develops an extensive new network of blood vessels. This is the proliferative phase of the cycle and lasts about a week. If a fertilized egg later implants and develops, the blood vessels of the embryo will grow close to those in the wall of the uterus to form the placenta, a structure that allows nutrients and oxygen to diffuse from the maternal to the fetal circulation. Glands also develop in the uterine lining, producing either mucus or nutrients for the embryo. Dur-ing the proliferative phase, the glands at the neck of the womb (the cervix) produce a watery mucus. This phase ends around day 14 with the release of the egg (ovulation) from the ovary. This marks the transition from the follicular half of the cycle to the luteal half. The follicle that is left behind continues to produce hormones, but over several days the levels of estrogen decline before rising once more, while the produc-tion of progesterone steadily increases. The progesterone causes the uterine lining

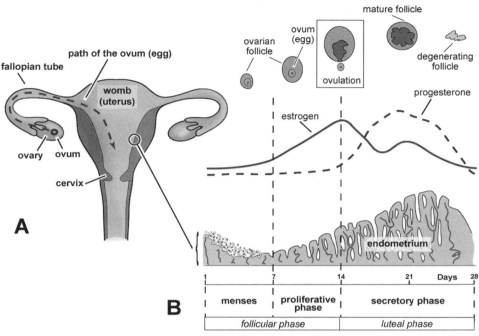

Figure 5-15. Hormonal fluctuations during the ovarian cycle. A. The ovaries and uterus. A human egg (ovum) develops in the ovary and is released into the fallopian tube by means of which it reaches the uterus. If fertilized by sperm, it will implant into the wall of the uterus and develop into a fetus; otherwise it is expelled through the neck of the womb (cervix) into the vagina. B. In preparation for implantation, the lining of the womb (the endometrium) changes in structure over the menstrual cycle under the influence of the hormones estrogen and progesterone, which are produced by the tissue that surrounded the egg (the follicle). This tissue remains in the ovary when the egg is released. The onset of menstruation (menses) is designated as day 1 of the menstrual cycle. At this time, tissue from the endometrium that developed during the previous cycle is lost. At the end of menses, levels of estrogen start to rise. The endometrium thickens and its blood supply develops. When estrogen levels peak, ovulation takes place and progesterone levels start to rise, further preparing the endometrium for implantation. If this does not happen, the levels of progesterone and estrogen begin to fall as the follicle degenerates until menses is initiated once more.

to develop further in preparation for implantation and the mucus from the cervix to become thicker. This is the secretory phase of the cycle, and unless an egg is fertilized and implants into the endometrium, it lasts for about a fortnight, after which the follicle degenerates and ceases to produce hormones.

At puberty, an increase in the level of sex hormones causes other changes in the body. Estrogens stimulate breast development and the typical female pattern of fat deposition, particularly on the hips and thighs. Fatty tissue is itself a minor source of estrogens. However, "male" hormones (androgens) are also present in women and are secreted from glands (the adrenals) that sit on top of the kidneys. These stimulate the growth of pubic and armpit hair and control female libido. High levels of androgens, for example due to adrenal tumors, can cause the vocal pitch of young girls to fall, but there is no evidence that these hormones normally have a role in the changes in the female voice at puberty. Rather, this is correlated with the rise in circulating estrogens (Pedersen et al. 1990).

Armed with this information, we are ready to consider the effects of female sex hormones on the voice. Hormones are signal molecules and the body tissues on which they act must contain proteins known as receptors, which will bind to them if they are to have any effect. If the hormones are the keys, the receptors represent the locks. When the two come together, this triggers changes in the behavior of the cells that make up the tissue. As the female larynx contains receptors that can bind estrogens, progesterone, or androgens, all of these hormones have the potential to affect the voice. Not all singers experience obvious vocal changes related to the monthly fluctuations in hormone levels, but in about one-third it causes some problems with the voice. The effects of estrogen and progesterone on the larynx are in some ways similar to the effects that they have on the uterus (Abitbol, Abitbol, and Abitbol 1999). For example, the rise in levels of estrogen prior to ovulation may thicken the mucosa of the larynx and increase its watery secretions. This can alter voice quality to a small degree around the time of ovulation, but this is usually minor and causes few problems. The most troublesome changes in the voice occur in the four to five days prior to menstruation (see table 5-3). The rising levels of progesterone reduce the amount of fluid secreted by the laryngeal mucosa. This thickens its consistency with the result that the surfaces of the vocal folds become drier. At the same time, there is an increase in the amount of fluid retained within the folds and a fall in the tone (tension) of the laryngeal muscles. This causes a reduction in the fundamental frequency of the voice and can lead to a curtailment of its upper range. The small blood vessels on the upper surface of the folds become distended and are prone to rupture. It is advisable that singers should avoid using aspirin or ibuprofen to treat premenstrual pain or discomfort as both inhibit blood clotting and consequently will worsen the effects of any bleeding that arises within the vocal folds. Painkillers such as acetaminophen or codeine do not have this effect. Where treatment is required for premenstrual vocal problems, this may be purely to provide symptomatic relief (e.g., anti-inflammatory drugs to reduce edema); however, hormone fluctuations can also

Table 5-3.   Physical and Vocal Symptoms of Premenstrual Syndrome

Physical Change	Vocal Consequence
Dryness and loss of vocal fold suppleness Thickened laryngeal mucus	Reduced amplitude of vocal fold movement (reduced volume)
Loss of muscle tone in larynx (opening of glottal chink)	Vocal fatigue Reduced vocal power Breathiness
Enlarged veins on vocal folds	Increased chance of bleeding (especially if taking aspirin)
Edema (water retention) of vocal folds, reducing amplitude of vibration and increasing mass	Loss of upper range of the voice Loss of upper harmonics Reduced fundamental frequency

be eliminated by using oral contraceptives (which may present their own problems, as described below).

Contraceptives

In the 1960s, investigations into the effects of the first oral contraceptives revealed that some had adverse effects on the voice, and this led to the recommendation that they should be avoided by professional singers (Wendler et al. 1995). Many oral contraceptives contain two components, one a synthetic estrogen and the other a synthetic progesterone. These have three main actions: 1) to prevent ovulation, 2) to thicken the mucus at the entrance to the womb, which makes it difficult for sperm to enter, and 3) to make the lining of the womb unable to support an implanted embryo. The problem for singers is that one class of progesterone-like compounds used in some of these early contraceptive pills (the 19-norsteroids) mimics to some degree the action of androgens (male hormones) on the larynx. These compounds can potentially masculinize the larynx by inducing it to grow, which causes the average pitch of the voice to fall slightly. Even when present in the small amounts found in certain modern contraceptives that are not expected to affect the voice, 19-norsteroids can cause hoarseness or discomfort in the throat (Wendler et al. 1995). In many pills, however, they are replaced by synthetic hormones that not only mimic progesterone, but block androgenic effects. As a result, they can also reduce other unwelcome actions of androgens such as greasy skin, acne, and excessive growth of body hair. Studies of women using low-dose contraceptives that contain such alternatives to the 19-norsteroids strongly suggest that they do not have adverse effects on the voice (Amir, Kishon-Rabin, and Muchnik 2002) and may even have beneficial properties, such as reducing jitter and shimmer (irregularities in frequency and amplitude of the voice, respectively) (Amir and Kishon-Rabin 2004; Amir et al. 2003). Though the results presented in these studies agree with what one would predict, it should be noted that they involved only small numbers of women, none of whom were trained singers. However, a recent study has examined the effects of a third-generation combined pill (ethinylestradiol/drospirenone) on the singing voices of a small group of classically trained, semiprofessional singers (La et al. 2007). During the luteal half of the menstrual cycle, hormone levels were similar in the placebo and the pill group but during the follicular half, levels of follicle-stimulating hormone, leutinizing hormone, and testosterone were reduced, and though no change was observed in jitter, shimmer was also reduced. It was suggested that the effect on shimmer in the pill group might be due to a reduction in the incidence of menstrually related abdominal cramps, which can interfere with support, and the absence of vocal fold edema. Nonetheless, as masculinization of the larynx is largely irreversible, any decision about the use and choice of contraceptives should be taken under the guidance of a physician with experience both in vocal function and in the formulation of different contraceptive preparations.

Menopause and Hormone Replacement Therapy

The onset of menopause typically occurs around the age of fifty and can have a significant effect on voice quality. At this time, ovulation ends and the ovaries cease to produce estrogen and progesterone. Though the levels of sex hormones in the blood-stream decline significantly, they do not fall to zero. At this time, fat cells become the dominant source of estrogens, though the quantities generated are relatively small. The raw material for the production of estrogens is androgens, for which the adrenal glands are the major source, just as they were prior to menopause. Though the quantities are quite small, the levels of enzymes in fat tissue that are responsible for converting androgens to estrogens are higher in postmenopausal women (Misso et al. 2005). The changes in circulating hormone levels have a number of consequences. We have already seen that fluctuations in hormone levels during the menstrual cycle affect the secretions of the mucosal lining of the larynx, and their decline at menopause leads to a thinning of the mucosa and a reduction in the glands that keep it moist (Abitbol, Abitbol, and Abitbol 1999). This contributes to a reduction in the suppleness of the vocal folds, which limits their ability to vibrate freely. There is also a reduction in muscle strength, not only in the larynx, but throughout the body (Greeves et al. 1999), including the respiratory muscles, and this, in conjunction with the changes in the mucosa, can lead to a reduction in vocal intensity and range. These symptoms are accompanied by a decline in the speed of articulation (Meurer et al. 2004). In many women there may be no significant change in the pitch of the voice, but in others it may fall (Lindholm et al. 1997; Abitbol, Abitbol, and Abitbol 1999). Whether this occurs depends on the relative levels of estrogens and androgens circulating in the blood and is correlated with body type. Abitbol et al. (1999) explain this in terms of two types of female figures. The Rubenesque figure has considerable subcutaneous fat, and as the cells that make up this tissue produce estrogens, the ratio of estrogens to androgens remains high, helping to ensure that the pitch of the voice remains at its premenopausal level. In women with a thinner Modigliani-type figure, the much smaller amount of subcutaneous fat means that the balance of circulating hormones swings in favor of the androgens. These can consequently have a masculinizing effect on the voice by triggering growth of the larynx and a fall in vocal pitch after menopause. In addition, the change in the hormonal balance may contribute to dryness of the vocal fold edges (Lindholm et al. 1997; Abitbol, Abitbol, and Abitbol 1999). Though it does not affect the voice directly, the decline in estrogen causes a reduction in the retention of calcium by the bones (osteoporosis), which makes them weaker and more prone to collapse or breakage. One consequence of osteoporosis of the spine is that the shoulders may become rounded and the body stooped, both of which tend to reduce lung capacity.

Many of the changes caused by menopause can be prevented or reversed by hormone replacement therapy (HRT), which is frequently used to combat osteoporosis and other unpleasant symptoms of menopause such as hot flashes, vaginal dryness, mood changes, and insomnia. It may also reduce the likelihood of conditions such as cardiovascular and Alzheimer's disease, though this remains controversial. HRT is often prescribed for women who have entered menopause prematurely, for example, as a consequence of surgical removal of the ovaries or of a hysterectomy. Though where possible the ovaries are left in the body during the latter operation, the loss of the womb can still lead to early menopause. HRT does carry a small increased risk of blood clots and certain types of cancer (notably of the breast and womb) and so is not generally recommended for women with a family history of these conditions, but many women consider that the small risk is outweighed by the benefits in quality of life. As with contraceptives, the effect of HRT on the voice depends on the precise formulation prescribed. In general the treatment should aim to return the concentration of circulating sex hormones to premenopausal levels. Some forms of HRT include steroids with androgenic properties. These may be offered orally or by injection for such conditions as endometriosis, fibrocystic breast disease, or the low energy and decreased libido that may follow hysterectomy. At any age, these androgens can cause irreversible masculinization of the voice. Over a period of only a few weeks, such treatment can alter the pitch of the voice to a degree that would abruptly terminate the career of a professional singer (Baker 1999). In the eventuality that a singer notices any voice changes with such medication, she should seek medical advice immediately and in general should avoid this type of treatment where at all possible because of the permanent nature of the vocal changes.

The Musici

No discussion of the effects of hormones on the voice would be complete without a consideration of the castrati, or, as they were rather more flatteringly known in Italy, the Musici. Records of the castrati performing in the churches and great private houses of Italy first appear in the mid-sixteenth century (Jenkins 1998; Pain 2006). Around a hundred years later they began to feature in performances of opera, where they reached the peak of their popularity in the first half of the eighteenth century (Somerset-Ward 2004). Though they performed all over Europe, the greatest demand for castrati during this period was in London, where the best performers could command immense fees. Leopold Mozart reports that in order to secure the services of the famous castrato Manzuoli for the 1764–1765 London season, it was necessary to guarantee him a fee of £1,500 in advance before he would even leave Italy and that in a single benefit concert in London on March 7, 1765, he made a profit of 1,000 guineas (Anderson 1990). Two of the best known castrati who spent time in London were Carlo Broschi (who went under the stage name of Farinelli) and Gaetano Majorano (Cafarelli). Cafarelli sang there for Handel during the 1737–1738 season. The fourteen-year-old Mozart met both of these musici when he visited Italy in 1770; Farinelli at his estate near Bologna and Cafarelli in Naples, where he had bought himself a dukedom and built an opulent villa. With the irreverence of youth, Mozart described Cafarelli as "a very rich castrato who goes around singing in churches to scrape up a few coins" (Anderson 1990). With the increasing involvement of female singers, public taste for the singing of the castrati declined toward the end of the eighteenth century. Rossini and Meyerbeer were among the last major composers who composed parts for them. Wagner toyed briefly with the idea of writing the role of Klingsor in *Parsifal* for a castrato singer called Mustafa, who is regarded as the last of the virtuoso castrati (Scammell 1987), but in the end discarded the idea.

Despite documentary evidence for castrati in Vatican choirs from 1589 until the retirement of the last one (Alessandro Moreschi) in 1913, castration for nonmedical reasons was always against the law of the church but was conveniently ignored, partly because of the interdiction against female singers in church choirs. Castrato singers were never popular in France, and between 1807 and 1815, Napoleon briefly effected a ban on them when he held control of the Papal States, but it was not until Garibaldi's forces entered Rome in 1870 and the Catholic Church lost all temporal power that the law against it was finally enforced.

The potential wealth that successful castrati could earn in the eighteenth century was a powerful incentive for many poor families to encourage one of their sons to undergo the operation, though the chances of reaching the heights of the profession, or even making a good living from it, were relatively small (Somerset-Ward 2004), as neither the ultimate quality of the voice nor the singer's dedication for the intense training that the profession demanded could be predicted. Castration was usually carried out on boys between seven and nine years of age so that when the normal time of puberty was reached there was little change in the size of the larynx and their voices remained relatively high. During the teenage years, their bodies grew in height as they would normally, and indeed for their time they often became taller than their peers because the absence of male hormones delayed the end of the growth of the long bones. However, they developed no facial hair and subcutaneous fat was deposited in the female pattern. Their skin was smooth and their hair fine and abundant, as they did not suffer from testosterone-dependent male-pattern baldness. Though a few of the castrati, notably Farinelli, had a voice that reached into the upper soprano range, most had what we would now regard as mezzo-soprano (e.g., Cafarelli) or alto voices (Somerset-Ward 2004).

Joachim Quantz heard Farinelli sing in Milan in 1726 and described his voice as follows: "Farinelli had a penetrating, full, rich, bright and consistent soprano voice, whose range extended from the A below middle C to the D three octaves above. . . . His intonation was pure, his trillo beautiful, his breath control remarkable and his throat very flexible, so that he performed the widest intervals quickly and with the greatest ease and certainty. Passage work and runs were of no difficulty to him and in the adagio his ornamentation was very extensive" (Quantz 1754).

A range of this size was highly unusual among the castrati, for whom two octaves or less was more typical. The castrato voice was said by some to have the clarity and purity associated with that of a choirboy, but, as it was produced by a body with the resonant qualities and lung development of an adult, was a great deal more powerful (Jenkins 2001). Its properties were enhanced by a formidable training regimen. Cafarelli's daily eight-hour schedule included practice of technically difficult passages, expressive singing, and deportment while performing. Their technical abilities were described as prodigious. It was reported that Farinelli could hold a single note for over a minute without taking a breath, and though this may have been an exaggeration, one contemporary score indicates a single note held for thirty seconds and ending in a sustained fortissimo (Depalle, Garcia, and Rodet 1995). Though many eighteenth-century castrati were notorious for their extravagant exhibitions of pyrotechnical coloratura singing and elaborate improvisation, many were famed for their mellifluous and expressive performances.

The last surviving castrato was Alessandro Moreschi, who became a member of the choir of the Sistine Chapel in 1883 and its conductor in 1889. He continued to sing in the choir until his retirement in 1913. In 1902 and 1904, sound recordists from the London division of the Gramophone and Typewriter Company visited Rome to record the voice of the nonagenarian Pope Leo XIII; however, today they are remembered not for this, but for their recordings of Moreschi (Moreschi 1987). Moreschi was never one of the great virtuoso castrati, and by 1902 he was already past his prime as a singer; nevertheless, these recordings, which are available commercially, do give a hint of the quality of this otherwise lost sound world.

The Aging Voice

If one compares recordings of the same singer at different periods over a long career, it is immediately apparent that there are significant changes in voice quality over time. Though some of this will reflect a maturation of technique, it will also partly be due to physical changes in the body and larynx. At the latter end of a career, these changes may start to interfere noticeably with performance. Voice tremor, loss of range, vocal stamina, and breath control, and difficulty in regulating pitch may start to become evident. Some of these problems arise from changes in the vocal folds, which with age become thinner and less elastic and their edges less smooth (Sataloff, Spiegel, and Rosen 1998). Other changes are related to a decline in the efficiency of the muscles of the larynx and of the respiratory system. The consequences of menopause aside, some deterioration in the voice is inevitable in both sexes; however, it is possible to exert considerable influence over the rate at which this happens. One outcome of recent research in the field of human aging has been the appreciation that the rate of physical decline varies greatly between individuals; that is, some people age much more successfully than others. Though partly genetic, it is to a considerable degree related to lifestyle and attitude. For example, though the muscles gradually grow weaker, muscle bulk is strongly dependent on exercise regardless of age. If an arm or leg is immobilized following a fracture, its muscles waste rapidly even in the young. In older people, muscle strength and resistance to fatigue can be retained to a great degree through regular exercise. Maintaining a reasonable level of fitness through activities such as walking, swimming, or sports will help condition the respiratory muscles required for singing, while vocal exercises can be used to counter newly arising technical problems such as vocal tremor. Older singers can also use the skills developed over a professional lifetime to enable them to perform closer to the limit of their abilities and thus compensate for some loss of facility. In putting into effect strategies that will allow the extension of a performing career, attitude is all-important. When young, we tackle technical obstacles confidently because we have an expectation that we will be able to overcome them. A similar level of self-belief is needed for a satisfactory outcome in later years. One should not expect necessarily to continue singing the same repertoire; indeed, opera singers see the changing roles they perform during their careers as part of a logical progression. For those in whom singing is recreational, the physical nature of performing can itself be seen as part of an exercise regimen that will not only provide physical benefit, but through its social dimension will contribute to mental health. For further information on this subject the reader is referred to Sataloff et al. (1997) and Sataloff, Spiegel, and Rosen (1998).

REFERENCES

Abitbol, J., P. Abitbol, and B. Abitbol. 1999. Sex hormones and the female voice. *J Voice* 13 (3):424–46.

Amir, O., T. Biron-Shental, C. Muchnik, and L. Kishon-Rabin. 2003. Do oral contraceptives improve vocal quality? Limited trial on low-dose formulations. *Obstet Gynecol* 101 (4):773–77.

Amir, O., and L. Kishon-Rabin. 2004. Association between birth control pills and voice quality. *Laryngoscope* 114 (6):1021–26.

Amir, O., L. Kishon-Rabin, and C. Muchnik. 2002. The effect of oral contraceptives on voice: Preliminary observations. *J Voice* 16 (2):267–73.

Anderson, E. 1990. *The letters of Mozart and his family.* 3rd ed. London: Macmillan.

Andreatta, R. D., E. A. Mann, C. J. Poletto, and C. L. Ludlow. 2002. Mucosal afferents mediate laryngeal adductor responses in the cat. *J Appl Physiol* 93 (5):1622–29.

Baker, J. 1999. A report on alterations to the speaking and singing voices of four women following hormonal therapy with virilizing agents. *J Voice* 13 (4):496–507.

Benninger, M. S., M. A. Carwell, E. M. Finnegan, R. Miller, and H. L. Levine. 1989. Flexible direct nasopharyngolaryngoscopy in association with vocal pedagogy. *Med Prob Perform Artists* 4:163–67.

Blatt, I. M. 1983. Training singing children during the phases of voice mutation. *Ann Otol Rhinol Laryngol* 92 (5 Pt 1):462–68.

Bouhuys, A., D. F. Proctor, and J. Mead. 1966. Kinetic aspects of singing. *J Appl Physiol* 21 (2):483–96.

Bradley, R. M. 2000. Sensory receptors of the larynx. *Am J Med* 108 (Suppl 4a):47S–50S.

Brandon, C. A., C. Rosen, G. Georgelis, M. J. Horton, M. P. Mooney, and J. J. Sciote. 2003. Staining of human thyroarytenoid muscle with myosin antibodies reveals some unique extrafusal fibers, but no muscle spindles. *J Voice* 17 (2):245–54.

Dana, P. 2000. Orofacial problems. In *Medical problems of the instrumental musician*, ed. R. Tubiana and P. C. Amadio. London: Martin Dunitz.

Davies, D. G., and A. F. Jahn. 2004. *Care of the professional voice.* 2nd ed. London: A & C Black.

Davis, P. J., and B. S. Nail. 1987. Quantitative analysis of laryngeal mechanosensitivity in the cat and rabbit. *J Physiol* 388:467–85.

Depalle, P., G. Garcia, and X. Rodet. 1995. The re-creation of the castrato voice, Farinelli's voice. Proceedings of the 1995 workshop on applications of single processing to audio and acoustics, IEEE, New York.

Elias, M. E., R. T. Sataloff, D. C. Rosen, R. J. Heuer, and J. R. Spiegel. 1997. Normal strobovideolaryngoscopy: Variability in healthy singers. *J Voice* 11 (1):104–7.

Gould, W. J., and H. Okamura. 1974. Interrelationships between voice and laryngeal mucosal reflexes. In *Ventilatory and phonatory control systems*, ed. B. Wyke. London: Oxford University Press.

Gray, H., and P. L. Williams. 1989. *Gray's anatomy.* 37th ed. Edinburgh: C. Livingstone.

Greeves, J. P., N. T. Cable, T. Reilly, and C. Kingsland. 1999. Changes in muscle strength in women following the menopause: A longitudinal assessment of the efficacy of hormone replacement therapy. *Clin Sci (Lond)* 97 (1):79–84.

Han, Y., J. Wang, D. A. Fischman, H. F. Biller, and I. Sanders. 1999. Slow tonic muscle fibers in the thyroarytenoid muscles of human vocal folds; a possible specialization for speech. *Anat Rec* 256 (2):146–57.

Hanson, D. G., and J. J. Jiang. 1998. Laryngitis from reflux: Prevention for the performing singer. *Med Prob Perform Artists* 13:51–55.

Heman-Ackah, Y. D., C. M. Dean, and R. T. Sataloff. 2002. Strobovideolaryngoscopic findings in singing teachers. *J Voice* 16 (1):81–86.

Hillel, A. D. 2001. The study of laryngeal muscle activity in normal human subjects and in patients with laryngeal dystonia using multiple fine-wire electromyography. *Laryngoscope* 111 (4 Pt 2 Suppl 97):1–47.

Hirano, M., W. Vennard, and J. Ohala. 1970. Regulation of register, pitch and intensity of voice. An electromyographic investigation of intrinsic laryngeal muscles. *Folia Phoniatr (Basel)* 22 (1):1–20.

Hirayama, M., T. Matsui, M. Tachibana, Y. Ibata, and O. Mizukoshi. 1987. An electron microscopic study of the muscle spindle in the arytenoid muscle of the human larynx. *Arch Otorhinolaryngol* 244 (4):249–52.

Hollien, H., and G. P. Moore. 1960. Measurements of the vocal folds during changes in pitch. *J Speech Hear Res* 3:157–65.

Holmberg, E. B., R. E. Hillman, B. Hammarberg, M. Sodersten, and P. Doyle. 2001. Efficacy of a behaviorally based voice therapy protocol for vocal nodules. *J Voice* 15 (3):395–412.

Hurme, P., and A. Sonninen. 1995. Vertical and saggital position of the larynx in singing. Proceedings of the XIII International Congress of Phonetic Sciences, ed. K. Elenius and P. Branderud. http://users.jyu.fi/~hurme/Sthlm.html (accessed April 23, 2008).

Iwarsson, J. 2001. Effects of inhalatory abdominal wall movement on vertical laryngeal position during phonation. *J Voice* 15 (3):384–94.

Iwarsson, J., and J. Sundberg. 1998. Effects of lung volume on vertical larynx position during phonation. *J Voice* 12 (2):159–65.

Jenkins, J. 2001. The voice of the castrato. *Trans Med Soc Lond* 118:37–42.

Jenkins, J. S. 1998. The voice of the castrato. *Lancet* 351 (9119):1877–80.

Joliveau, E., J. Smith, and J. Wolfe. 2004. Acoustics: Tuning of vocal tract resonance by sopranos. *Nature* 427 (6970):116.

Keene, M. F. 1961. Muscle spindles in human laryngeal muscles. *J Anat* 95:25–29.

Kirchner, J. A., and B. Wyke. 1964a. Electromyographic analysis of laryngeal articular reflexes. *Nature* 203:1243–45.

———. 1964b. Laryngeal articular reflexes. *Nature* 202:600.

Koufman, J. A. 1992. Voice disorders. *Visible Voice* 1:16–19.

———. 1993. Vocal nodules. *Visible Voice* 2 (4):74–76.

Koufman, J. A., and P. D. Blalock. 1991. Functional voice disorders. *Otolaryngol Clin North Am* 24 (5):1059–73.

La, F. M., W. L. Ledger, J. W. Davidson, D. M. Howard, and G. L. Jones. 2007. The effects of a third generation combined oral contraceptive pill on the classical singing voice. *J Voice* 21 (6):754–61.

Laukkanen, A. M., R. Takalo, M. Arvonen, and E. Vilkman. 2002. Pitch-synchronous changes in the anterior cricothyroid space during singing. *J Voice* 16 (2):182–94.

Levin, T. C., and M. E. Edgerton. 1999. The throat singers of Tuva. *Sci Am* 281 (3):80–87.

Lindholm, P., E. Vilkman, T. Raudaskoski, E. Suvanto-Luukkonen, and A. Kauppila. 1997. The effect of postmenopause and postmenopausal HRT on measured voice values and vocal symptoms. *Maturitas* 28 (1):47–53.

Lundy, D. S., R. R. Casiano, P. A. Sullivan, S. Roy, J. W. Xue, and J. Evans. 1999. Incidence of abnormal laryngeal findings in asymptomatic singing students. *Otolaryngol Head Neck Surg* 121 (1):69–77.

Meurer, E. M., M. C. Wender, H. von Eye Corleta, and E. Capp. 2004. Phono-articulatory variations of women in reproductive age and postmenopausal. *J Voice* 18 (3):369–74.

Misso, M. L., C. Jang, J. Adams, J. Tran, Y. Murata, R. Bell, W. C. Boon, E. R. Simpson, and S. R. Davis. 2005. Adipose aromatase gene expression is greater in older women and is unaffected by postmenopausal estrogen therapy. *Menopause* 12 (2):210–15.

Moreschi, A. 1987. *The last castrato: Complete Vatican recordings.* Wadhurst, UK: Pavilion Records, Opal CD 9823.

Nagai, T. 1987. Encapsulated nerve structures in the human vocal cord. An electronmicroscopic study. *Acta Otolaryngol* 104 (3–4):363–69.

Pain, S. 2006. Histories: Superstar sopranos. *New Scientist* 189 (March 25):52.

Pedersen, M. F., S. Moller, S. Krabbe, P. Bennett, and B. Svenstrup. 1990. Fundamental voice frequency in female puberty measured with electroglottography during continuous speech as a secondary sex characteristic. A comparison between voice, pubertal stages, oestrogens and androgens. *Int J Pediatr Otorhinolaryngol* 20 (1):17–24.

Peterson, G. E., and H. L. Barney. 1952. Control methods used in a study of the vowels. *J Acoust Soc Am* 24 (2):175–84.

Pontes, P., L. Kyrillos, M. Behlau, N. De Biase, and A. Pontes. 2002. Vocal nodules and laryngeal morphology. *J Voice* 16 (3):408–14.

Quantz, J. J. 1754. Johann Joachim Quantzens Lebenslauf, von ihm selbst entworfen [The course of Johann Joachim Quantz's life as outlined by himself]. In *Historisch-kritische Beiträge zur Aufnahme der Musik* [*Historical critical essays on the perception of music*], ed. F. W. Marpurg. Berlin: G. A. Lange.

Reilly, J. S. 1997. The "singing-acting" child: The laryngologist's perspective—1995. *J Voice* 11 (2):126–29.

Rossing, T. D., J. Sundberg, and S. Ternstrom. 1986. Acoustic comparison of voice use in solo and choir singing. *J Acoust Soc Am* 79 (6):1975–81.

Sampson, S., and C. Eyzaguirre. 1964. Some functional characteristics of mechanoreceptors in the larynx of the cat. *J Neurophysiol* 27:464–80.

Sanders, I., Y. Han, J. Wang, and H. Biller. 1998. Muscle spindles are concentrated in the superior vocalis subcompartment of the human thyroarytenoid muscle. *J Voice* 12 (1):7–16.

Sanders, I., and L. Mu. 1998. Anatomy of the human internal superior laryngeal nerve. *Anat Rec* 252 (4):646–56.

Sanders, I., S. Rai, Y. Han, and H. F. Biller. 1998. Human vocalis contains distinct superior and inferior subcompartments: Possible candidates for the two masses of vocal fold vibration. *Ann Otol Rhinol Laryngol* 107 (10 Pt 1):826–33.

Sataloff, R. T. 1987. Common diagnoses and treatments in professional voice users. *Med Prob Perform Artists* 2:15–20.

——. 1995. G. Paul Moore Lecture. Rational thought: The impact of voice science upon voice care. *J Voice* 9 (3):215–34.

——. 1998. Common medical diagnoses and treatments in professional voice users. In *Vocal health and pedagogy*, ed. R. T. Sataloff. San Diego: Singular Publishing Group.

——. 2006a. *Science and assessment.* Vol. 1 of *Vocal health and pedagogy.* 2nd ed. San Diego: Plural Publishing.

——. 2006b. *Advanced assessment and treatment.* Vol. 2 of *Vocal health and pedagogy.* 2nd ed. San Diego: Plural Publishing.

Sataloff, R. T., D. C. Rosen, M. Hawkshaw, and J. R. Spiegel. 1997. The aging adult voice. *J Voice* 11 (2):156–60.

Sataloff, R. T., J. R. Spiegel, and D. C. Rosen. 1998. The effects of age on the voice. In *Vocal health and pedagogy*, ed. R. T. Sataloff. San Diego: Singular Publishing Group.

Scammell, E. 1987. Alessandro Moreschi. *The last castrato: Complete Vatican recordings* (sleeve notes). Pavilion Records, Opal CD 9823.

Scherer, R. C. 2006. Laryngeal function during phonation. In *Vocal health and pedagogy*, ed. R. T. Sataloff. San Diego: Plural Publishing.

Shiba, K., T. Miura, J. Yuza, T. Sakamoto, and Y. Nakajima. 1999. Laryngeal afferent inputs during vocalization in the cat. *Neuroreport* 10 (5):987–91.

Shiba, K., K. Yoshida, and T. Miura. 1995. Functional roles of the superior laryngeal nerve afferents in electrically induced vocalization in anesthetized cats. *Neurosci Res* 22 (1):23–30.

Shiba, K., K. Yoshida, Y. Nakajima, and A. Konno. 1997. Influences of laryngeal afferent inputs on intralaryngeal muscle activity during vocalization in the cat. *Neurosci Res* 27 (1):85–92.

Shipp, T. 1987. Vertical laryngeal position: Research findings and application for singers. *J Voice* 1 (3):217–19.

Shipp, T., E. T. Doherty, and P. Morrissey. 1979. Predicting vocal frequency from selected physiologic measures. *J Acoust Soc Am* 66 (3):678–84.

Shipp, T., and K. Izdebski. 1975. Letter: Vocal frequency and vertical larynx positioning by singers and nonsingers. *J Acoust Soc Am* 58 (5):1104–6.

Sjolander, P., and J. Sundberg. 2004. Spectrum effects of subglottal pressure variation in professional baritone singers. *J Acoust Soc Am* 115 (3):1270–73.

Smith, L. A., and B. L. Scott. 1980. Increasing the intelligibility of sung vowels. *J Acoust Soc Am* 67 (5):1795–97.

Solomon, N. P., G. N. McCall, M. W. Trosset, and W. C. Gray. 1989. Laryngeal configuration and constriction during two types of whispering. *J Speech Hear Res* 32 (1):161–74.

Somerset-Ward, R. 2004. The castrato ascendancy. In *Angels and monsters: Male and female sopranos in the story of opera, 1600–1900*. New Haven, Conn.: Yale University Press.

Sonninen, A., P. Hurme, and A. M. Laukkanen. 1999. The external frame function in the control of pitch, register, and singing mode: Radiographic observations of a female singer. *J Voice* 13 (3):319–40.

Spiegel, J. R., R. T. Sataloff, and K. A. Emerich. 1997. The young adult voice. *J Voice* 11 (2):138–43.

Sundberg, J. 1972. Production and function of the singing formant. In the Report of the 11th congress of the International Musicological Society, ed. H. Glahn, S. Sorenson, and R. Ryom. Wilhelm Hansen edition, 679–688.

———. 1977. The acoustics of the singing voice. *Sci Am* 236 (3):82–91.

———. 1987. *The science of the singing voice*. DeKalb: Northern Ilinois University Press.

———. 1999. The perception of singing. In *The psychology of music*, ed. D. Deutsch. San Diego: Academic Press.

Sundberg, J., J. Iwarsson, and A. H. Billstrom. 1995. Significance of mechanoreceptors in the subglottal mucosa for subglottal pressure control in singers. *J Voice* 9 (1):20–26.

Tellis, C. M., C. Rosen, A. Thekdi, and J. J. Sciote. 2004. Anatomy and fiber type composition of human interarytenoid muscle. *Ann Otol Rhinol Laryngol* 113 (2):97–107.

Tepe, E. S., E. S. Deutsch, Q. Sampson, S. Lawless, J. S. Reilly, and R. T. Sataloff. 2002. A pilot survey of vocal health in young singers. *J Voice* 16 (2):244–50.

Titze, I. R. 1994. *Principles of voice production*. Englewood Cliffs, N.J.: Prentice Hall.

———. 2000. *Principles of voice production*. 2nd printing. Iowa City, Iowa: National Center for Voice and Speech.

———. 2008. The human instrument. *Sci Am* 298 (1):78–85.

Tsunoda, K., Y. Ohta, Y. Soda, S. Niimi, and H. Hirose. 1997. Laryngeal adjustment in whispering magnetic resonance imaging study. *Ann Otol Rhinol Laryngol* 106 (1):41–43.

Wendler, J., C. Siegert, P. Schelhorn, G. Klinger, S. Gurr, J. Kaufmann, S. Aydinlik, and T. Braunschweig. 1995. The influence of microgynon and diane-35, two sub-fifty ovulation inhibitors, on voice function in women. *Contraception* 52 (6):343–48.

Williams, R. G., and R. Eccles. 1990. A new clinical measure of external laryngeal size which predicts the fundamental frequency of the larynx. *Acta Otolaryngol* 110 (1–2):141–48.

Wyke, B. D. 1974. Proceedings: Laryngeal myotatic reflexes and phonation. *Folia Phoniatr (Basel)* 26 (4):249–64.

Wyke, B., and J. A. Kirchner. 1976. Neurology of the larynx. In *Scientific foundations of otolaryngology*, ed. R. Hinchcliffe and D. F. N. Harrison. London: Heinemann Medical.

Yanagisawa, E., J. Estill, L. Mambrino, and D. Talkin. 1991. Supraglottic contributions to pitch raising. Videoendoscopic study with spectroanalysis. *Ann Otol Rhinol Laryngol* 100 (1):19–30.

Yoshida, Y., Y. Tanaka, M. Hirano, and T. Nakashima. 2000. Sensory innervation of the pharynx and larynx. *Am J Med* 108 (Suppl 4a):51S–61S.

Chapter Six

The Embouchure and Wind Playing

In this chapter we will consider not only the embouchure in its narrowest sense (the muscles surrounding the opening of the mouth), but also structures such as the jaw and teeth that support it. We will also investigate the involvement of the larynx and the throat (pharynx) in wind playing. Finally, we will explore a range of problems that can afflict wind players, either as a result of a failure of the mechanism of the embouchure itself or the consequence of generating high pressures in the airway.

THE SKULL AND JAW

During embryonic life, the skull is formed from a number of separate bones that fuse to form a single structure. Here we need only concern ourselves with some aspects of the basic structure of the face and jaw, which provide the bony attachments of the muscles that contribute to the embouchure. Most of the region of the skull that makes up the face below the eyes is formed by a bone called the maxilla. The upper teeth arise from sockets that develop in the spongy (alveolar) bone on its lower edge. What are commonly called the cheekbones (the zygomatic bones) form the lateral edge of the eye socket. Together with a forward-directed spur from the temporal bone, which provides part of the side wall of the skull, the zygomatic bone forms an arch (the zygomatic arch) that runs backward as far as the temporomandibular (jaw) joint (fig. 6-1). Through the space that lies between the zygomatic arch and the side of the skull runs the temporalis muscle, which is attached at its upper end to the side of the skull and at its lower end, to the inside of the jawbone (the mandible). Another muscle, the masseter, runs from the outside of the zygomatic arch to the lower corner of the outer surface of the jaw. Both of these muscles raise the jaw to close the mouth. The mandible is made up of two bones, one on the left and one on the right, that are fused in the middle of the chin. On each side it articulates with the skull via the temporo-mandibular joint. The saddle-shaped surfaces of this joint also allow the jaw to slide forward (protract) or backward (retract) and to move from side to side. The joint is a synovial one (see chapter 1), but unusually it contains a sheet of cartilage, called the

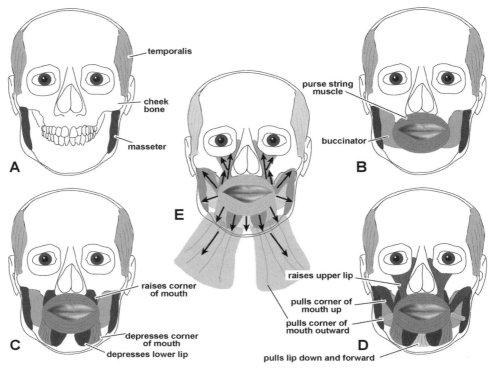

Figure 6-1. The muscles contributing to the embouchure are labeled according to their actions on the embouchure. Anatomists and doctors use the Latin names, which can be found in another version of the figure on the accompanying disc. Here they have been translated into English. The central component of the embouchure is the purse-string muscle that surrounds the lips. The other muscles radiate outward from this, and the direction of pull exerted by each is shown in the central figure (E).

articular disk, which sits between the two articular surfaces. The muscles that cause these movements are the medial and lateral pterygoids, which lie deep in the cheek behind the jaw. In order to allow this freedom of movement, the capsule and ligaments that surround the joint and hold it in place are relatively lax. As a result, if the jaw is opened very wide, or if the chin is struck when open, it can become dislocated, particularly in those individuals who have loose ligaments in the joint capsule. The forward and backward movement of the jaw is important for adjusting the airstream in the playing of many wind instruments. The jaws of some people naturally protrude more than others, so the degree of protraction or retraction required for different playing tasks will vary from individual to individual.

How the head is positioned on the neck influences how wide open the pharynx (or throat) is held. The head is supported by a number of muscles attached to the base of the skull (see chapter 5). On each side a sternocleidomastoid muscle runs from just behind the ear to the junction of the collarbone (clavicle) and the breastbone (sternum). Each rotates the head upward and to the opposite side. When they act together they pull the head forward, flexing the neck. Other small muscles running from the

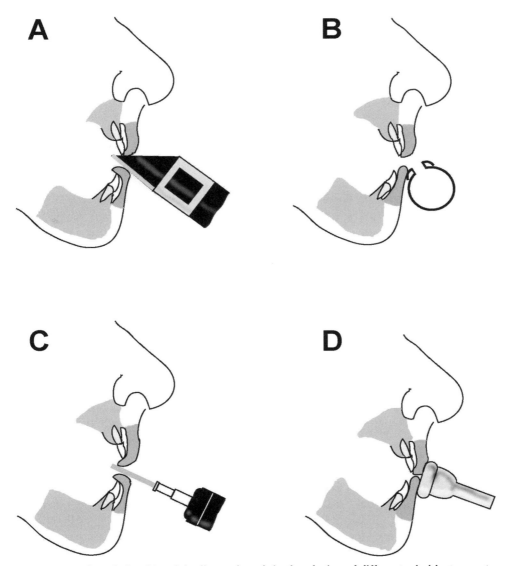

**Figure 6-2. The relationship of the lips and teeth in the playing of different wind instruments.
A. Single reed (clarinet). B. Flute, piccolo. C. Double reed (oboe, cor anglais, bassoon). D. Brass
instruments.**

base of the skull to the front of the vertebral column also pull the head forward. All
of these muscles may be active to resist the force of the mouthpiece against the lips.
They are opposed by a number of muscles that run up the back of the neck and pull on
the lower surface of the skull. The head is tilted from side to side by muscles that run
like guy ropes from the sides of the upper vertebrae of the neck to the shoulder blade
and to the upper ribs (the scalenes and levator scapuli; see chapter 2). Damage to any
of the major muscles that do this interferes markedly with wind instrument playing

because of the difficulty in maintaining the throat in an optimum open configuration. Excessive pressure of the mouthpiece on the embouchure will lead to chronic tension in the muscles, which may cause pain and discomfort.

THE TEETH

In the playing of wind instruments, the front teeth, particularly the incisors, are used to grip the mouthpiece (woodwind instruments) or support the embouchure (brass instruments) (fig. 6-2). For single-reed instruments, the reed is gripped between the upper incisors, which make contact with the top of the mouthpiece, and the lower lip, which is curled over the lower incisors. For double-reed instruments, both lips are curled over the incisors to apply the pressure to the reed. The teeth are inserted into the spongy alveolar bone of the upper and lower jaw. Though this forms a rigid platform in the short term, bone can be remolded over time in response to pressure. This property allows orthodontists to straighten or adjust tooth position using tooth braces. To do this, braces are used to generate forces of between 36 and 60 grams over periods of six hours or more at a time. The pressure applied directly to the teeth by wind instruments can be much higher. Average pressures of 211 grams have been reported for the flute, 270 grams for reed instruments, and 500 grams for brass instruments (Engelman 1965); however, one should treat these values with some caution as they were made on very young players (ten to seventeen years) with as little as one year's experience on their instrument. As we will see later, a study of the pressures applied to the mouthpiece by the lips of adult trumpeters revealed values four to ten times as high (Barbenel, Kenny, and Davies 1988). Though it is clear that wind instrument playing has the potential to affect tooth alignment, studies of this in adult players have been inconclusive. It may be that the duration of the practice sessions typical of adult amateur musicians is too short to have a major effect on the teeth, though there is some evidence for changes in tooth alignment in musicians under the age of fifteen. Indeed, a suitable choice of instrument can apparently aid orthodontal treatment for those in this age group (Yeo et al. 2002)! When the surfaces of the molars come together, the cutting surfaces of the upper front teeth (incisors and canines) overlap slightly over those of the lower front teeth. The vertical overlap of these edges is called the overbite, and the horizontal overlap (the margin by which the top teeth project over the bottom teeth) is called the overjet (fig. 6-3). If the lower incisors overlap the ones on the upper jaw, this is called underjet or underbite. Single-reed instruments can increase overjet and overbite, while double-reed instruments tend to reduce overjet and increase overbite, and brass instruments reduce both overjet and overbite (Herman 1981).

Irregularities and sharp or chipped edges on the anterior teeth can pose particular problems for reed players. The contact between the lower incisors and the lip is the main source of trauma for players of single-reed instruments, while for players of double-reed instruments, both the upper and lower lips may be affected. In the short term, tenderness and ulceration may result. Over time, the soft lining of the inside of the lip will change its characteristics so that the cell layers at the point of contact acquire more granules of keratin (a structurally strong protein), forming a protective

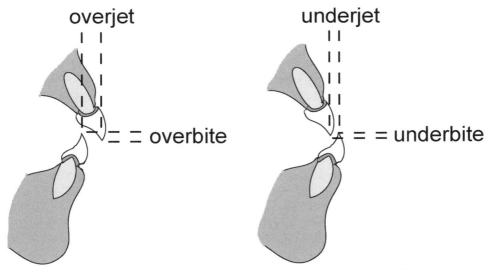

Figure 6-3. A diagram with an explanation of the terminology used for describing the relative position of the upper and lower incisor teeth.

callus. This quickly develops in all players who practice consistently; however, serious problems with the lips in professional players can be alleviated by having chips or sharp edges on the teeth rounded or repaired. A lip shield can also be used to reduce the discomfort. In single-reed players, the upper incisors may become worn due to friction against the mouthpiece. The application of rubber patches to the top surface of the mouthpiece is now common practice, and acrylic shields can be made to cover the upper incisors and canines in order to protect both natural teeth and vulnerable dental work such as crowns (Herman 1974).

MUSCLES OF THE MOUTH, JAW, AND EMBOUCHURE

The muscles around the mouth (oral cavity) that are associated with singing and wind playing can be divided into two groups. The first group contains the deep muscles that move the jaw or form the inner wall of the cheek and the second, the superficial muscles that insert into the lips (fig. 6-1).

Deep Muscles

Two large muscles are responsible for closing the mouth. These are the masseter and temporalis muscles. If you clench your teeth tightly and put your fingers on the angle of the jaw, a couple of centimeters below the ear, you will feel a tense ball of muscle. This is the masseter, which links this part of the jaw to the cheekbone (the zygomatic arch). If you repeat the action of clenching your teeth but this time place your fingers on the side of the head above the cheekbone but behind the eye, you will feel the contraction of another large muscle, the temporalis. This descends behind the zygomatic arch and attaches to a sheet of bone (the coronoid process) that rises upward from the jaw. The fibers of the temporalis muscle fan out from the coronoid process so that although those running straight upward close the jaw, others run backward almost horizontally so that parts of the muscle pull the jaw backward (i.e., retract it). The jaw is pulled forward by muscles (the pterygoids) that run from the back of the lower jaw to a region of the skull behind the upper teeth. The jaw may be protracted and retracted during playing when changing registers, for example, in brass instruments such as the trumpet (Ridgeon 1986)—while in the flute, the lower jaw may be retracted in the lower register.

Deep to the temporalis and masseter is another sheet of muscle that attaches at one end to the bone above the upper teeth, and at the other end to the outer surface of the lower jaw below the teeth roots. This muscle is called the buccinator (its name is derived from the Latin word for a trumpeter). It forms the inner wall of the cheek and extends forward to the opening of the mouth, where it contributes to the embouchure. At the back it merges with the outer muscle layer of the pharynx (the superior constrictor—see chapter 5) so that the muscular wall of the throat is continuous all the way to the lips. This ensures that the airway can resist the high pressures generated in the playing of many wind instruments. In some trumpeters who allow their cheeks to puff out, the buccinator is stretched and can become ever thinner until it reaches a state in which it is easily damaged. The muscles that move the jaw are all supplied by branches of the trigeminal nerve, which is responsible for sensation on the face. By contrast, the buccinator and the muscles of the embouchure, described below, are supplied by the facial nerve.

Superficial Muscles

The embouchure, per se, is formed by muscles of the superficial group. Figure 6-1 describes them by their actions, in English. A version of this figure with the muscles named in Latin can be found on the accompanying disc. The Latin names are the ones that are used in the reports of studies into embouchure function in wind players. The superficial muscles are known as muscles of facial expression. They are attached to the overlying skin, and we use them to give conscious or unconscious indications of recognition and of mood or to provide signals that reveal how we feel about what is going on around us. Their Latin names indicate their relationship to the opening of the mouth (oris) or the lip (labium). The central muscle of the embouchure is one called the orbicularis oris because its fibers encircle (or orbit) the mouth. Some of its fibers are attached to the bones of the upper and lower jaw and others to the deep layers of the skin. The muscle has a purse-string action, which is most graphically demonstrated in pouting. The other muscles that control the shape of the embouchure radiate out from the orbicularis oris (to which they are attached) to various anchor points on the bones of the face and jaw. The upper lip can be raised by a muscle that runs up to the bone under the eye and on the side of the nose (hence its name—levator labii superioris). The corner of the mouth is raised by a small, deep triangular muscle (levator anguli oris) and pulled upward and backward by muscles that run from the zygomatic arch of the cheek (zygomaticus major and minor). A comparable set of muscles act on the lower lip. These all run from the lower jaw and they can depress the lip (depressor labii inferioris and mentalis) or the corner of the mouth (depressor anguli oris). The region at the corner of the mouth where the levator and depressor anguli oris and the zygomatic muscles all merge with the orbicularis oris is called the modiolis. In addition to these muscles, a much smaller one, the risorius (smiling muscle), contributes to the embouchure by pulling the corner of the mouth backward. In this it is aided by the buccinator and by the platysma. As its name suggests, platysma is a thin, flat sheet of muscle that runs beneath the skin of the neck, to which it is attached. Its upper fibers pass over the lower edge of the jawline and interleave with the muscles that contribute to the embouchure. The branches of the facial nerve, which supply the muscles of the embouchure, radiate out from under the largest of the salivary glands (the parotid gland), which lies beneath the skin over the angle of the jaw.

THE EMBOUCHURE IN WIND PLAYING

The role of the embouchure varies depending on the instrument being played, but in all cases its shape must be precisely regulated using not only the orbicularis oris, but also the other muscles that surround it. Sometimes when trying new embouchure configurations, fatigue and stiffness may be detectable in individual muscular elements of the embouchure. In the case of reed instruments the first role of the embouchure is to maintain a seal around the mouthpiece or reed(s), often against high intraoral pressures. It is also necessary to apply a variable pressure to the reed depending on the sound being produced, and this may involve the muscles that raise the lower jaw (temporalis and masseter) as well as those controlling the lips. In the flute, the airhole is always open but the precise shape of the embouchure is adjusted to direct the air jet and control its length. In brass instruments, the basic pursing of the lips is also achieved by the orbicularis oris. Players of these instruments generate extreme intraoral pressures in the upper registers (see chapter 4). The tension in the orbicularis oris will determine the frequency at which the lips vibrate to generate the sound. This involves not just contraction of the fibers of the orbicularis oris itself, but of the muscles radiating out from it. Indeed it is the activity of this latter group that dominates in expert players. In order to gain the degree of control over the embouchure needed to allow precise control over pitch in all registers, the muscles that contribute to it must be strengthened over time and be kept in good physical condition by constant training to maintain good performance standards. In an active player this may noticeably alter the shape of the face. In the French horn, where the overtones of the instrument used for the notes in the upper register are very close together, the control of the embouchure is particularly critical. For brass players, the precise shape of the embouchure depends not only on register but also on the instrument, as mouthpieces vary greatly in size and shape (Ridgeon 1986). It is not just the shape of the mouth aperture that is used to control the airflow. The position and shape of the tongue also play a crucial role. For example, it may be raised to reduce the area of the air jet (and presumably increase its pressure) in the upper register (Ridgeon 1986). In the flute, the opening of the embouchure itself is reduced as pitch increases, for similar reasons (Cossette, Sliwinski, and Macklem 2000).

The question of the optimal pattern of muscle activity in the embouchure is central to the teaching of brass technique; however, only a few studies have examined this directly and all have focused on trumpet players (White and Basmajian 1973; Basmajian and White 1973; Heuser and McNitt-Gray 1991, 1993, 1998). Basmajian and White recorded the electrical activity in embouchure muscles using small wires that were inserted directly into them through the skin. They monitored the upper and lower regions of the orbicularis oris and the levator and depressor anguli oris muscles, as they considered these to be the most crucial elements of the embouchure for this instrument. The results demonstrated that despite being considered as a single muscle from an anatomical standpoint, the fibers of the orbicularis oris in the upper and lower lip could be controlled separately. Muscle activity was compared in players with a wide range of expertise ranging from teenage beginners to adult professionals. In all players, there was greater muscle activity when playing in the upper registers than the lower, and when playing loudly as opposed to softly. When playing a note, muscle activity was first seen in the preparatory period before its onset. This more closely matched the activity required during the note in experienced players than in beginners, a finding confirmed by other investigators (Heuser and McNitt-Gray 1991). This presumably reflects a greater accuracy in note placement. Basmajian and White found that in all players, the end of the note coincided precisely with an abrupt and complete cessation of all muscle activity, though other studies have suggested that this is more marked in those with most experience (Heuser and McNitt-Gray 1991). In advanced players, the activity in the muscles surrounding the lips (i.e., levator and depressor anguli oris) was greater than in the lips themselves (the orbicularis oris) and there was no difference in activity between the upper and lower lip. In beginners, there was generally more activity in the upper lip. The players in the study were asked to carry out a number of simple exercises including small-interval lip slurs and both slurred and tongued arpeggios and repeated notes. The advanced players showed very little variation in muscle activity during the small-interval slurs, suggesting that they were using some other method to manage the transition between the notes. It was proposed that mouthpiece pressure, pressure distribution on the lips, air pressure, airflow, tooth aperture, and tongue position might be candidates for this, but the question was not investigated further. The experienced players also showed much smaller differences in the pattern of muscle activity used for slurred and tongued arpeggios than the novices. Electrical recordings from muscles of the embouchure can be made less invasively using electrodes that are applied to the surface of the skin. Though less accurate than making recordings via wires inserted into the muscle, this technique does not involve breaking the skin and so can be used much more easily in a nonclinical context (Heuser and McNitt-Gray 1991). Heuser and McNitt-Gray recorded from the zygomaticus major and the depressor anguli oris. Surface recording of embouchure muscles may have a role in normal teaching aimed at correcting or refining embouchure technique. For example, in some players, poor tone production was associated with a lack of synchronization of muscle activity within the embouchure or an imbalance in the activity of equivalent muscles on the left and right sides (Heuser and McNitt-Gray

1998). In addition, players with a history of attack difficulties showed poor control of the onset and offset of muscle activity. Resolution of these difficulties is accompanied by a clearly observable change in the pattern of electrical activity of the muscles. Brass teachers generally recommend that the mouthpiece be placed centrally on the lips because this is thought to be optimal for tone quality; however, some experienced players do perform with it displaced to one side. This can be due to irregularities in the upper incisors that make central positioning uncomfortable (Nixon 1963). One might expect that this would be associated with some asymmetry in embouchure muscle activity, but a comparison of three such players with a group that used the more normal configuration showed no observable differences between them over a range of playing tasks (Heuser and McNitt-Gray 1993).

The pressures applied to the mouthpiece by lips of trumpet players has been thoroughly investigated by Barbenel, Kenny, and Davies (1988), who tested sixty performers, half of whom were top-level professional orchestral, jazz, or band musicians and half of whom were less-accomplished players with at least six years of playing experience. For all subjects, mouthpiece pressure rose increasingly more rapidly with rising pitch (i.e., rose in a nonlinear fashion). For notes in the middle to upper part of the range there was little difference between the two groups in terms of the forces used. For example, for the note G5 played at 95 decibels using a normal level of force, the mean range was 2–2.7 kilograms (kg) (20–27 newtons [N]). When players were asked to produce notes at the upper extreme of the range (C6–G6), less than half were successful. Those who were could typically tolerate a mouthpiece pressure of 7.7 kg, while those that were not could support only 4.5 kg. This contradicts the popular myth that virtuoso performers can play when exerting almost no pressure on the mouthpiece. Reducing the pressure by as little as 0.3 kg in this study was sufficient to render it impossible to continue playing a note at the same intensity. A smaller study of college-level trumpeters confirmed that while similarly high pressures were sometimes used for short periods, the average pressures exerted were relatively low—in this case about half those measured by Barbenel (Devroop and Chesky 2002). The perception that proficient or virtuoso players use very little force may stem from the fact that when it comes to estimating visually how much force is being used, both professional performers and nonmusicians do rather poorly (Barbenel, Davies, and Kenny 1986). What watching players does reveal is how much effort they are using to produce the tone—in other words, how close they are to their physical limits. Hence, highly proficient players give the illusion of using low mouthpiece pressures because they are playing well within their capabilities. Interestingly, it also proved difficult for players of all proficiencies to estimate how much pressure they were applying to the mouthpiece themselves. Both groups tended to think they were using a greater range of pressures than they actually were.

THE ROLE OF THE LARYNX AND PHARYNX

Several studies involving direct visualization of the larynx have been directed at the role of the glottis in wind playing (Rydell et al. 1996; King, Ashby, and Nelson 1989;

King, Ashby, and Nelson 1988; Brown 1976). Though these studies present rather brief and incomplete descriptions of laryngeal function, some general features were observed consistently. The larynx appears to be used to control airflow in all wind instruments, though this varies in degree and in context between instruments. In the flute, the glottis is kept wide open during playing, but rhythmic movements of the vocal folds were consistently seen to contribute to the production of vibrato. In reed and brass instruments, the contribution of the glottis to the production of vibrato varies considerably between players and is sometimes absent entirely. During the playing of these instruments, the two vocal folds are actively brought into close proximity (though not into contact). In brass players this is more marked in instruments that require high pressure and low airflow, such as the trumpet, than in larger-bore instruments that require higher flow rates at lower pressure, such as the tuba. It is has been proposed that in the trumpet this may be a first stage in which fine control may be exerted on the pressure being generated. This may be aided by a depression of the epiglottis and by use of the tongue. In brass and reed instruments it was noted that the reduction in the opening of the glottis was most marked in heavy tonguing, during which the arching of the back of the tongue may have also contributed to the reduction in airflow. Complete closure of the glottis in this situation is seen most commonly in the trumpet and reed instruments. Whether this closure was functional or represented an inappropriate engagement of the valsalva maneuver was not discussed in any of the above-mentioned studies (see chapter 4).

The height of the larynx may also be manipulated during woodwind playing. A lowering of the larynx has been noted during playing of the flute, saxophone, and oboe (Rydell et al. 1996; King, Ashby, and Nelson 1988). In the flute it is maintained in this low position, and changes in tonal quality are brought about by altering the embouchure and the direction of the air jet. It has been suggested, however, that the resonance of the cavity of the pharynx may be used, particularly by advanced woodwind players, to contribute to the timbre of the sound (King, Ashby, and Nelson 1988; Benade 1986). The resonant properties of the pharynx are affected in part by the height of the larynx, to which of course it is attached, and are greatest when the glottis is held nearly closed during playing. When the glottis is opened, the resonances are weakened by being dissipated into the lungs. In the teaching of brass players, the instruction to play with an "open throat" refers to the pharynx; playing with a tight throat is said to produce a pinched tone, suggesting that resonance in the cavity of the pharynx contributes to the quality of the sound. In the oboe it has been proposed that a maintained low position of the larynx is necessary for the development of the harmonic structure typical of this instrument, presumably as a result of the effect this has of increasing the volume of the pharynx, though the validity of this has not been tested experimentally. In single-reed instruments, the movement of the larynx varies considerably between individual players and can be difficult to quantify. Some reports suggest that it tends to rise with pitch (King, Ashby, and Nelson 1988), while others state that it remains in a stable position (Weikert and Schlomicher-Thier 1999). It has been proposed that the diversity in technique may be related to individual variability in the physical dimensions of the vocal tract.

In the past, technical difficulties in making measurements of the acoustic impedance of the airway during playing had resulted in considerable disagreement concerning the importance of vocal tract resonances in woodwind playing; however, recent advances in measuring equipment have made accurate analysis a more realistic possibility (Fritze and Wolfe 2005). In the case of clarinet players, it appears that the vocal tract resonances remain fairly constant throughout most of the range; however, they may be manipulated to a considerable extent in the highest register and for special effects such as glissandi and slurring. Some players report that they move the tongue and facial muscles between positions that are similar to those typical of certain vowels (e.g., "ee" for the top register versus "aw" for a full sound in the low register). Of course, any change in jaw or lip configuration that accompanies these configurations may also alter the loading on the reed and so the results require careful interpretation; however, it at least appears feasible that the magnitude of changes in vocal tract resonances might be capable of affecting the quality of the sound, and certainly many players believe this (Fritze and Wolfe 2005).

One instrument in which the major contribution of vocal tract resonances to the sound produced is unequivocal is the Australian aboriginal didgeridoo (Amir 2004). This is an unusual instrument both structurally and acoustically. Its bore varies randomly along its length and it has no mouthpiece or narrowing at the playing end. The fundamental frequency is strong though very low (typically around 70 Hz) where the auditory system is not particularly sensitive. In good instruments, the lowest harmonics (typically the second to ninth) are weak or absent. The vocal tract is strongly coupled (though in a complex way) to the instrument through the lips, which act as the reed. The frequencies generated from the tenth harmonic upward appear to be dominated by the formant frequencies of the vocal tract; the sound can be modulated by using vowel-like conformations of the mouth, while the vocal folds remain open and free of vibration. This manipulates the relative frequencies of the formants (see chapter 5) and strongly influences the timbre of the note produced by the instrument.

PROBLEMS ASSOCIATED WITH THE EMBOUCHURE IN WIND PLAYERS

Dental Problems

Clarinet and saxophone players who have a pronounced overbite may experience excessive wear on the incisors (Yeo et al. 2002). The overbite results in the frictional wear being applied to the back of the edge of the tooth. If the wear extends beyond the outer layers of the tooth, the central pulp, which contains its nerve and blood supply, can be affected and the tissue may die as a result. A number of dental interventions can be used to treat this. If the wear has not already affected the pulp, a surface coating to the back of the tooth will provide useful protection; however, if the pulp dies, a root canal filling with a post and crown would be necessary to preserve the tooth. This involves removing the pulp and inserting a rigid post to support the crown, but the tooth is weakened as a result.

The effect of backward pressure exerted by the mouthpiece on the teeth remains uncertain. One study reported that in single-reed and brass players the incisors were inclined backward twice as frequently as in the general population (Gualtieri 1979), while another noted only minor differences (Rindisbacher et al. 1990). The pressure on the teeth does, however, produce significant problems for those with false front teeth. Absence of any natural teeth presents almost insuperable obstacles for anchoring removable dentures sufficiently to support the embouchure, while retention of even a small number (e.g., two to five) can provide enough support for dentures if properly designed (Fine 1986). Surgical implanted supports for the dentures can be effective where there are no teeth to support the dentures. If any front teeth must be removed, a cast should be made so that the replacement dental prosthesis will match them as closely as possible in order to minimize the adjustments needed in playing. Indeed, for professional players with sound teeth, it is a sensible insurance policy to have casts made to facilitate reconstruction in case of future accidents. Even loss of the teeth at the back of the mouth can result in difficulty in controlling the airstream and so their replacement should not be neglected.

High Pressure in the Airway

The possible effects of high pressure in the lungs of wind players is discussed in chapter 4. Though the tissues within the lungs might theoretically be compressed, the chest cavity is well supported against high internal pressures by the rib cage; however, other regions of the airway in the pharynx and oral cavity (mouth) do not have skeletal support and may undergo distension and damage due to high internal pressures. We will start by considering problems due to weakness of the soft palate. The high pressures that are required in playing brass and reed instruments can only be supported if the passageway from the throat to the back of the nose is efficiently blocked off by the raising of the soft palate against the back of the nasopharynx (see fig. 4-14). Occasionally this mechanism fails in wind players, a situation that is known as loss of seal or, more technically, velopharyngeal insufficiency (Ziporyn 1984; Gilbert 1998). The symptoms are either an inability to generate enough pressure to play certain notes, or noise coming from the nose when certain notes are played. It would be logical to assume that this is particularly associated with the instruments that require the highest maximum pharyngeal pressures, for example, oboe, horn, and B-flat and piccolo trumpets when playing in the upper registers. To some extent this is true, but it is not the whole story as it does not explain why clarinetists are among the wind players most commonly affected. Though the maximum pressures generated when playing the clarinet are far outstripped by the other instruments mentioned above, it does require among the highest minimum pressures to initiate notes (Schwab and Schultze-Florey 2004). Put more simply, to initiate the notes in the lower and middle registers, which is the part of the range in most constant use, requires higher pressures than notes in the equivalent range of the horn and trumpet. As a result, the muscles of the soft palate in clarinetists must on average do more work than those in players of small-bore brass instruments. Though not the sole cause of loss of seal, fatigue in the muscles of the soft palate (the tensor and levator palatini muscles) is the major one. The problem frequently arises as a result of a period of intense playing maintained over a number of days or weeks. It may also occur following a break from playing (such as a holiday), because the muscles have lost some of their condition, or be experienced during a cold infection or during a time of emotional stress (Schwab and Schultze-Florey 2004). Loss of seal is most common in young players (particularly in females), either because the muscles of the soft palate are not fully developed or, less often, because the soft palate as a whole is too short to make unobstructed contact with the back of the throat. Depending on circumstances, complete rest or a return to less-demanding repertoire, followed by a program of progressive exercise for the muscles of the palate, is generally sufficient to resolve the problem. It can also arise following tonsillectomy, after which it is not unusual for wind players to experience difficulties for three to six weeks or more. During this period, great care should be taken not to damage muscle and other tissues around the site of the tonsils (Hart and Logemann 1986). The presence of enlarged adenoids (tonsils), which is common in children and teenagers, may in itself prevent the formation of an efficient seal. If loss of seal for whatever reason is persistent in professional players, a prosthesis (a physical support), typically a plastic plate similar to one used to hold dentures but extending backward beyond the hard palate, is one option to keep the soft palate in position during playing. This is not worn constantly but is slipped in only for playing. Alternatively, if this fails or interferes with playing, it may be possible to enlarge the soft palate by surgical means (Dibbell, Ewanowski, and Carter 1979). The least major form of surgery is to inject some inert material under the surface of the soft palate where it fails to make adequate contact with the back of the throat. This material can be fat taken from the player's own body (Klotz et al. 2001), or a man-made material such as Teflon (Gordon, Astrachan, and Yanagisawa 1994). Though players who have had a cleft palate repair early in life sometimes report problems with seal following periods of increasingly intensive playing, there is no reason to assume that they are more prone to this type of problem than other wind players.

Pharyngoceles and Laryngoceles

The pharynx (the throat) is a muscular tube whose walls, unlike those of the trachea or the thorax, are not supported by a skeleton of cartilage or bone. The high pressures required for playing double-reed and small-bore brass instruments can cause the pharynx to become chronically distended (Levine 1986). Young players are likely to be most at risk because its muscular walls are less well developed at this stage than in adults. Consequently, it may be advisable to limit the volume of sound and amount of playing that young musicians carry out in parts of the range where the pressures are highest (Stasney, Beaver, and Rodriguez 2003). For brass instruments, this will be the extreme upper end of the range, but the same is not true for all woodwind instruments (Fuks and Sundberg 1999). Certain conditions in which the supporting connective tissue of the pharynx is weak may increase the risk of distension, which can lead to the formation within its walls of pocketlike folds called pharyngoceles (fig. 6-4D). When these develop, swallowing can become difficult and food can be trapped within them. As a result, food fragments may appear again in the mouth during playing when the throat expands, even though some time has elapsed since eating. A small amount of distension of the neck during playing is generally regarded as normal and often makes it necessary to keep the top shirt button undone or to wear shirts with a larger

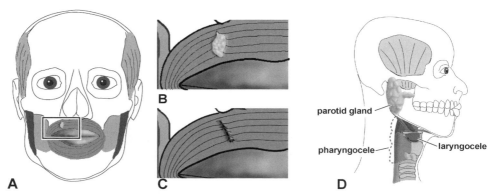

Figure 6-4. **A–C. Rupture of the orbicularis oris muscle, commonly known as Satchmo's syndrome. The tear in the muscle (the purse-string muscle of the mouth) is typically at right angles to the direction of its fibers. The affected part of the muscle, indicated by the box in A, is seen at higher magnification in B. Underlying fatty tissue may push out through the tear. Nowadays this can be treated surgically by stitching the tear closed (C). D. This diagram shows symptoms of several problems that may arise as a result of the high pressure generated in the airway during playing. Air may be forced into the parotid salivary gland, causing it to swell (pneumoparotitis). The muscular wall of the pharynx may become distended (dashed line), forming a pharyngocele. A small sac that is in communication with the central space of the larynx may become inflated so that it appears on the outside of the thyroid cartilage. This is called a laryngocele.**

collar size. Where distension is extreme, a medical opinion should be sought. In former times, some players used to strap the neck during playing, and even today a soft cervical collar may be recommended (Smith and Levine 1986). An intensive program to strengthen the superficial muscles of the neck (trapezius, sternocleidomastoid, and platysma) is also likely to be suggested even though none of these lie directly in contact with the pharynx. If there is a persistent and significant problem, switching to another instrument is advisable.

Within the larynx there are also spaces that can become enlarged by pressurized air (Levine 1986; Gallivan and Gallivan 2002). The gap between the vocal folds and the vestibular folds is known as the ventricle. This is a slitlike opening that enlarges into a blind-ended pouch the extends forward and is a weak point in the wall of the larynx, which is otherwise supported by cartilage. It can become enlarged to form what is known as a laryngocele, a cavity that pushes outward to emerge above the thyroid cartilage (fig. 6-4D). The first clinical description of laryngoceles is thought to be from Napoleon's surgeon, Baron Larrey, who described them in army drill manuals in 1829 (Gallivan and Gallivan 2002), but they appear to be very common in wind players, in whom they are generally asymptomatic. They are an occupational hazard for glassblowers, who also generate high airway pressures. Problems only arise when the fluid that collects in them becomes infected.

Pneumoparotitis (Wind Parotitis)

Three sets of salivary glands empty into the mouth. The largest is the parotid gland, which lies on the cheek over the angle of the jaw (fig. 6-4D). The saliva it produces runs along a duct that opens through the muscular wall of the cheek at the level of the second upper molar tooth. Though large, the gland is not usually prominent unless it becomes swollen, for example, during an attack of mumps. The high pressures in the mouth during the playing of brass and woodwind instruments can drive air into the duct, causing the gland to inflate. This has been recorded in wind players for hundreds of years, beginning with medieval cornet players. French Foreign Legionnaires who wanted to avoid duty were known to induce this condition so they appeared to have the mumps (Levine 1986). High air pressure in the mouth can drive saliva as well as air into the duct of the parotid gland. This can carry bacteria that may precipitate infection and a blockage of the duct, leading to swelling of the gland. The swelling is painful because the gland is enclosed in a tough sheath. Such infections are treated with antibiotics but are not easily prevented (Yeo et al. 2002)

Syncope

Syncope is a lack of blood flow to the brain that may cause dizziness and fainting. It can be caused by the very high pressures that are produced in the thoracic cavity during the playing of brass instruments such as the trumpet. When players generate pressures that exceed the peak (systolic) blood pressure, the vessels in the thorax become compressed and the flow of blood to the brain is reduced or temporarily halted. Syncope is most likely to occur in players of small-bore brass instruments, at the end of long passages of high-intensity playing in the upper registers (Tucker, Faulkner, and Horvath 1971).

Eye Problems

Some accounts of brass playing technique suggest that generating high pressure in the airway may cause bleeding within the eye. This is not likely unless the player has an existing eye problem such as diabetic retinopathy or age-related macular degeneration (wet type), which are associated with the growth of new blood vessels that are fragile and therefore at risk of rupture (Marmor 1986). Raised pressure in the blood vessels of the head that occurs when playing some instruments has been demonstrated to lead to a transient increase in the pressure within the eyeball together with an increase in the thickness of a layer beneath the retina (choroid) that contains most of the blood vessels (Schuman et al. 2000). Both of these increases last only for as long as high lung pressure is maintained and fall immediately when the player takes a breath. Chronic raised intraocular pressure is symptomatic of glaucoma, a condition in which the production of the fluid within the eyeball exceeds its ability to drain away into the venous system of the eyeball. It can ultimately lead to blindness due to compression of the head of the optic nerve; however, for this to happen the high pressure must be maintained for prolonged periods of time (many days). As the paper by Schuman appears to be the only rigorous study of its type performed to date, it is worth describing in more detail. Only three subjects were involved. One was a seventy-two-year-old oboist and the second a seventy-eight-year-old trumpeter, both of whom had been playing for fifty years or more, while the third was a forty-six-year-old player of various wind instruments who had thirty-six years' playing experience. Each had a different type of glaucoma though this had little or no effect on their visual acuity, and their intraocular pressures when not playing were close to normal (10–20 mmHg). In the oboist, intraocular pressure rose from 16 to 40 mmHg over a period of twenty seconds when playing high and loud. For another of the subjects, playing the saxophone or clarinet as loud and as high as possible raised intraocular pressure only from 10 to 21 mmHg, though for neither instrument is this the range where peak pressures are generated (Fuks and Sundberg 1999). When playing the trumpet, intraocular pressure in the same individual rose to over 30 mmHg. Other studies have provided no evidence that intraocular pressure is more sensitive to raised thoracic pressure in individuals with existing glaucoma than in those without, so these values are probably typical for such instruments. In order to increase the scope of the study, the authors carried out detailed visual field tests in an additional forty-six professional musicians but did not measure their intraocular pressure during playing. These were nine players of high-pressure wind instruments, twelve of low-pressure instruments, and twenty-three players of nonwind instruments. These players had on average more than thirty years' playing experience. The high-pressure wind players had an extremely small but statistically significant increase in what could be regarded as glaucomatous damage, but at a level that was unlikely to be clinically significant. Clearly this subject would benefit from investigation of a much larger pool of players in which various aspects of lifestyle were also taken into consideration.

Rupture of Orbicularis Oris (Satchmo's Syndrome)

The orbicularis oris muscle can be physically damaged in brass instrumentalists through the demands of playing in very high registers or with great intensity. Rupture of the muscle is commonly known as Satchmo's syndrome because just such an injury was sustained by Louis Armstrong in 1935, with the result that he had to cease playing for a considerable period. The injury is often triggered by a player switching to a new mouthpiece requiring a modification of the embouchure (Papsin, Maaske, and McGrail 1996). The most commonly reported symptoms are weakness of the embouchure, followed by pain, loss of tone, and loss of seal against the mouthpiece. The damage to the muscle is typically a tear that lies at right angles to the direction of the muscle fibers (fig. 6-4A, B). If left untreated, this may heal only incompletely, leaving a rigid scar, or may result in a thinning of the muscle at the site of injury. If the tear remains open, the underlying fatty tissue may push through the gap as a small hernia. Before the advent of surgical treatments, the only remedy was either to stop playing and hope that it would heal naturally, to avoid extreme registers, or to try to continue playing using a small-bore mouthpiece. Recovery was rarely complete. Nowadays, simple surgical methods can be used to repair the damage, apparently with a reasonable degree of success (fig. 6-4C). The operation is generally carried out with the patient awake, as the incisions are superficial. Under such circumstances, asking the patient to buzz the embouchure during the procedure makes it easier to identify the damaged area. In addition, when the muscle is stitched but before the wound in the skin is closed, the surgeon can check that the sutures will hold when the muscle is contracted to form the embouchure. Playing can generally recommence three to twelve weeks after the operation, and players are said to return to their full level of proficiency (Papsin, Maaske, and McGrail 1996; Planas 1988).

Focal Dystonia of the Embouchure

Focal dystonia is a loss of muscle control that can affect either the embouchure or the hand in musicians. A full account of its nature and origin will be found in chapter 8. The overall incidence of dystonia among musicians as a whole is difficult to quantify; however, in a group of over 1,300 players with neuromuscular or musculoskeletal problems that affected their playing, about 8 percent were given a diagnosis of dystonia (Lederman 2003). The most detailed account to date of embouchure dystonia is a review of twenty-six cases among brass and woodwind players (Frucht et al. 2001). Because of the number of cases covered in this study, it is possible to draw some preliminary conclusions concerning the incidence of different forms of embouchure dystonia in players of a range of instruments, as well as to assess the outcomes of various therapies. The dystonia manifests itself as a lack of embouchure control, which may include symptoms such as lip tremor or fatigue, or involuntary activity of facial muscles contributing to the embouchure or of those moving the jaw. In individuals with lip tremor, this symptom appears with the onset of playing and is usually associated not with the entire range of the instrument, but with a particular register. The abnormal muscle activity often involves a lateral pulling on one corner of the lip. Among the musicians studied by Frucht, this was reported only in players of high-register brass instruments, most commonly the French horn. In players of low-register brass instruments, involuntary lip closure was a more typical symptom. Like focal dystonia elsewhere, the typical age of onset for embouchure dystonia is the mid- to late thirties, on average around twenty-five years after the musician first started to study the instrument. It is rarely associated with pain, though some discomfort is not unusual. A variety of treatments have been tried for embouchure dystonia, such as retraining, the use of dental prosthetic devices, and various alternative therapies, but none has a satisfactory success rate. Botox injections are often advocated for reducing the strength of the troublesome muscle contractions. These are rarely effective, as not only do they not treat the root of the problem, but it is extremely difficult to deliver the precise quantity needed to reduce the level of contraction to the correct degree in such small muscles. As with other forms of dystonia, the symptoms are typically context dependent (i.e., they are associated only with playing) and only rarely do they spread to other activities involving the mouth. This is exemplified by a case quoted by Frucht in which a player who gave up the trumpet because of dystonia successfully switched to playing the bassoon without reactivating the symptoms.

Damage to Nerves in the Face

The muscles that contribute to the embouchure are supplied by branches of the facial nerve. These emerge from under the parotid salivary gland, whose position is shown in figure 6-4. The fine branches of the nerve are vulnerable to deep cuts to the face.

As the nerves run predominantly horizontally, vertical cuts are likely to be the most dangerous. If nerve branches are severed, the muscles will be paralyzed. If the ends of the nerves can be brought together, the motor neurons supplying the muscles may be able to regrow to supply the muscles. Alternatively, nerve grafts can be used to aid regrowth. Paralysis of the facial nerve also occurs in a condition known as facial nerve (or Bell's) palsy. This condition is usually of unknown origin but may arise following exposure to cold or be associated with dental treatment (perhaps as a result of injection of anesthetic) or a middle ear infection. The outcome depends on how severely the nerves are damaged. Complete recovery may occur over a period of months, particularly if only the ends of the nerve branches have lost function. However, recovery sometimes brings changes to the pattern of nerve supply so that attempts to activate one muscle or set of muscles cause abnormal twitches in others.

Sensation to the face is supplied by the branches of the trigeminal nerve. Trigeminal neuralgia, another condition that is usually of unknown cause, results in severe stabbing pain in the face. It is often triggered by gentle touch, by chewing, or by brushing the teeth. Though each bout of pain lasts only a short time, it can nonetheless be debilitating. The symptoms, although not the underlying cause, are usually controllable with drugs. More drastic treatments involving surgical intervention to cut nerve fibers have varying levels of success and of course will result in loss of sensation, which is crucial for wind players. It has recently been discovered that compression of the base of the trigeminal nerves by blood vessels within the skull can be a source of trigeminal neuralgia, in which case it can be relieved by invasive surgical treatment. Burning mouth syndrome (a painful sensation of heat within the mouth) may be related to trigeminal neuralgia in the sense that it also affects this nerve; however, if anything it is even more enigmatic (Wall, McMahon, and Koltzenburg 2006). It is most commonly reported in postmenopausal women but is not confined to this group. Emotional stress is often cited as a trigger, though there is a danger that this conclusion is reached only as the last stage in a process of elimination and is therefore a tacit admission that an organic cause cannot be found. Changes in the properties of the nerve endings within the mouth have recently been demonstrated in one group of patients, but it is still not known why this occurs (Yilmaz et al. 2007).

REFERENCES

Amir, N. 2004. Some insight into the acoustics of the didgeridu. *Applied Acoustics* 65:1181–96.

Barbenel, J. C., J. B. Davies, and P. Kenny. 1986. Science proves musical myths wrong. *New Scientist* 110 (1502):29–32.

Barbenel, J. C., P. Kenny, and J. B. Davies. 1988. Mouthpiece forces produced while playing the trumpet. *J Biomech* 21 (5):417–24.

Basmajian, J. V., and E. R. White. 1973. Neuromuscular control of trumpeters' lip. *Nature* 241 (5384):70.

Benade, A. H. 1986. Interactions between the player's windway and the air column of a musical instrument. *Cleve Clin Q* 53 (1):27–32.

Brown, A. F. D. 1976. A cinefluorographic pilot study of the throat while vibrato tones are played on flute and oboe. *J Int Double Reed Soc* no. 4.

Cossette, I., P. Sliwinski, and P. T. Macklem. 2000. Respiratory parameters during professional flute playing. *Respir Physiol* 121 (1):33–44.

Devroop, K., and K. S. Chesky. 2002. Comparison of biomechanical forces generated during trumpet performance in contrasting settings. *Med Prob Perform Artists* 17:149–54.

Dibbell, D. G., S. Ewanowski, and W. L. Carter. 1979. Successful correction of velopharyngeal stress incompetence in musicians playing wind instruments. *Plast Reconstr Surg* 64 (5):662–64.

Engelman, J. A. 1965. Measurement of perioral pressures during playing of musical wind instruments. *Am J Orthod* 51 (11):856–64.

Fine, L. 1986. Dental problems in the wind instrumentalist. *Cleve Clin Q* 53 (1):3–9.

Fritze, C., and J. Wolfe. 2005. How do clarinet players adjust the resonances of their vocal tracts for different playing effects? *J Acoust Soc Am* 118 (5):3306–15.

Frucht, S. J., S. Fahn, P. E. Greene, C. O'Brien, M. Gelb, D. D. Truong, J. Welsh, S. Factor, and B. Ford. 2001. The natural history of embouchure dystonia. *Mov Disord* 16 (5):899–906.

Fuks, L., and J. Sundberg. 1999. Blowing pressures in bassoon, clarinet, oboe and saxophone. *Acustica* 85:267–77.

Gallivan, K. H., and G. J. Gallivan. 2002. Bilateral mixed laryngoceles: Simultaneous strobovideolaryngoscopy and external video examination. *J Voice* 16 (2):258–66.

Gilbert, T. B. 1998. Breathing difficulties in wind instrument players. *Md Med J* 47 (1):23–27.

Gordon, N. A., D. Astrachan, and E. Yanagisawa. 1994. Videoendoscopic diagnosis and correction of velopharyngeal stress incompetence in a bassoonist. *Ann Otol Rhinol Laryngol* 103 (8 Pt 1):595–600.

Gualtieri, P. A. 1979. May Johnny or Janie play the clarinet? The Eastman Study: A report on the orthodontic evaluations of college-level and professional musicians who play brass and woodwind instruments. *Am J Orthod* 76 (3):260–76.

Hart, C. W., and J. A. Logemann. 1986. Tonsils and adenoids and the professional musician. *Med Prob Perform Artists* 1:58–60.

Herman, E. 1974. Dental considerations in the playing of musical instruments. *J Am Dent Assoc* 89 (3):611–19.

———. 1981. Influence of musical instruments on tooth positions. *Am J Orthod* 80 (2):145–55.

Heuser, F., and J. L. McNitt-Gray. 1991. EMG potentials prior to tone commencement in trumpet players. *Med Prob Perform Artists* 6 (4):51–56.

———. 1993. EMG patterns in embouchure muscles of trumpet players with asymmetrical mouthpiece placement. *Med Prob Perform Artists* 8:96–102.

———. 1998. Enhancing and validating: Pedagogical practice. The use of electromyography during trumpet instruction. *Med Prob Perform Artists* 13 (4):155–59.

King, A. I., J. Ashby, and C. Nelson. 1988. Laryngeal function in wind instrumentalists: The woodwinds. *J Voice* 1:365–67.

———. 1989. Laryngeal function in wind instruments: The brass. 3 (1):65–67.

Klotz, D. A., J. Howard, A. S. Hengerer, and O. Slupchynskj. 2001. Lipoinjection augmentation of the soft palate for velopharyngeal stress incompetence. *Laryngoscope* 111 (12):2157–61.

Lederman, R. J. 2003. Neuromuscular and musculoskeletal problems in instrumental musicians. *Muscle Nerve* 27 (5):549–61.

Levine, H. L. 1986. Functional disorders of the upper airway associated with playing wind instruments. *Cleve Clin Q* 53 (1):11–13.

Marmor, M. F. 1986. Vision and the musician. *Med Prob Perform Artists* 1:117–20.

Nixon, G. 1963. Dental problems in brass instrumentalists. *Br Dent J* 105:160–61.

Papsin, B. C., L. A. Maaske, and J. S. McGrail. 1996. Orbicularis oris muscle injury in brass players. *Laryngoscope* 106 (6):757–60.

Planas, J. 1988. Further experience with rupture of the orbicularis oris in trumpet players. *Plast Reconstr Surg* 81 (6):975–81.

Ridgeon, J. 1986. *The physiology of brass playing*: Manton, UK: Brass Wind Educational Supplies.

Rindisbacher, T., U. Hirschi, B. Ingervall, and A. Geering. 1990. Little influence on tooth position from playing a wind instrument. *Angle Orthod* 60 (3):223–28.

Rydell, R., M. Karlsson, A. Milesson, and L. Schalen. 1996. Laryngeal activity during wind instrument playing: Video endoscopic documentation. *Logoped Phoniatr Vocol* 21:43–48.

Schuman, J. S., E. C. Massicotte, S. Connolly, E. Hertzmark, B. Mukherji, and M. Z. Kunen. 2000. Increased intraocular pressure and visual field defects in high resistance wind instrument players. *Ophthalmology* 107 (1):127–33.

Schwab, B., and A. Schultze-Florey. 2004. Velopharyngeal insufficiency in woodwind and brass players. *Med Prob Perform Artists* 19:21–25.

Smith, R., and H. Levine. 1986. Hypopharyngeal dilatation in musicians. *Med Prob Perform Artists* 1:20–23.

Stasney, C. R., M. E. Beaver, and M. Rodriguez. 2003. Hypopharyngeal pressure in brass musicians. *Med Prob Perform Artists* 14:153–55.

Tucker, A., M. E. Faulkner, and S. M. Horvath. 1971. Electrocardiography and lung function in brass instrument players. *Arch Environ Health* 23 (5):327–34.

Wall, Patrick D., S. B. McMahon, and Martin Koltzenburg. 2006. *Wall and Melzack's textbook of pain*. 5th ed. Philadelphia: Elsevier/Churchill Livingstone.

Weikert, M., and J. Schlomicher-Thier. 1999. Laryngeal movements in saxophone playing: Video-endoscopic investigations with saxophone players. A pilot study. *J Voice* 13 (2):265–73.

White, E. R., and J. V. Basmajian. 1973. Electromyography of lip muscles and their role in trumpet playing. *J Appl Physiol* 35 (6):892–97.

Yeo, D. K., T. P. Pham, J. Baker, and S. A. Porters. 2002. Specific orofacial problems experienced by musicians. *Aust Dent J* 47 (1):2–11.

Yilmaz, Z., T. Renton, Y. Yiangou, J. Zakrzewska, I. P. Chessell, C. Bountra, and P. Anand. 2007. Burning mouth syndrome as a trigeminal small fiber neuropathy: Increased heat and capsaicin receptor TRPV1 in nerve fibers correlates with pain score. *J Clin Neurosci* 14 (9):864–71.

Ziporyn, T. 1984. Pianist's cramp to stage fright: The medical side of music-making. *JAMA* 252 (8):985–89.

Chapter Seven

The Structure and Organization of the Brain

The human brain manages to compress a phenomenal amount of computing power into a very small volume. Its main task is through our senses, to analyze the world around us and as a result to generate appropriate behavior. In so doing it routinely carries out computations in real time that the most powerful computers have difficulty in matching. On the other hand, before we start to feel too self-satisfied, it must also be admitted that it has difficulties with simple arithmetic operations that the cheapest of calculators can manage with ease. Nevertheless, complex sensory tasks such as our ability to identify objects regardless of the angle of view, to recognize individual faces or voices instantly or a piece of music from a phrase lasting a couple of seconds, are remarkable feats that we perform effortlessly. Not only do we take these complex tasks for granted, but the ability to lead a normal life is entirely dependent on their being achieved with almost total reliability. Any lapses would immediately be detected by our companions, who would quickly alter their behavior toward us as a result. The brain's achievements in controlling the movement of the body are equally impressive. Think of a cricketer diving at full stretch to catch a ball. The three-dimensional trajectory of the ball must first be calculated in a fraction of a second and its subsequent motion predicted. The body is then moved toward a point where the ball can be intercepted. If time is short the player may throw his body down along its own predicted trajectory with an arm extended to reach the intercept point with millisecond accuracy. While all this is happening the brain is also occupied with maintaining normal body functions (breathing, temperature regulation, metabolic control, etc.), providing emotional responses to the situation, matching the experience with previous memories, and predicting how success or failure with the catch will affect the outcome of the match!

The brain weighs approximately 1.5 kilograms. Forty percent of this is made up of the nerve cells involved in carrying out computations or memory storage, while 60 percent represents the cabling that links its different regions together. It contains approximately 100 billion (10^{11}) nerve cells (or neurons), each of which is connected to hundreds or thousands of other nerve cells. The structure of typical nerve cells in the brain is shown in figure. 7-1. Each has a cell body at the center of which lies the

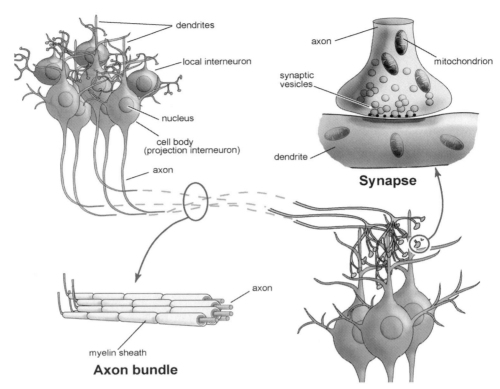

Figure 7-1. The main features of nerve cells in the brain. Each nerve cell has a cell body that contains the nucleus, a spherical structure that carries all the information the cell requires to maintain its normal functions. The cell body receives information from other nerve cells, either via contacts (synapses) made directly onto it or via its many branching dendrites. The cell body also has a single long axon that carries information to other nerve cells. Axons are often sheathed in myelin, which is composed of spirally wrapped glial cell membranes, and this speeds the passage of information along them. Axons end in synapses, which contact other neurons. Synapses contain many small vesicles that carry the chemical neurotransmitters that the nerve cells release in order to communicate with each other. They also contain mitochondria, which generate the energy needed to operate the synapse. In addition to projection interneurons, which carry information over long distances, the nervous system contains very large numbers of small local interneurons, which are responsible for the information processing that takes place within the computational units of the brain.

nucleus, the repository of the genetic instructions that are necessary for the development and normal functioning of the cell. These instructions carry the blueprints for the manufacture not only of the proteins that contribute to the structure of the nerve cells, but also those that control the chemical reactions and signaling processes that take place between and within the nerve cells (enzymes, receptors, and signal molecules). The proteins are manufactured almost entirely within the cell body and so when needed elsewhere, they must be transported, sometimes over considerable distances, to these sites. Many branches emerge from the cell body. Most of these are dendrites, whose role is to receive information through contacts (synapses) with other nerve cells in the nervous system. Each nerve cell also has a single branch, the axon, which carries information to other nerve cells. In some neurons it can be a meter or more in length, though in others it may terminate quite close to the cell body. The axon ends in a series of terminal branches carrying the synapses that contact other nerve cells in the circuit (fig. 7-1).

The nerve cells of the brain can be classified into four main categories. Sensory neurons (fig. 1-3) carry information from the skin, muscles, and joints and are responsible for sensations such as touch, pain, and temperature. Sensory cells, albeit of a rather different form, are also found within the special sense organs and are responsible for the sensations of taste, smell, vision, hearing, and balance. We interact with the world through our verbal and physical responses to it, and our behavior is ultimately manifested by the action of muscles, which are controlled by motor neurons (fig. 1-3). Between the sensory neurons and the motor neurons lie the great computational centers of the brain. Within these, the analysis and interpretation of the information received by the nervous system are carried out by what are known as interneurons—neurons that link one nerve cell to another (figs. 1-3, 7-1). There are two classes of interneurons. Those in one group (projection interneurons) have long axons that carry information over considerable distances from one part of the brain to another. The second group contains local interneurons, which are much smaller and confined to small, well-defined regions of the brain devoted to a particular task. The local interneurons are the ones that carry out the complex computations of the brain; the more advanced the animal, the greater the proportion of its total population of nerve cells that are of this type.

Each nerve cell is linked to hundreds or thousands of others, and the connections between pairs of nerve cells typically comprise tens or hundreds of individual synaptic connections. It has been estimated that a typical neuron receives 1,000–10,000 synapses, though for some neurons the figure may be as high as 200,000. The total number of synapses in the cortex of the brain alone is conservatively estimated at 60 trillion (6×10^{15})! The nerve cells communicate with each other by releasing chemicals called neurotransmitters, which are stored in vesicles that are found at the synapse (fig. 7-1). The neurotransmitters may excite or inhibit a neuron, or alter its sensitivity to other inputs. There are many tens of different types of neurotransmitters and each can have several quite distinct effects on nerve cell activity. All of this serves to increase the subtlety of the interactions between neurons. In addition, the connections do not remain immutable throughout life but can be broken and re-formed over time to change the properties of brain circuitry so that it can adapt to different situations. From this battery of statistics it will be obvious that the brain is literally unimaginably complex; one might be forgiven for wondering if there is any hope at all for attempts to unravel how it operates. We have in fact made quite a good beginning in the last century and a half toward revealing its secrets. In the last fifty years progress has become increasingly rapid through the development of a constantly expanding range of new investigative techniques that modern science has made available. However, it would be naive to imagine that we have done more than make a respectable start to our exploration of the brain. Today, the brain is studied at many different levels. It is possible to examine individual connections between nerve cells in order to reveal their properties or to look at how small groups of neurons interact with each other. This

information may be useful in the search for drugs to treat illness or to gain an insight
into how information is coded within the nervous system, but it does not often reveal a
great deal about how the brain achieves what it does in analytical or behavioral terms.
At the other end of the spectrum, it is possible to see which areas of the brain are active during particular types of behavior or when we are carrying out certain mental
tasks; however, it has not been revealed how this is achieved at a cellular level or how
the outcome is incorporated into normal behavior. Finally, one can also simply treat
the brain as a black box and study our psychological responses to different situations,
but once again this will not reveal the underlying mechanisms. Because of the incredibly complex nature of the interactions between nerve cells, bridging the gap between
these different approaches raises enormous challenges, and in any attempt to describe
how the brain responds in a particular context (such as music), these gaps in the fabric
of our understanding soon make their presence felt only too clearly.

Strange as it may seem, neurons are not the most abundant type of cell in the nervous system. They are outnumbered ten to fifty times by another class of cell called
glia. There are several types of glial cells, whose basic role is to support the function
of the nerve cells—to make the brain a "land fit for neurons." One class of glial cell
(astrocytes) regulates the environment of the neurons. Within the brain, the small
spaces between the nerve cells are filled with a salty fluid through which nutrients,
oxygen, neurotransmitters, ions, and other chemicals required for nerve cell survival
can diffuse freely. The glial cells control the composition of the salts in this fluid to
optimize it for nerve cell performance. They also break down some neurotransmitters
that would become toxic if they were not quickly removed after they had performed
their function. They help to provide general structural support for brain tissue and
maintain the integrity of key elements such as the synapses. Astrocytes also play a
role in regulating blood flow so that this is matched to the level of activity in regions
of brain tissue on a second-by-second basis.

Another class of glial cell (the oligodendrocytes or Schwann cells) produces sheets
of membrane that wrap around the long axons that link the nerve cells together. This
covering, known as the myelin sheath, acts as an insulator and has the effect of increasing the speed at which signals can pass along the axon (fig. 7-1). It is found only
in vertebrates and is particularly important in large animals. One reason it is so hard
for us to catch or swat a fly with our hand is that because the fly is so small, the axons
of its nerve cells are much shorter than ours. Even with the aid of myelination, the
time taken for signals to travel from the brain to the muscles used to move the hand is
much longer than the time it takes for a signal to travel from the brain of the fly to the
muscles that move its legs and wings, and we can only hope to outwit it using guile.
Bundles of myelinated axons appear white in brain tissue and as a result are referred to
as white matter (fig. 7-4). This therefore represents the cabling of the nervous system.
The areas of the brain that contain groups of nerve cell bodies and dendrites are darker
and as a result are referred to as gray matter (fig. 7-4). The gray matter areas are the
computational centers of the brain and it is here that the incoming streams of information are passed via synapses to the local interneurons, which integrate and manipulate
the signals before forwarding the data for further analysis elsewhere. Gray matter
areas may appear as solid masses or as thin sheets, depending on their location.

A third class of glial cell (microglia) is involved in fighting disease and removing the remnants of brain cells that have become damaged or have died. Very few nerve cells are produced beyond the first few months after birth, but glial cells continue to be replaced throughout life. As a consequence, brain tumors (which form as a result of uncontrolled cell division) never develop from nerve cells but arise either from glial cells or from the membranes that enclose the brain (the meninges).

Though the brain represents only about 2 percent of total body weight, it is a very active tissue; it uses 15–20 percent of the oxygen supply to the body and receives a similar proportion of the total blood supply. This varies little, whether we are trying to solve a difficult mathematical or chess problem or learn a complex new piece of music or are simply watching television or sleeping in our favorite armchair. There are many reasons for this. First, a considerable amount of brain activity is concerned with housekeeping functions. We can regard the body rather like an astronaut's spacesuit, which is responsible for life support; much of the brain is devoted to regulating such activities. These include the control of breathing, heart rate, temperature regulation, water balance, digestion, excretion, metabolism, and so forth. Second, as we have already seen, many perceptual and motor control functions that we take for granted require considerable brain activity, and these are constantly ongoing. Even when we are sleeping, the brain is busy and not only in dreaming. The role of sleep is still only partly understood, but we all know the consequences of going without it. These include loss of perceptual skills, decreased reaction times, and ultimately even disorientation and hallucination coupled with an increasing tendency to lapse into unconsciousness as sleep finally becomes irresistible.

The substance that makes up the living brain is very soft, with a consistency similar to that of blancmange. This potentially creates something of a problem because if unsupported, the lower surface of the brain would be compressed against the skull by its own weight. This would be sufficient to collapse blood vessels, cutting off the supply of oxygen and nutrients, and death of the tissue would rapidly ensue. The reason this does not happen is that the brain floats in a salty liquid called cerebrospinal fluid (CSF). As a consequence, its effective weight is reduced from 1.5 kilograms to about 50 grams. The CSF also resists the tendency of the brain to move within the skull and make contact with the bone. This is very effective unless we receive such a forceful blow to the head that buffering by CSF cannot prevent the brain from striking the skull. Such an impact may result in a partial or complete loss of consciousness, bleeding, or other damage that can cause the brain to swell and to become compressed. The brain and spinal cord are also protected by being wrapped in three layers of membranes known as meninges. The inner layer (the pia) is stuck to the surface of the brain and gives it some support. The CSF lies between this layer and a second layer (the arachnoid) that is very fine but impervious to fluid. This layer lies in contact with a very tough outer layer (the dura) that has the consistency of parchment and is fused to the inside of the skull. All three layers extend down through the central cavity in the vertebral column that contains the spinal cord. If it is suspected that the meninges have become infected (meningitis), CSF may be sampled by collecting it from the space within the vertebrae of the back (lumbar puncture, or spinal tap) so that it can be examined to determine the nature of the infection or damage.

The object of this chapter is to provide an overview of the structure of the brain. It will focus particularly on the structures that are important for an understanding of the ideas presented in the subsequent chapters on the brain's adaptation to music, the auditory system, and the role of the nervous system in stress responses. As a consequence, it should not be regarded as a general summary of brain organization, as many important and interesting features that are not directly relevant to these ends will be omitted.

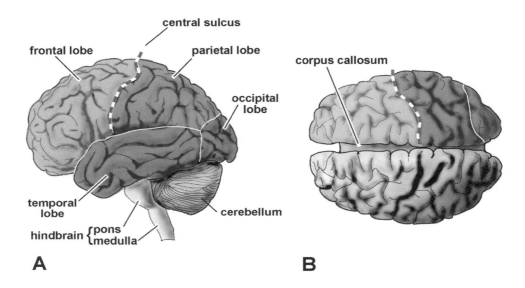

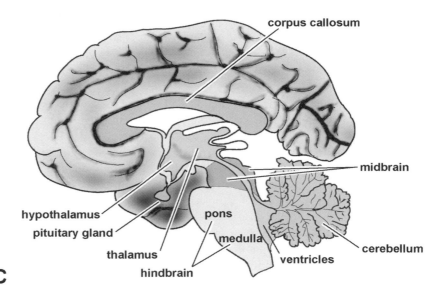

Figure 7-2

The brain originates in the embryo as a hollow tube, and in the mature brain the core of this tube is represented as a series of cavities called ventricles (fig. 7-2C). These are filled with cerebrospinal fluid, which is produced in the ventricles but which is able to find its way out of the brain into the spaces between the layers of the meninges. When we view it from the side, our impression of the intact brain is dominated by the two cerebral hemispheres (fig. 7-2A), a pair of highly infolded masses of nervous tissue that sit side by side, filling the upper part of the skull. At the back, beneath the cerebral hemispheres, sits a single unpaired structure called the cerebellum (literally, the little brain), which also has a highly folded surface. This is attached to the stalk, known as the brain stem, that connects the hemispheres to the spinal cord. For the purposes of anatomical description, the brain is usually divided into three parts: the forebrain (which includes the cerebral hemispheres), the midbrain, and the hindbrain (fig.7-2C). The latter two divisions together constitute the brain stem. The hindbrain is made up of three components, the medulla oblongata (which is continuous with the spinal cord), the pons, and the cerebellum. The pons is broader than the rest of the hindbrain because it contains several massive bundles of axons that connect it to the cerebellum. Traditionally, the cerebellum has been thought to be almost exclusively concerned with the control of movement; however, this idea is beginning to change as evidence accumulates for its involvement in a much broader range of functions, including the analysis of musical sound. The cerebellum receives information from three main sources: 1) the vestibular system, which is the part of the inner ear concerned with balance, 2) the specialized sensory structures within muscles and tendons that provide information on muscle contraction and loading, and 3) regions of the cortex involved in muscle control. The core of the cerebellum is composed mainly of the bundles of axons that connect it to the rest of the brain (i.e., white matter). The computational part is a thin sheet of gray matter that is tightly folded to pack as much of it as possible into the space available. Nerve cells of different types lie in a highly organized array within this sheet. The basic principles of its design have been known for decades; however, working out how it is used in the maintenance of equilibrium

Figure 7-2.   **The general architecture of the brain. A. The cortex is divided into regions called lobes, which are named after the overlying bones of the skull. Its surface is made up of a complex but relatively standardized series of ridges (gyri) separated by deep grooves (sulci). One of these grooves, the central sulcus (broken line), is an important landmark, forming the boundary between the frontal lobe and the parietal lobe. The occipital lobe lies at the back of the brain, and the temporal lobe runs along the side, partly beneath the lower edges of the frontal and parietal lobes. Underneath the cortex lies the brain stem. The parts of the brain stem visible here are the cerebellum, which is connected to the pons, and the medulla. Together these three structures form the hindbrain. B. The cortex as seen from above. Its two halves are called the cerebral hemispheres and they are linked by a very thick bundle of nerve fibers known as the corpus callosum. C. Here the brain has been cut in two by sectioning the corpus callosum and dividing the brain stem along the midline, revealing a series of fluid-filled spaces called ventricles that lie at its core. It is now possible to see the midbrain, which sits in front of the hindbrain. The forebrain is composed of the cortex and a number of structures that lie just beneath it (see fig. 7-4). Two of these (the thalamus and the hypothalamus) lie just beneath the wall of one of the ventricles. The hypothalamus controls the pituitary gland, a structure that influences many important bodily functions by releasing hormones into the bloodstream.**

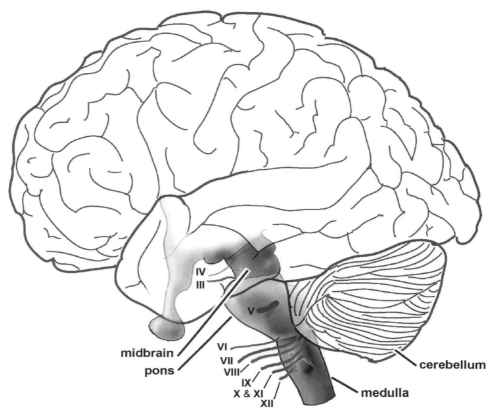

IV
III

V

VI
VII
VIII
midbrain
IX
pons
X & XI
XII

cerebellum

medulla

Figure 7-3. **The brain stem contains the control centers for the life support systems of the body. It exerts much of its influence via a series of ten cranial nerves. Two other cranial nerves (the olfactory and the optic) arise from the forebrain. This diagram shows the position of the other cranial nerves that emerge from the brain stem. Their names and a summary of their major functions are given in table 7-1. Each cranial nerve is assigned a Roman numeral that is often used as a shorthand label.**

and in motor learning has proved a difficult problem to resolve. In front of the cerebellum and pons lies the midbrain, which in humans is almost completely hidden under the back of the cortex. The midbrain roof is composed of two pairs of swellings called colliculi (Latin for "little hills"), which are involved in visual and auditory reflexes. These cause us to turn our head very quickly to look toward a novel source of sound or toward something that has appeared in the periphery of our visual field, actions that were very important for the survival of our vertebrate ancestors.

The brain stem contains many axon bundles that carry information between the spinal cord and the cortex, but its major role is as a control center for many of the body's life support systems. Even if all activity within the cortex ceases (as happens in some forms of brain death), the basic functions required for the body to survive can be maintained if the brain stem remains intact and continues to operate. It does this through signals distributed via a series of cranial nerves that emerge from each

Table 7-1. Cranial Nerve Function

No.	Name	Major Roles	Main Functions in Music
I	Olfactory	Smell	
II	Visual	Sight	Score reading
III	Oculomotor	Eye movement (all); focus, control of pupil (III)	
IV	Trochlear		
VI	Abducens		
V	Trigeminal	Sensory to face, jaw movement, tenses soft palate	Lip and tongue sensation, jaw position, helps maintain seal of palate
VII	Facial	Facial muscle control, taste, salivary glands	Embouchure control, moistens mouth
VIII	Vestibulocochlear	Hearing and balance	Hearing
IX	Glossopharyngeal	Salivary glands, taste, monitors blood composition	Moistens mouth, supplies one throat muscle
X	Vagus	Innervation of gut, larynx, heart, airway, pharynx, palate	Laryngeal sensation, control of laryngeal muscles, control of shape of vocal tract and (with V) seal of palate
XI	Accessory	Vagus + controls some neck muscles	Affects head/neck posture and assists deep breathing
XII	Hypoglossal	Supplies tongue muscles	Control of tongue

side. There are twelve cranial nerves in total, and all but two arise from the brain stem. These are shown in figure 7-3 and their names and functions are summarized in table 7-1. Three of them control the movement of the eyes, plus the focusing of the lens and the opening and closing of the pupils in response to light. One large nerve (the trigeminal nerve) carries sensation from the face and controls the muscles used in chewing; another (the facial nerve) controls the muscles of facial expression, which are also responsible for forming the embouchure. The auditory nerve (more correctly known as the vestibulocochlear nerve) carries both auditory sensation and information from the vestibular apparatus of the inner ear, which is important for maintaining balance. Several of the nerves contribute to the sensation of taste and the control of the salivary glands, while another (the hypoglossal nerve) is dedicated to the control of the muscles of the tongue. One cranial nerve with a particularly large sphere of influence is the vagus nerve. This controls the larynx and some of the muscles of the throat (pharynx) and has an influence over how easily air can flow into the lungs through the bronchioles. It contributes to the regulation of heart rate, controls the movement of the esophagus, stomach, and much of the gut, and promotes digestion. The core of the brain stem therefore contains centers involved in all of these functions and more. It will be clear from this account that a number of cranial nerve functions are crucial to musical performance (see table 7-1). Many tasks require the coordination of activity in several cranial and other nerves through these brain stem centers. A prime example of this is the apparently simple act of swallowing. This requires closure of the mouth (trigeminal nerve), backward movement of the tongue (hypoglossal nerve) and lifting of the soft palate (glossopharyngeal and trigeminal nerves), raising of the larynx (spinal nerves in the neck) and closure of the vocal and vestibular folds (vagus nerve), and contraction of the pharyngeal muscles (vagus) to push food or liquid down the esophagus. Swallowing must also be coordinated with breathing—we make a short intake of breath just before it starts so that there is a positive pressure in the lungs in case stray material has to be expelled from the airway. The act of swallowing therefore requires the orchestrated activity of many different centers within the brain

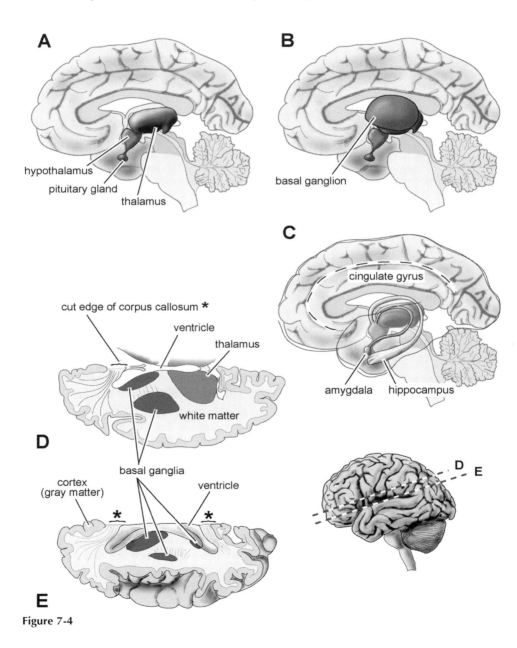

Figure 7-4

stem. Failure of this system can lead to material ending up in the lungs or trachea, with possibly fatal consequences.

Sensory information from the cranial nerves and from the spinal cord is sent to the forebrain. In addition, however, the forebrain receives information directly from two other cranial nerves: the optic and olfactory nerves, which carry visual information from the eye and the sense of smell from the inside of the nose. These nerves differ fundamentally from the other cranial nerves in that they arise from two complex structures that are derived from the brain during embryonic development. These are the retina, which lines the back of the eyeball, and the olfactory bulb. The olfactory bulb sits on the floor of the skull just above a specialized area at the back of the nose that contains nerve cells that respond to odor. The retina and olfactory bulb contain many interneurons, which process the raw visual and olfactory information before sending it to the brain.

The forebrain has two main divisions. The first lies in continuity with the brain stem and contains two major structures, the thalamus and the hypothalamus (figs. 7-2C and 7-4A). These are both paired structures, one of each lying on either side of the slitlike third ventricle, which is found at the midline of the forebrain. Both structures are composed of many separate clusters (or nuclei) of nerve cells, each with its own particular function. The thalamus has three main roles. First, it is the main gatekeeper controlling the flow of sensory information into the cortex. When we are asleep, for example, the thalamus can block the inflow of sensation. Second, the thalamus contains nuclei that are part of the complex network of brain areas that control movement. Finally, another set of nuclei plays a role in emotional responses to sensation, instinctive behavior, and general levels of awareness (arousal).

The hypothalamus lies beneath the thalamus and is another element of the life support system of the brain. It monitors body temperature and substances carried by the blood such as circulating hormones like androgens and estrogens. It controls cellular and whole body metabolism in two main ways: 1) It regulates the release of hormones

Figure 7-4. These diagrams show some of the large structures that lie deep in the forebrain, beneath the cortex. In A, the far side of the brain is shown intact, together with the thalamus and hypothalamus of the near side. The thalamus has several distinct regions with very different roles. Some control the flow of sensory information to the cortex, while others are involved in the control of muscle activity or of general levels of awareness. The hypothalamus monitors vital functions both by analyzing the properties of the blood that passes through it and by receiving sensory information from elsewhere in the body. It exerts its influence on metabolism and homeostasis through the nervous system (e.g., via some of the cranial nerves and the sympathetic nervous system) and through the release of hormones from the pituitary gland. In B we see one of a group of structures collectively known as the basal ganglia, which play a key role in motor control. In C are the principal components of the limbic system (see chapter 10); the hippocampus and amygdala sit near the tip of the temporal lobe, while the cingulate gyrus lies immediately above the corpus callosum. In D and E the positions of the structures shown in A and B can be seen in two horizontal sections through one cerebral hemisphere. The asterisks mark where the corpus callosum has been cut in order to separate the two hemispheres. The planes of these sections are shown by the broken lines on the small image of the brain. The corpus callosum and the other areas of white matter represent the cabling that links different parts of the brain. The thin outer layer of the cortex and the thalamus and basal ganglia are examples of the gray matter areas in which the brain carries out computations.

from the pituitary gland. This large gland hangs by a stalk from the underside of the brain just beneath the hypothalamus. 2) It activates the nerves that make up what is called the autonomic nervous system. We will consider this division of the nervous system in more detail when we deal with stress in chapter 10. At present it suffices to say that it regulates such important functions as heart rate, blood flow, and digestion. Some of the cranial nerves belong partly or entirely to the autonomic nervous system, but other autonomic nerves arise from the spinal cord. The control exercised by the hypothalamus operates over several time scales. It adjusts body temperature on a minute-by-minute basis through its influence on activities such as sweating and shivering and by switching blood flow to or from the skin. On a longer time scale, it regulates the mobilization of stored energy reserves and the rate at which cells burn energy-rich molecules, and influences food and water intake through the sensations of hunger and thirst. It is influenced by the daily fluctuation of light levels to adjust metabolic rate so that this is greatest during the day and lowest at night. When we travel rapidly across several time zones, we suffer the consequences of putting this system out of kilter. We may experience high body temperature during the night, which makes sleep difficult, and low body temperature during the day, with the result that we feel cold and shivery. As we adjust to the new time zone, our body temperature (a reflection of metabolic rate) becomes synchronized with the local cycle of light and dark. On a still longer time scale, the hypothalamus regulates the monthly cycle of female hormone release and controls the pattern of growth during childhood and adolescence through its influence on the release of growth hormone from the pituitary gland.

The second division of the forebrain is composed of the cortex together with some other large masses of nervous tissue that lie beneath it and which constitute a major part of what is known as the basal ganglia. As will be seen in the next chapter, the basal ganglia are involved predominantly in the control of movement and comprise a network of nuclei that also includes masses in another part of the forebrain and in the midbrain. The midbrain component is called the substantia nigra and is the region of the brain that degenerates in patients with Parkinson's disease.

The cortex is made up of two hemispheres, one on each side of the brain, that are linked together by a very large bundle of axons called the corpus callosum (fig. 7-2B), which will feature significantly in the next chapter. The cortex is divided into four major areas or lobes that are named after the bones of the skull under which they lie (fig. 7-2A). Lying just behind the forehead is the frontal lobe, and moving progressively farther back we encounter first the parietal lobe and finally the occipital lobe. Projecting downward from the parietal lobe rather like the thumb of a boxing glove is the temporal lobe. The surface of the cortex is thrown into a series of folds called gyri, separated by grooves known as sulci. If we were to make a horizontal cut through the cortex, we would see that it is composed of a thin sheet of gray matter sitting on a large mass of white matter (fig. 7-4). The sheet of gray matter has an organized structure composed of six sandwichlike layers, each of which has a different function and pattern of connections. The white matter wires these to other areas of the cortex, as well as to the rest of the brain and the spinal cord. The amount of white matter required for this is indicative of the extent and complexity of the connections that the cortex makes. The cortex is folded into sulci and gyri in order

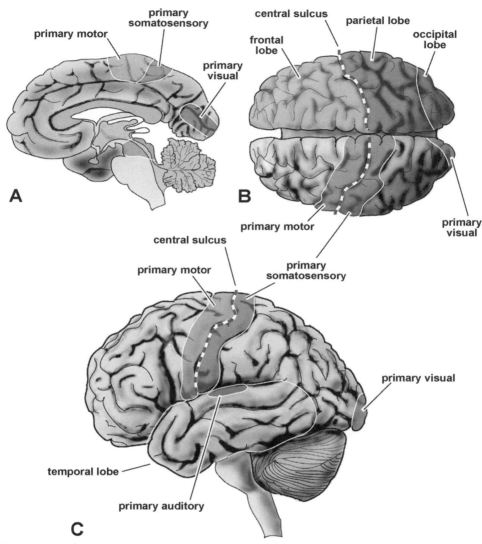

Figure 7-5. The primary motor and sensory areas of the cortex are here shown from three different viewpoints. It is through these regions that information from the eyes (the primary visual cortex) and the ears (primary auditory cortex) and sensation from the skin and muscles (somatosensory cortex) are distributed for higher-level processing. The somatosensory area lies in the parietal lobe, immediately behind the central sulcus, while the primary motor cortex (frontal cortex), which is the main center directing the conscious control of the muscles, lies just in front.

to pack as much of the thin sheet of gray matter as possible into the limited volume afforded by the skull.

The pattern of sulci and gyri is quite consistent between brains, and some of them mark important boundaries between different functional areas of the cortex. The most significant in this regard is the central sulcus, which lies at the boundary between the

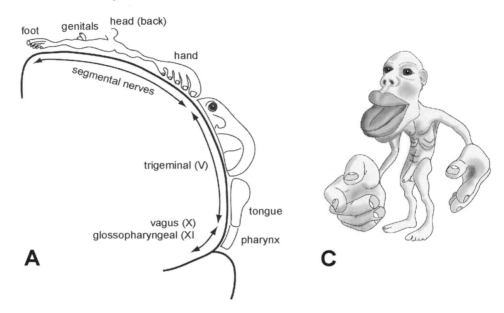

Sensory Homunculus

foot genitals head (back)

hand

segmental nerves

trigeminal (V)

tongue

vagus (X)
glossopharyngeal (XI)

pharynx

A

C

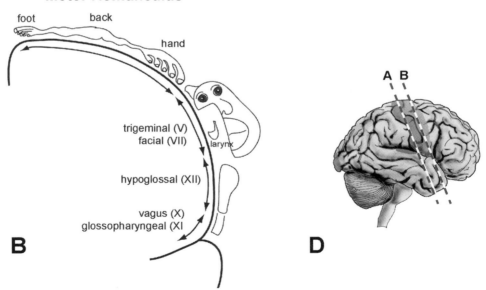

Motor Homunculus

foot back

hand

trigeminal (V)
facial (VII)

larynx

hypoglossal (XII)

vagus (X)
glossopharyngeal (XI)

B

A B

D

Figure 7-6

Figure 7-6. The organization of sensory and motor maps in the cortex. A. This image represents a slice through the primary sensory cortex along the line marked A in the diagram of the brain (D). Though the map of the body is clearly recognizable, it is distorted because proportionately more of the cortex is devoted to the areas of the body that contain the greatest density of sensory nerve endings. This is shown more graphically in C, which is a three-dimensional view of what is known as the sensory homunculus. The overall organization of the motor map is shown in B. In both panels A and B, the cranial nerves that contribute to the maps are indicated by name and number (see fig. 7-3 and table 7-1). Those who are familiar with drawings of the homunculi will notice some differences between this figure and standard representations, which have remained virtually unchanged since first presented by Penfield and Rasmussen (1950): 1) the size of the tongue is increased (in accord with the original observations of Penfield and Boldrey (1937), 2) the genitals are shown in somatotopic order and the foot does not lie on the medial face of the cortex (this derives from recent observations [Kell et al. 2005]), 3) the distal joint of the finger has a larger representation and the palm a smaller one, 4) in C, the representation of the dominant hand (here the right) is larger (Amunts et al. 1996), and 5) the unaccountably large representation of the ears on the standard version of this figure is reduced. It should be noted, however, that while the sensory homunculus is a reasonable interpretation of the organization of the primary sensory cortex, there are problems in depicting the primary motor cortex in this way (as Penfield and Rasmussen pointed out), and these are discussed in the next chapter.

frontal and parietal cortices (fig. 7-5). The different regions of the cortex have different functions, and the central sulcus marks the boundary between the areas involved in muscle or motor control (which lie in the frontal cortex) and those processing sensory information (which lie in the parietal cortex and beyond). The ridge or gyrus immediately in front of the central sulcus is called the primary motor cortex (figs. 7-5, 7-6). This contains a more or less orderly map of the muscle groups of the body but on the opposite side. Hence the right motor cortex controls the movement of the left side of the body and vice versa. The region of the primary motor cortex that lies just above the temporal lobe is associated with movement of the face. Above this lies a large area controlling the hand followed by areas controlling the arm, the trunk, and the leg (fig. 7-6). In front of the primary motor cortex are some other motor areas with more complex functions, which will be discussed in the next chapter. These include Broca's area, which is involved in generation of the motor program required for speech, which is then "played" through regions of the primary motor area responsible for the muscles of the mouth, tongue, larynx, and pharynx.

The ridge or gyrus immediately behind the central sulcus contains the primary sensory cortex. This has a sensory map of the surface of the body that sits in register with the primary motor map that lies on the other side of the sulcus (fig. 7-6A). Thus, the face is represented on the most lateral surface, with the hand represented just above, followed by the arm, trunk, and leg. The primary sensory cortex is the gateway through which the sensory information from the body first enters the cortex, and as with the primary motor cortex, the map represents the opposite side. Other discrete primary sensory areas receive visual and auditory input (fig. 7-5). The primary auditory area lies on the upper surface of the temporal lobe, while the primary visual area is found at the back of the brain in the occipital lobe. Each also contains a sensory map. In the case of the auditory cortex, this is one of sound frequency, and for the visual cortex, it is a map of the visual field.

Now that we have identified the main primary motor and sensory areas of the cortex, it is clear that most of the cerebral hemispheres remain unaccounted for in terms of function. The information reaching the primary sensory areas is presented in a very basic form. We do not just look, hear, touch, or see; we interpret, analyze, and integrate this information. Sound may represent an object, an animal, or a person. It may be music and be analyzed as such or be treated as language and broken down and interpreted according to grammatical rules. We also combine information from the different senses, bringing together texture, form, color, smell, movement, and sound to generate a holistic view of the world. We may recognize an individual person, animal, thing, or place by any one or by several of these features when we encounter them or when we recall them from memory. This all takes place in the areas between the primary cortical regions for the different senses; for this reason they are described as association areas. It is possible to assign a particular role to some of these areas. For example, a region known as Wernicke's area, which lies just behind the primary auditory cortex, contributes to our understanding of language as well as our ability to generate it. Though the speech of patients with damage to this region sounds fluent and grammatical, its content is often meaningless. One must be careful not to be too prescriptive in assigning function to cortical regions, however, as our knowledge of what they do (often based on the symptoms of brain damage) may be incomplete. Broca's "speech motor" area, though located in a region known primarily to be associated with the generation of movement, is also involved in grammatical construction of spoken and written language as well as in verbal fluency. In the last two decades it has also been discovered that Broca's area contains what are known as mirror neurons: neurons that are active both when an action is being performed by the brain's owner or when it is seen or even heard being performed by others. This may reflect an important role in the learning by imitation not only of speech, but also of other cultural or noncultural types of movement.

The way in which various aspects of sensation are analyzed by the brain can be surprising. Though we have a clear holistic visual impression of, for example, a person walking across a room, different aspects of the scene are analyzed in discrete areas of the visual system before being recombined. This task specificity of computational units is common in sensory systems and indeed is often also a feature of complex computer systems. The higher processing of visual information is sometimes described as following two streams within the cortex. The first flows upward from the primary visual cortex into the parietal cortex and beyond into the motor regions. This is concerned primarily with the spatial relationships between objects: the "where" of vision, which plays a role in the visual guidance of movement. The second stream flows down into the temporal lobe and is more concerned with the identity of objects: the "what" of vision. For example, there are regions involved in identifying not only individual faces, but also what constitutes a face, so strange as it may seem, damage to this region may make it impossible to distinguish a face from a roundish physical object such as a hat (Sacks 1998). The primary visual cortex is interested mainly in the angles of the lines that make up the contours of shapes. Color is analyzed elsewhere, and it is possible (though rare) for brain damage to lead to loss of this aspect of vision alone. A description of the surreal consequences this has is given in a fascinating book by the neurologist Oliver Sacks (Sacks 1995). Interestingly, not only is the ability to see in color lost, but the ability to remember in color (i.e., to extract color information from replayed memories) disappears as well. To take another example, subjectively we would expect that some part of the visual system would be interested in the form of objects, animate or otherwise, and in this we would be correct. However, it is not so intuitive to suspect that the form of moving objects would be treated as a separate category for analysis, which is actually the case (Zeki 1992). Damage to the region of the cortex responsible for this function leads to a bizarre inability to see objects or people when they are moving but not when they are stationary (Sacks 1995). This raises an important question when we begin to consider how the brain responds to music: does the brain always use the same strategies that we apply subjectively to the analysis of music, or does it sometimes employ a different approach? If we fail to answer this correctly and design our experiments accordingly, our investigations may yield conflicting or ambiguous results. For many elements of musical interpretation this question remains unresolved.

We now come to a system within the brain that is ancient and which is involved in controlling drive-related behaviors that are crucial for survival, such as maternal behavior and self-defense, but which as a result is also the seat of fear and anxiety (see chapter 10). This is the limbic system. It comprises a number of areas of specialized cortex with links to the thalamus and hypothalamus, through which it initiates autonomic responses to stress and fear. Its main cortical areas are the cingulate gyrus, a band of gray matter that lies immediately above the corpus callosum, and the hippocampus and amygdala, which lie near the tip of the temporal lobe (fig. 7-4C), in the floor and at the end of the lateral ventricle, respectively. The latter two regions are concerned with memory. The hippocampus is responsible for the laying down of associative memory (factual learning), though it is not the repository of memories once they have been established. The amygdala, on the other hand, gives memories their emotional flavor. Merely thinking about a stressful event can start the heart racing and make us break out in a cold sweat; that is the responsibility of the amygdala. As we will see in chapter 9, the amygdala is also involved in emotional responses to music.

It may come as a surprise for the reader to learn that though the two hemispheres appear generally similar in form, they are not identical in function. Most people consider themselves right or left handed; that is, they have greater control over one hand or the other and consequently use it for the tasks that are most demanding, such as writing. This difference between the two sides of the brain arises during embryonic development and in part is a consequence of exposure to circulating testosterone. As each hemisphere is responsible for the opposite side of the body, it is the left hemisphere that controls the right hand and is thus dominant in those who are right handed. The side controlling the most "dextrous" hand is generally known as the dominant hemisphere. This is a rather misleading term as the hemisphere does not dominate the other hemisphere in any meaningful way, though it is certainly different in terms of some of its other abilities. Linguistic function provides a particularly dramatic example. In 95 percent of right handers, linguistic function is largely confined to the left hemisphere, that is, it is only on this side that one finds Wernicke's and Broca's areas (Springer and Deutsch 1997). The situation for left handers is not so clear. Seventy percent show this pattern; however, in the remaining 30 percent, language is bilaterally represented. The lateralization of linguistic functions obviously has major implications for the cortex. If it is damaged in adulthood, for example, as the result of a stroke (a loss of blood supply to part of the brain), the ability of the opposite hemisphere to compensate for lost language function is extremely limited. The one aspect of language that is represented in the nondominant hemisphere is prosody, that is, the inflection or lilt of speech. This not only makes speech interesting to listen to, it also imparts meaning. Consider the short-word sentence "This is your book." Switching the stress from one word to another produces four different statements, or, by giving the sentence a rising inflection, four different questions. So prosody provides eight shades of meaning. This may be linked to the observation that some aspects of music analysis, in nonmusicians at least, appear to be largely carried out in the auditory association cortex on the nondominant (usually right) hemisphere. In more general terms it has been suggested that the dominant hemisphere is involved particularly with serial analytical functions, while the nondominant hemisphere deals with more holistic, integrative functions, such as visuospatial operations like face recognition. Indeed, it has further been proposed that language and visuospatial tasks compete for cortical space (i.e., for computational resources), as in normal individuals who are blindfolded for a number of days, linguistic function starts to invade the visual areas of the cortex. This underlines the fact that the cortex is a dynamic and competitive environment. This is seen most starkly when a region of cortex loses its input or target, for example, when a finger or limb is amputated. The areas of the primary sensory and motor cortices associated with the missing region do not cease operation; instead, they are rapidly invaded by links from adjacent areas. As a result, stimulating a limb stump can produce a phantom sensation of the missing region because the brain still has it assigned to the amputated part. On a less draconian scale, it is this competition for resources that allows us to develop new skills.

In the music world today, both genders are well represented, so in studies of the central nervous system of musicians, it is important to consider whether there are significant differences between the sexes in cognitive and other abilities or in brain structure. There is in fact ample evidence for this (Kimura 1999), which supports the general impression that, as far as motor skills are concerned, men are better at targeting (throwing) and interception (catching). On the other hand, women are in general superior at fine manipulations of the fingers and the copying of hand postures. In the area of spatial skills, men are superior at map reading and when finding their way in this fashion tend to use direction and distance as guiding parameters, while women navigate more with reference to landmarks. Men are also superior at complex visualization tasks such as imagining the effects of rotating two- and three-dimensional objects. Women, on the other hand, are better at remembering the relative positions of objects. When it comes to mathematics, women tend to be better at calculation, while men are better at applying reasoning or math to real problems. In the realms of perception, women outperform men in reading the emotional content of facial expression. They are also more fluent verbally, though there is no gender difference in vocabulary size.

Studies comparing the size and morphology of particular brain regions in different groups of people can be difficult to carry out due to the degree of individual variation, which may reflect underlying factors not detected by the experimenters. Nonetheless, there is some evidence that structural differences also exist between the brains of men and women (Cahill 2005). Overall, the male brain is slightly heavier when corrected for body size, but the cerebellum and parts of the corpus callosum are proportionately larger in females. It has also been suggested that on average the degree of hemispheric asymmetry is less in right-handed women than it is in right-handed men. There appear to be gender differences in the size of some of the nuclei within the hypothalamus and, as this part of the brain is responsible for hormonal control of the menstrual cycle, clear functional differences also. This means that in searching for changes in brain organization that may be brought about by musical training, gender is one of the factors that must be taken into consideration. We will see from the next chapter that some studies that have pooled data from the two sexes have reached conclusions that on more careful examination have not proved equally applicable to both.

REFERENCES

Amunts, K., G. Schlaug, A. Schleicher, H. Steinmetz, A. Dabringhaus, P. E. Roland, and K. Zilles. 1996. Asymmetry in the human motor cortex and handedness. *Neuroimage* 4:216–222.

Cahill, L. 2005. His brain, her brain. *Sci Am* 292 (5):40–47.

Kell C. A., K. von Kriegstein, A. Rosler, A. Kleinschmidt, and H. Laufs. 2005. The sensory cortical representation of the human penis: Revisiting somatotopy in the male homunculus. *J Neurosci* 25:5984–5987.

Kimura, D. 1999. *Sex and cognition.* Cambridge, Mass.: MIT Press.

Sacks, O. W. 1995. The case of the colorblind painter. In *An anthropologist on Mars: Seven paradoxical tales.* New York: Knopf.

———. 1998. *The man who mistook his wife for a hat and other clinical tales.* 1st Touchstone ed. New York: Simon & Schuster.

Penfield, W., and E. Boldrey. 1937. Somatic motor and sensory representation in the cerebral cortex of man as studied by electrical stimulation. *Brain* 60:389–443.

Penfield, W., and T. Rasmussen. 1950. *The cerebral cortex of man; a clinical study of localization of function.* New York: Macmillan.

Springer, S. P., and G. Deutsch. 1997. *Left brain, right brain: Perspectives from cognitive neuroscience.* 5th ed. New York: Freeman.

Zeki, S. 1992. The visual image in mind and brain. *Sci Am* 267 (3):68–76.

Chapter Eight

How the Performance of Music Affects the Brain

With the knowledge we have gained from the preceding chapter, we can now move on to consider how the performance of music alters the brain and its responses. We will deal here mainly with the regions of the brain involved in the physical performance of music, concentrating particularly on sensory function and on the control and coordination of muscle activity. This will lead us to a consideration of how expert skills are developed during practice. Finally, we will examine a disturbing and intractable condition called focal dystonia, which sometimes drastically curtails the professional life of musicians in midcareer and which appears to be a consequence of maladaptive changes in brain organization. The response of the brain to musical sound will be dealt with in the next chapter.

DIFFERENCES IN BRAIN STRUCTURE
BETWEEN MUSICIANS AND NONMUSICIANS

Just as a muscle becomes larger and stronger with use and the bone to which it is attached grows thicker under continuous loading, the circuitry of the central nervous system adapts to the demands that are made upon it. The ability of the brain to be molded by experience is called plasticity and is greatest during childhood, when it may be capable of compensating almost completely for damage that, if incurred later in life, would cause catastrophic loss of function. Much of this plasticity we take for granted. The ability to lay down new memories and acquire new skills throughout life is a necessity of normal existence. Musicianship is a particularly potent driving force for plasticity. One would hardly consider starting to train a child under school age in the skills required for most other occupations; however, it is regarded as perfectly socially acceptable (and even desirable) to do so in an activity that has the higher cultural overtones possessed by certain forms of music. Quite young children may already be spending regular periods each day developing the very specialized perceptual and motor abilities that musical performance demands, and the exceptional standard that some of these children achieve by their teenage years is to a considerable degree a testament to the early plasticity of the central nervous system.

The advent of techniques for scanning the bodies of living subjects has opened up the possibility of analyzing the structure and activity of the brain while it is carrying out a variety of cognitive and motor tasks. The large and very expensive machines used for this are increasingly widely available in hospitals and research centers, where they have rapidly taken on a major role, not only in the diagnosis of disease, but also in the study of normal brain function. The most widely used scanning technique for studying the effect of music-related activity on the brain is magnetic resonance imaging (MRI). This can generate images of a series of virtual slices through the brain or combine them to produce a three-dimensional reconstruction of its entirety. When it is used to reveal patterns of brain activity, it is known as functional MRI (fMRI). Blood flow is enhanced in active areas of brain tissue in order to bring in more oxygen and nutrients to support the higher levels of metabolism they require. With fMRI it is possible to obtain a blood oxygen level–dependent (BOLD) signal because the scanner can distinguish between oxygenated and deoxygenated hemoglobin. The information this yields allows a detailed analysis of cortical and subcortical activity patterns underlying musical tasks, as well as making it possible to compare these patterns in different individuals (e.g., to compare brain activity in musicians and nonmusicians). One limitation of fMRI is that it cannot track very rapid changes in activity, as it takes several seconds for the data in a single scan to be collected. To record the fleeting changes typical of normal brain function, it is necessary to measure the electrical activity of the brain more directly. At one time the principal method of doing this was electroencephalography, but today this has been largely superseded by magnetoencephalography (MEG). Sensors placed close to the scalp monitor the magnetic fields that are generated by electrical activity. Computer analysis of the data can be used to determine the likely location of the source of the signals with a fair degree of accuracy. The spatial resolution is greatest for sources near the surface of the brain (i.e., the cortex) but falls off when the center of activity lies deep below the surface. It is therefore less useful for signals arising from the basal ganglia, for example. There is also the possibility that by using this type of analysis, two separate foci will be interpreted as a single source lying in an intermediate position. The increased availability of fMRI and MEG has stimulated a flurry of scientific activity; however, the complexity of the brain and its circuitry means that interpreting the results is far from straightforward. It is important to avoid leaping to conclusions from patterns of activity that we do not yet properly comprehend. In most cases it is not possible to attribute a single function to a given brain region (even if we were able to define clearly the discrete functional elements of the brain). It is becoming increasingly clear that the same region may be involved in the processing of many different types of information and in most cases it will be some time before we understand what fundamental aspects of information processing underlie this.

The same caveat applies to the analysis of differences in the structure of the brain between individuals. The foundation for our understanding of the functional geography of the brain was laid in the nineteenth century from observations of the consequences of traumatic head injuries in survivors of wars and industrial accidents, or of natural accidents such as strokes (a loss of the blood supply to regions of the brain due to damage to or blockage of blood vessels). The results were collated to produce a crude map of cerebral function that still forms the basis of most standard textbook descriptions today. We are only now beginning to learn that these are often only a partial reflection of the physiological properties of the brain regions concerned. In addition, some functions are not strongly localized to a discrete location in the cortex, but are instead the properties of diffuse networks covering large areas. Many years were spent in a fruitless search for the location of the engram—the imprint of memory. This is now regarded as a distributed function, probably residing within a network in which many memories are superimposed. Each memory may be represented as a different pattern of activity within the network, in the same way that multiple views of an image can be stored within a holographic crystal. Nevertheless, there are many features of brain maps that have stood the test of time, though there remain numerous pitfalls for the unwary.

Though the "science" of phrenology, which purported to be able to deduce character from the shape of the head, has long been discredited, there is some evidence that individual experience can leave a physical imprint on the structure of the brain, particularly if the shaping influences are present early enough in life. Modifications in brain circuitry that occur later, while highly significant for brain function, do not in general result in gross anatomical changes. As a result, when searching for anatomical consequences of musical training, it is usually necessary to treat individuals whose training started before the age of about seven as a separate group from those who, though they may have spent many years or even decades playing intensively, began their training at a more advanced age. Most of the plasticity observed to date is in the cortex and its connections. The major anatomical features of the cortex observable to the naked eye are the ridges (gyri) and grooves (sulci) on its surface, and comparisons between musicians and nonmusicians based on these features depend on there being a consistent relationship between topography and cortical function. While this does seem valid in broad terms, one should nevertheless be cautious, particularly when only subtle differences are reported, as the difficulties of defining the boundaries of cortical areas could render them meaningless. Another factor that must be taken into consideration is that there is considerable variation in brain size between individuals, and so the volumes or areas to be compared must be scaled according to the overall dimensions of the brain.

Though most changes in the functional organization of the brain are not reflected in modifications to its gross anatomy, they can nevertheless be demonstrated with the imaging methods we have just encountered. Of course, when a music-related task is being studied, not all (or even most) of the activity in the brain will be associated with music alone. It is therefore common practice to monitor the signal from a neutral activity not associated with music and to subtract this from the experimental pattern in an attempt to isolate the areas that are specifically linked to the task in question. This is called masking. Another technique is to compare activity patterns when subjects are asked explicitly or implicitly to analyze different aspects of patterned sound. A third method is to compare activity between different groups of subjects carrying out the same task. For example, one can subtract the signals obtained from expert musicians with those from amateurs or nonmusicians to identify the effects of training. The range of different subtraction methods used, together with the consequences of other differences in experimental design, can make comparisons between fMRI studies of the same phenomena frustratingly difficult; as a result, the published literature is often rather confusing. If this was not enough, there are additional constraints imposed by the scanners themselves. The first is that they are noisy machines, which can create difficulties for investigations of auditory processing. The second is that the space available for the subject within the machines is very restricted, which means that only small movements can be made. In addition, it is important that the head remain as stationary as possible. Finally, because these machines use very strong magnetic fields, metal objects cannot be placed near them. All of these place practical limitations on the activities that can be studied.

Musicians are no more a homogeneous group than any other human population, and the degree of individual variation means that conclusions about how the brain may be modified by musical experience can only be drawn from comparisons of large populations of musicians (amateur and professional) and nonmusicians. It is also important to consider the possibility that the differences observed between the brains of musicians and nonmusicians may not just be a consequence of musical experience, but may also reflect inherited characteristics that predispose some individuals to success in music. For example, one study has suggested that male musicians have lower levels of testosterone in their bloodstream than male nonmusicians, while female musicians have higher levels than female nonmusicians (Hassler 2000). At the present time the consequences of this are not clear, but during embryonic development testosterone levels have an effect on structural and functional asymmetry in the cortex of the forebrain (i.e., on hemispheric dominance). If these levels are elevated at crucial times or if the brain has a high sensitivity to testosterone, the development of the left hemisphere may be held back, while that of the right hemisphere is enhanced. This shifts the balance between the ability to process verbal and nonverbal information and may favor the emergence of musical and other abilities. Those carrying out morphological brain studies of musicians must therefore try to distinguish features that might have arisen in this way from those that reflect the result of musical experience. This may not be an easy call, and often relies on reasoning based on rather circumstantial evidence.

Musical perception involves the analysis of many different parameters such as melody, rhythm, harmony, and timbre, and how our brains have been shaped to respond to these depends to some extent on expectations based on our previous experience. This causes us to formulate certain rules of syntax and to react particularly strongly to events that disobey these rules, for example discords or unexpected chord progressions. The rules, and hence the expectations, are culture dependent, and even within the Western musical tradition, what is harmonically acceptable has changed throughout history. Consequently, some of the details of the observations made on the functional organization of the brains of musicians raised in the Western classical tradition (who are the main subjects of published studies to date) may not be entirely applicable to all musical cultures.

We will now turn our attention to the areas of the brain that are involved in the acquisition of the skills necessary for musical performance. In each case, we will first consider the general organization of the system, and then how this is modified by musical training. The music-related changes discussed are summarized in table 8-1. We will

Table 8-1.   Changes in Brain Structure Related to Musical Experience

Brain Region	Change	Instrument	Correlation	Gender Factors	Source
Heschl's gyrus (primary auditory cortex)	Increased gray matter volume up to 130%	Not specified	Musical aptitude/experience (professional > amateur > nonmusician)	Not known	Schneider et al. 2002
Left PT	Greater leftward asymmetry (smaller right PT)	Mainly string and keyboard players	Absolute pitch, early musical training	Males only	Schlaug et al. 1995 Zatorre 1998 Luders et al. 2004
Primary sensory cortex	Greater left-hand map area (right cortex)	String players	Early musical training?	Not known	Elbert et al. 1995 Hashimoto et al. 2004
Primary motor cortex	Intrasulcal length greater in right-hand region	Keyboard players	Early musical training	Only males tested	Amunts et al. 1997
Corpus callosum	Enlargement especially in anterior part	Keyboard and string players	Musical experience	Males only?	Schlaug et al. 1995 Ozturk et al. 2002 Lee et al. 2003
Corpus callosum	Increased organization/ myelination?	Keyboard players	Musical training tested	Only males	Bengtsson et al. 2005
Broca's area	Increased gray matter	Various orchestral players	Total years of playing, not early musical experience*	Only males tested	Sluming et al. 2002
Cerebellum	Increased gray matter volume	Keyboard players	Lifelong practice intensity, not early musical experience or total playing years	Males only	Schlaug 2001 Hutchinson et al. 2003

PT = planum temporale
? = some contradictory evidence
* = few of the musicians in this study started playing at an early age, so correlations unlikely

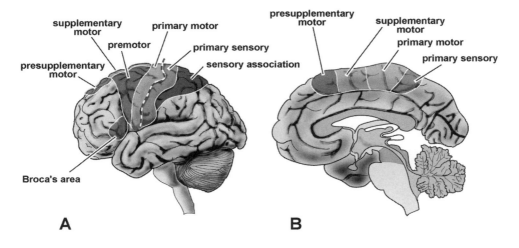

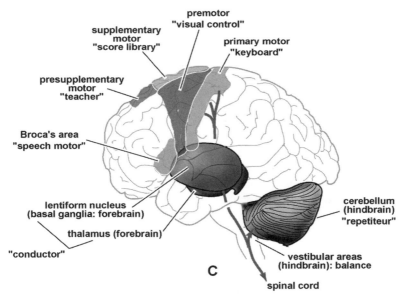

Figure 8-1. Cortical and subcortical motor areas of the brain. A, B. The primary motor area of the cortex is driven by input from the supplementary and premotor areas. These make important contributions to the planning and initiation of movements and the establishment and storage of learned motor patterns. Sensory feedback from primary somatosensory and sensory association areas is necessary for these operations. Broca's area is a speech motor area (left hemisphere only) that not only contributes to the control of the muscles used in speech, but is also involved in the analysis of grammar in language. C. The accurate execution of movement is also dependent on processes that take place in the spinal cord and in regions of the brain outside the cortex. These include the thalamus and elements of the basal ganglia that lie in the forebrain and midbrain. The cerebellum is involved in the maintenance of equilibrium and plays a central role in motor learning. It receives sensory information from the muscles and the balance organs of the ears as well as input from the cortex. In order to make it easier to come to terms with the diverse functions of these different areas, they have been given metaphorical subtitles here and in figure 8-2.

start with a consideration of the regions of the brain that receive sensory information from the body, in particular from the hands, and the motor areas that control and co-ordinate the actions of the muscles used in performance. For reasons that will become apparent, these are among the most extensively studied systems from the viewpoint of music-related plasticity.

SENSORY AREAS OF THE BRAIN

In the first chapter we discussed the different types of sensation that sensory nerve cells carry. From this it will be remembered that information coming from the skin is said to be exteroceptive because it monitors events that originate in the external world, such as temperature, touch, and vibration. We also receive information from the muscles, tendons, and joints that tells us about the position of limbs and the loading of muscles. This is called proprioceptive information and is very important for the control of movement. Both of these types of sensation are central to performance.

The axons of exteroceptive sensory nerve cells enter the spinal cord and contact interneurons that ascend to the brain stem before terminating in the thalamus on the opposite side of the brain. Here they contact other nerve cells that send their axons to the primary sensory cortex. The left sensory cortex therefore receives information from the right side of the body and vice versa. The primary sensory cortex is a narrow strip of gray matter that runs parallel to the central sulcus (fig. 8-1; see also previous chapter). Projected onto this strip is a map of the surface of the body called the sensory homunculus (literally, the "little sensory man"). In figure 7-6C, he is shown in three dimensions, from which it can be seen that though the map is complete, it is distorted so that regions such as the hands, lips, and tongue are disproportionately large. The areas that are most strongly represented in the map are those with the highest concentration of sensory nerve endings. The sensory homunculus does not therefore represent how we see ourselves, but what it feels like to be us. We are mostly unaware of this distortion, but if you have ever had a filling fall out of a tooth you will know that when you explore the hole with your tongue, the hole seems much larger than it looks in the mirror. This is because the tongue is overrepresented on the sensory map due to the high concentration of sensory endings on its surface. The densely distributed sensory endings in the skin on different parts of the body can be compared by using a pair of dividers to measure how far apart two points of contact must be to be perceived subjectively as separate. On the fingertips, the lips, or the tongue, this is on the order of a couple of millimeters, but on the palm it increases to a centimeter and on the arm to four centimeters, while on the back it can be as much as 40 centimeters (try it!).

The proprioceptive sensory information from the muscles and tendons also contributes to the map in the sensory cortex and is represented in a strip of cortex that runs parallel to the band receiving information from the exteroceptors. Proprioceptive information goes not only to the cortex, but also to the cerebellum where it plays a role in the feedback control of movement. However, instead of being passed to the half of the cerebellum on the opposite side of the brain as happens with the cortex, it runs to the half that lies on the same side of the body as the muscle, tendon, or joint from which the information originates. Sensory information from the left side of the body therefore generates activity in the left cerebellum but the right sensory cortex. This has to be borne in mind when interpreting the results of research into patterns of brain activity produced by musical activities.

Sensory feedback is clearly important for monitoring the physical processes involved in the playing of a musical instrument. Sensory signals from the skin on fingers provide information about the position of the pads on the keys, the vibration of strings, and the effects of movements that may be used to generate vibrato. Signals from the muscles, tendons, and joints provide information about the position assumed by the hands and arms and the forces being generated by movement. For many instruments, one of the key early skills that must be developed is to be able to place the fingers in the correct position without having to look at them. For wind players, tactile and vibratory sensations from the lips and sensory input from the muscles of the embouchure are important for regulating the pitch and the quality of the sound.

Music-Induced Plasticity

The sensory maps in the brain are not immutable but can be remolded in the light of sensory experience. Though the changes in the map may be radical, this does not usually produce any change in the dimensions of the sulci or gyri of the primary sensory cortex, and so expansion of the representation of one region of the body must be at the expense of that of another. We have seen that if a limb or finger is lost, the region of the cortex that received information from it is quickly taken over by adjacent regions of the body. The map can also be modified in the opposite direction. Some people are born with their fingers fused together, and this is reflected in the sensory cortex where these fingers are represented as a single structure. If the fingers are surgically separated, the map adapts to this by dividing the representation into two distinct areas. These effects are rapid, taking place over a period of weeks and demonstrating that the map is highly dynamic, being maintained by constant competition between sensory signals from adjacent regions of the body surface. Changes in the cortical map can take place much faster than this, however, even over a period of only a few minutes (Noppeney et al. 1999). This implies that several mechanisms for plasticity exist that operate over different time scales. The short-term changes are probably the effect of alterations in activity within circuits, which act to block some connections and enhance others. The long-term changes, on the other hand, are likely to be the result of alterations to the structure of the circuit involving growth of nerve cell branches and the forming of new connections.

Two studies have been carried out on string players to see if it is possible to demonstrate changes to the representation of the hand that are consistent with theoretical expectations. Though the results differed somewhat in detail, both reported an enlarged cortical representation of the left hand compared to that of the right (Elbert et al. 1995; Hashimoto et al. 2004). The cortical representations of the left hand of the musicians were also proportionately larger than those in a group of nonmusicians. Both studies also revealed a shift in the position of the map within the cortex, though not in the same direction. This indicated that it was encroaching into areas that would normally map other regions of the body surface. However, while one of the studies (Elbert et al. 1995) found that the magnitude of the changes appeared to be correlated with the age at which musical training began, the other (Hashimoto et al. 2004) did not. Though currently unresolved, this discrepancy probably reflects the small number of musicians studied in each group and methodological differences in the experiments. In general, the degree of modification of the sensory maps does not appear to be solely a function of the pattern of sensory stimulation. It is not the repetition of the activity per se that leads to enhancement of the associated area of the map. The effect depends significantly on whether the attention of the subject is directed to the finger or fingers being stimulated (Noppeney et al. 1999). This, of course, is likely to be the case in musicians perfecting their playing technique and is a feature of what we will encounter as "deliberate" practice later in this chapter.

MOTOR AREAS OF THE BRAIN

The roles and interrelationships of the many areas within the brain that control the muscles are complex; to make it easier to understand what I will do is use a number of musical analogies (figs. 8-1, 8-2). While these can never be exact or truly reflect the full functionality of this system (to which a considerable proportion of the brain's

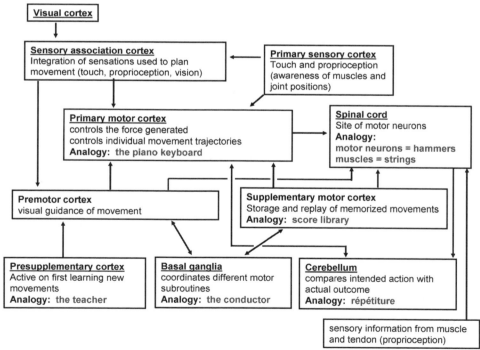

Figure 8-2. This diagram summarizes some of the relationships between the main regions of the cortex involved in motor activity shown in figure 8-1.

resources are devoted), I hope that by this means you will be better able to grasp the significance of the principal components of this intricate system.

Motor Areas Inside the Cortex

Running parallel with the primary sensory cortex and lying immediately in front of it on the other side of the central sulcus is the primary motor cortex (Kandel, Schwartz, and Jessell 2000). Like the primary sensory cortex, it also contains a map of the body—this time of the muscles on the opposite side. The motor map lies roughly in register with the sensory map, with the foot and leg lying close to the upper surface of the cortex, the trunk on the upper surface, the arm and hand on the lateral surface, and below that the face (fig. 7-6). As with the sensory representation, the motor map is distorted because small muscles that perform intricate or finely controlled movements (such as those moving the fingers or the muscles of facial expression that contribute to the embouchure) have a larger area of the cortex devoted to their control than postural muscles such as those of the thigh, which, though much larger, do not require such precise control. This is related to differences in the number of motor units within the muscles. A motor unit is the group of muscle fibers controlled by a single motor neuron (see chapter 1). If the force generated by a muscle is to be controlled very precisely, it must contain a large number of small motor units and will need more cortical neurons to control it than a muscle that has a smaller number of motor units. Nerve cells in the primary motor cortex run down through the brain and into the spinal cord and in many cases make direct contact with pools of motor neurons that supply the muscles. These motor neuron pools may lie either in the brain stem (if the motor neurons run in cranial nerves supplying muscles in the head and neck) or in the spinal cord, so the axons of the neurons in the motor cortex are often very long. The major bundle of axons that runs down from the motor cortex to the spinal cord is called the pyramidal tract and is particularly important for the control of fine hand movements. If it is damaged, motor control of much of the body may recover at least to some extent, but individual control of the fingers is lost.

The structure of the motor map was originally thought to be quite similar to the sensory map. If a brief electrical stimulation was applied to a single point on the primary motor cortex, a well-defined discrete movement was produced that appeared to be the result of activity in a single muscle. This was first observed in humans whose brains were exposed during surgery, but similar results can now be obtained in normal awake individuals by using magnetic field stimulation, which does not involve broaching the skull. This led to the notion that the map was a simple representation of individual muscles. To use a musical analogy, it was seen as representing a keyboard on which the rest of the brain could play. Pressing down a key activates a mechanism that leads to the sounding of a single note or, in this case, a single muscle. In this analogy, the motor neurons in the spinal cord act like the hammers of the piano and are responsible for sounding the strings (the muscles). However, this notion has proved to be a considerable oversimplification. Though the motor map initially appeared to run continuously from the toes to the fingers, when examined closely it was found to be fragmented. The nerve cells controlling a particular muscle do not all lie precisely in the same place but are scattered across a small area of the motor cortex. As a result, while the area of motor cortex controlling the hand is relatively easy to define, the representations of the individual muscles moving the fingers are to some extent intermingled. Furthermore, it now appears that single nerve cells in the primary motor cortex may supply several muscles that may even control more than one joint. Using pulses of electrical stimulation that are longer or more intense than those needed to produce twitches in single muscles evokes complex but well coordinated movements. It transpires that a given cortical neuron may drive a muscle or set of muscles only during one particular movement and remain silent when the same muscles are used in a different context. This has led to the idea that the cortical map may in fact represent movement trajectories (Graziano et al. 2002). To return to our musical analogy, the pressing of a key results not in the striking of a single note, but in the sounding of a chord. To produce a different chord, another key must be pressed, even though several of the same notes are present in both.

Activity in the primary motor cortex is driven or influenced by connections from a number of other cortical regions (figs. 8-1, 8-2). Not surprisingly, one of these is the primary sensory cortex. Additional connections arise from sensory association areas such as the superior parietal region, which sits behind the primary sensory cortex and plays a role in integrating the sensory information that is used in the planning of motor activity. In addition to these sensory streams, the primary motor cortex also receives inputs from several other motor areas that lie just in front of it (figs. 8-1, 8-2). These are principally the supplementary motor cortex (which lies on the top or superior surface of the hemisphere) and the premotor areas (which sit in front of the primary motor cortex). Both also have connections to the motor pools in the brain stem and spinal cord, so they can act on these directly as well as through the motor cortex. Like the motor cortex, they receive information from sensory association areas. Information from the primary visual cortex reaches the premotor cortex via the visual association areas along two processing paths. The more ventral stream carries information on the shape and position of objects and is used to direct reaching and grasping behavior. The more dorsal stream is active when visual and other sensory signals trigger a movement but do not guide it. The supplementary area, by contrast, is concerned with movement that is self-generated rather than triggered by external cues. Into this category fall the movements required for playing an instrument and the finger-tapping tasks discussed below in the context of motor learning. It also controls sequences of movements replayed from memory. We can therefore consider it as a "score library" for movement, though perhaps more of short "phrases" than of complete "pieces." When a new set of movements is first being learned, an area of the cortex that lies just in front of the supplementary motor cortex (imaginatively named the presupplementary motor area) is active. Though connected to it, the supplementary motor cortex is silent during this initial period, but once learning is complete it becomes active when the sequences are reenacted. With greater practice, the replaying of the movement sequences becomes fully automatic. The supplementary motor cortex may then fall relatively quiet again, and the activity becomes largely confined to the primary motor cortex. This drift in cortical activation during learning will be encountered again when we discuss the contribution of the different motor areas of the brain in the context of musical experience (fig. 8-3).

Motor Areas Outside the Cortex

In addition to the spinal cord, motor control involves many areas of the brain that lie outside the cortex (figs. 8-1C, 8-2). Substantial contributions are made by large masses of gray matter deep within the forebrain and midbrain that are collectively known as the basal ganglia, and by the cerebellum. The separate elements of the basal ganglia are linked to each other and to the various motor areas of the cortex through a series of loops that involve part of the thalamus. These pathways modulate the motor activity of the cortex and help to ensure that individual movements generated run smoothly into one another. Their corporate action can be regarded as being like that of an orchestral conductor. Not surprisingly, therefore, they are important in the learning of new motor tasks. Their role is perhaps best appreciated by observing what goes wrong when they cease to function effectively. Basal ganglion problems fall into two broad categories, those in which there is too little movement and those in which there is too much. A familiar example of the former is Parkinson's disease. Patients with this condition may find it difficult to initiate a movement and once started, a sequence of movements may cease partway through. The movements themselves may be abnormal; for example, when walking, the steps taken may be short and shuffling. At the other extreme are conditions where movements are exaggerated or appear spontaneously against the wishes of the patient. Movements in this category can be described as choreas (dancelike jerks—the word has the same origin as choreography). Huntingdon's chorea is a genetically inherited condition affecting the basal ganglia. Other abnormal movements are writhings (athetosis) and tics (twitching of single muscles or small groups of muscles).

The cerebellum is another major player in the control of movement. It is a complex structure that contains more than a quarter of all the nerve cells in the entire central nervous system. It receives information from the organs of balance within the inner ear (the vestibular system) and so one of its main functions is to maintain our equilibrium through the action of the muscles of the trunk and the big postural muscles at the base of the limbs, particularly the legs. As we stand upright on two rather small feet, maintaining our balance requires the constant intervention of the cerebellum, though we are almost entirely unaware of this. When a movement is initiated by the motor cortex, it sends information about what is intended to the cerebellum, which then compares this with what is actually taking place. We can consider this role to resemble that of the répétiteur who ensures that the words that are spoken or sung by the performers on stage match those in the script. The telemetry that allows it to do this is provided by the proprioceptors in the muscles and tendons, some of the sensory neurons supplying the skin (particularly the soles of the feet), the eyes, and the vestibular system. It then generates a signal that directs the motor cortex to make corrections to the movement even while it is still taking place. This ensures that the outcome matches the expectation, which is particularly important during the acquisition of motor skills. For example, when we learn to ride a bike, the challenge of maintaining balance at first seems insuperable, but rapidly becomes automatic. The importance of the cerebellum in everyday life is easily seen when its normal functions are compromised by overindulgence in alcohol!

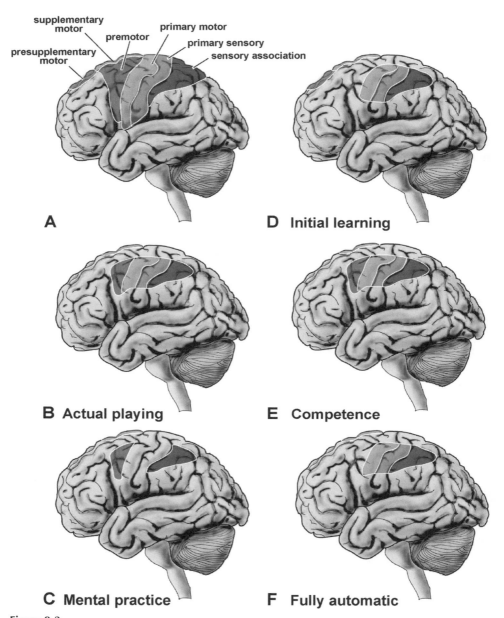

supplementary motor
premotor
primary motor
primary sensory
sensory association
presupplementary motor

A

D Initial learning

B Actual playing

E Competence

C Mental practice

F Fully automatic

Figure 8-3

Figure 8-3. This figure highlights the sensory and motor areas of the cortex that are involved in hand control, for example, in keyboard or string playing. It also shows their changing pattern of activation during skill learning. A. The regions of the cortex most involved in the control and coordination of muscle activity are shaded. Their major contributions and connections are summarized in figure 8-2. B. The regions particularly involved during keyboard or string playing are highlighted. Activity is focused in regions that control the hand. C. During mental practice, the pattern of activity is similar to that for playing except that the somatosensory cortex is not receiving information from the fingers, and the region of the motor cortex controlling the hand is silent. Panels D–F schematically illustrate the changes in cortical activation as performance skills are first learned then perfected. While new motor patterns are being laid down or when a piece is played for the first time, there is strong activity in the presupplementary cortex. As the movement sequences are repeated during learning, activity soon shifts to the premotor cortex (E). When playing becomes fully automatic and a high level of competence is achieved, premotor activity is greatly reduced, while activity in the primary motor and sensory cortex becomes intensified and more tightly focused within the hand area.

Within the spinal cord, the pools of motor neurons that supply individual muscles lie in the ventral horn of the gray matter (see chapter 1). Sensory information from the muscles, tendons, and skin flows into the cord and though, as we have seen, it is sent up to the brain, branches from the sensory neurons also end in the cord itself. As a result, all of the circuitry needed to control some simple forms of motor behavior is found here. Limb reflexes, for example, are mainly spinal. Tapping the large tendon below the kneecap causes a knee-jerk reaction—a spinal reflex over which we have no voluntary control. When we walk, as we swing one arm or leg forward, the other moves back. The nerve circuitry responsible is again confined in the spinal cord. Spinal circuitry also reduces interference between antagonistic muscles. If we use the triceps muscle to straighten the arm, the muscles that flex it relax. The presence of spinal reflexes simplifies the task required by the motor cortex in controlling many types of movement, though it also retains the option to override the spinal circuitry if this is appropriate.

PERFORMANCE-RELATED BRAIN ACTIVITY IN
AMATEUR AND PROFESSIONAL MUSICIANS

Patterns of brain activity differ considerably between professional and amateur musicians, even during the playing of quite simple pieces of music. In one study, professional violinists playing around thirty hours a week and with an average of thirty years' experience were compared with amateurs who played only one hour a week and had about ten years of training (Lotze et al. 2003). Their brain activity was recorded using fMRI while they performed the left-hand finger movements required to play a short extract of a Mozart concerto. Because the experiment was carried out within the limited confines of a brain scanner, the piece was memorized and the finger movements of the left hand made without the instrument. As would be expected, there were many similarities between the brain responses of the professionals and the amateurs; both showed activity in primary sensory and primary motor areas that represented the hand. However, the activity in the professional group was much more tightly focused and in the primary motor cortex was more intense and confined to the right side of the brain (the side that controls the left hand), whereas in the amateurs it was present on both sides. The stronger signal from the hand area of the cortex in the professional group may be a reflection of an increase in its cortical representation (Schlaug 2001; Amunts et al. 1997). The supplementary and premotor regions of the cortex were also active in both groups, though more so in the amateurs. These, together with some other frontal areas, and the left side of the cerebellum (as expected on the same side as the active hand), which were also active in amateurs, are involved in the acquisition of complex motor skills before they become fully automatic. In professional players, therefore, it appears that many of the complex motor programs required for playing have become fully integrated and refined so that they arise fully formed directly from the primary motor cortex. Activity in the basal ganglia, which is often seen at an early stage in the formation of motor programs, was found only in the amateurs, again reflecting their lower level of proficiency. This may also underlie a greater level of activity in the right side of the cerebellum in the amateurs. By contrast, in the professionals, particularly those who started their training in early life, there was an increased level of activity in a small region of the cerebellum on the same side as the active left hand. This may be correlated with the observed structural changes seen in the cerebellum of musicians (Schlaug 2001; Gaser and Schlaug 2003).

MUSIC-INDUCED STRUCTURAL CHANGES
IN THE MOTOR AREAS OF THE BRAIN

Because of the complexity of the demands made on their manual dexterity, keyboard players are among the most often studied in the search for changes in brain structure and function related to musical performance. The primary motor and sensory areas of the cortex are obvious places to search for such modifications because they contain topographical body maps in which distortions, should they exist, will be readily detectable. Most people show a greater dexterity with one hand or the other; that is, they are either right or left handed, and brain imaging studies have revealed that this is reflected in the depth of the central sulcus that lies along the edge of the primary motor cortex on the opposite side of the brain (Amunts et al. 1996). Because there are more cells in this sheet of gray matter on the side controlling the dominant hand, it bulges out more, making the sulcus deeper. As the strip of gray matter that makes up the primary motor cortex contains a map of the body in terms of muscles or movement, only part of it is concerned with control of the arm and hand. Left/right asymmetry is seen in this region only, and not in the region lying immediately below, which controls the muscles of the face. The playing of keyboard instruments requires an almost equal dexterity in both hands, so it can be hypothesized that the difference between the depth of the central sulcus on the left and right side should be less in keyboard players than in the general population. This indeed appears to be the case, at least for male players (who are the only group studied so far), and can be attributed to the sulcus being deeper in the pianists on the side controlling the nondominant hand (Amunts et al. 1997; Schlaug 2001). This anatomical observation correlates with a greater symmetry in finger dexterity in the two hands in pianists (Jancke, Schlaug, and Steinmetz 1997). The depth of the sulcus on both sides of the brain of keyboard players shows some correlation with the age at which the musicians started to learn to play. There is no correlation with the total number of years of playing at the time the study was carried out, indicating that the effect reflects a plasticity in brain structure present only early in life.

There is evidence that the extent of the gyrus may also be increased in the hand area of musicians (fig. 8-4). The region of the primary motor cortex controlling the hand is quite commonly folded into an omega (Ω) shape. Comparisons of the brains of sixteen violinists, sixteen pianists, and thirty-two nonplayers (all right handed) revealed that in the violinists the omega shape tended to be considerably more pronounced in the right primary motor cortex (which controls the left hand) than on the other side, which of course controls the bowing hand. In pianists, however, the opposite situation prevailed, and it was on the left side that the omega shape was more strongly marked (Bangert and Schlaug 2006). Though the most obvious conclusion is that this is a result of hand use, it is always possible that it is genetic and that musicians self-select an appropriate instrument, so long-term studies of brain development in children are currently in progress to clarify the issue (Schlaug 2006).

The two cerebral hemispheres of the brain are linked by an extensive sheet of nerve fibers called the corpus callosum, and it might be envisaged that the requirement to coordinate the two hands in instrumentalists such as pianists could lead to changes in its structure. The corpus callosum matures slowly. Though it grows most rapidly in the first decade of life, it continues to increase in size into the midtwenties. The period of

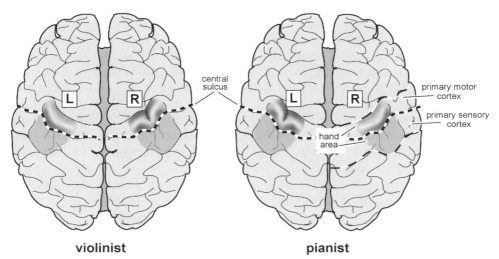

violinist　　　　　　**pianist**

Figure 8-4. Morphological features of the primary motor cortex associated with the complex hand movements required by musicians. These diagrams, based on observations by Bangert and Schlaug (2006), illustrate that the hand region of the right (R) primary motor cortex of violin players is more likely to exhibit a well-defined omega-shaped fold than the left. In pianists the opposite is true. The shaded area behind the central sulcus (dashed line) represents the hand area of the primary sensory cortex.

most rapid growth coincides with the time in early childhood when motor coordination is developing. Sensory deprivation during this period can result in a reduction in the size of parts of the corpus callosum. A comparison has been made of the size of the callosum between a population of musicians and one of nonmusicians in the eighteen-to-thirty-five age range. The musicians were classically trained keyboard and/or string players who were either professionals or music students, while the members of the control group were matched for age and educational status but did not play an instrument and had no musical training. In two separate studies of different groups of male musicians, the anterior part of the corpus callosum was found to have a greater area than in the control groups (Lee, Chen, and Schlaug 2003; Schlaug et al. 1995). This region of the corpus callosum carries connections between the primary sensory and primary motor areas of the two hemispheres, as well as between the premotor and supplementary motor regions. Its larger size in musicians might therefore be associated with the observed changes in the primary motor cortex already discussed. This is likely to be related to the importance of bimanual coordination in the playing of many instruments. Another study showed a higher degree of organization within the corpus callosum of male pianists than in age-matched controls (Bengtsson et al. 2005). This used an MRI technique called diffusion tensor imaging. The level of organization and the degree of myelination (as indicated by a parameter called functional anisotropy) was correlated with the amount of practice carried out during childhood and adolescence. One physiological manifestation of the enlarged callosum may be a reduction in the inhibition normally seen between the two sides of the brain that has been reported in pianists and guitarists (Nordstrom and Butler 2002; Ridding, Brouwer, and Nordstrom 2000). This is an inhibition that occurs in the primary motor cortex on one side of the brain during activity in the equivalent region on the opposite side, and it is mediated by nerve fibers in the corpus callosum. It has been hypothesized that its reduction may improve the ability to coordinate the precise timing of the movements of the two hands. Another investigation of the corpus callosum involving only string players confirmed the results obtained by Schlaug and colleagues and also found evidence of enlargement of the posterior part of the corpus callosum (Ozturk et al. 2002), which is known to carry fibers that link the auditory centers on each side of the brain.

In contrast to the situation seen in male musicians, one study has suggested that female musicians show no increase in the dimensions of the corpus callosum (Lee, Chen, and Schlaug 2003). Several possible explanations have been put forward to explain this. One is based on the suggestion that females show less asymmetry between the hemispheres than males. If the changes in the corpus callosum in males were related to the reduction in asymmetry of the motor cortex already described, then any change in females due to bimanual training might be much smaller. Another possible explanation relates to the higher incidence of absolute pitch seen in the female musician group than in the male group. Absolute pitch is associated with a greater degree of lateralization (a greater difference in structure between the two hemispheres) in the auditory regions, which might be reflected in fewer connections crossing between them. When averaged across a number of female subjects, any increase in size in the corpus callosum due to hand training may might be masked by its reduction in those with absolute pitch. On the other hand, though the study by Ozturk (2002) did not distinguish between male and female brains, the majority of his subjects were female and yet he still found an enlargement in the musician group. As there is considerable variability in both sexes in the size of the corpus callosum, the question of whether only male musicians show changes in its architecture deserves further investigation.

Since the middle of the nineteenth century, the cerebellum has been associated with the control of motor activity and motor learning, a relationship that was reinforced by studies of brain damage in soldiers during the First World War (Parsons 2003). This is clearly important in learning to play an instrument and in developing expert levels of performance. However, our ideas of cerebellar function are changing, and evidence is accumulating that it also makes a significant contribution to sensory discrimination. This includes a role in the comprehension and analysis of harmony, melody, and rhythm, where its activity appears to support the high-level processing of auditory information that takes place in various regions of the cerebral hemispheres (Parsons 2001). Imaging studies of the cerebellum in living subjects have revealed that its volume (as a percentage of total brain volume) appears greater in male musicians than in male nonmusicians (Schlaug 2001). Interestingly, unlike some other morphological changes, this is said to be related not to the age at which music training began but to the intensity of current long-term practice (Hutchinson et al. 2003). The time scale over which this volume change might take place is unknown. There is no comparable difference in cerebellar size between female musicians and nonmusicians; however, it appears that the female nonmusicians already have a relative cerebellar volume comparable to that of the male musician group. The computational part of the cerebellum is its thin but highly folded cortex, but most of its volume is made of white matter, which represents the cabling that links the cortex to other regions of the brain. However, it appears that the increased volume of the cerebellum in male musicians is not due to an increase in the white matter alone. The relative size of the region of the cerebellar cortex that is involved in control of finger movement in the left hand is also positively correlated with the degree of musical training (Gaser and Schlaug 2003). As all of the musicians in the study were right handed, this result, like the observation of the reduced asymmetry between the left and right motor cortex that we have already discussed, represents an increase in the development of brain regions controlling the nondominant hand.

MUSIC-INDUCED CHANGES IN
ASSOCIATION AREAS OF THE BRAIN

Comparisons between musicians and nonmusicians have also been made in cortical gray matter areas. One region where gray matter volume is enhanced in musicians is the superior parietal cortex, which lies just behind the primary sensory cortex on the upper surface of the brain (Gaser and Schlaug 2003). This forms part of the sensory association area shown in figure 8-1 and has been implicated as one component in a network that is active in sight-reading (Sergent et al. 1992). As we have seen, this area is involved in the spatial analysis of visual information, an ability required not only for guiding hand movements, but also for the interpretation of the position of notes on the stave of written music. Being connected to the primary sensory cortex and the primary, supplementary, and premotor areas, it is strategically placed to control visually guided precision motor tasks such as the placement of a finger on a string or key. Another region of the cortex that appears to be enhanced in musicians lies within Broca's area (Sluming et al. 2002), which is found in the left frontal cortex just above the tip of the temporal lobe. This area is traditionally regarded as having a role in the control of speech motor activity, but recent functional studies suggest that this general area may also be involved in a number of music-related functions (see chapter 9). It is, for example, implicated in the analysis of rhythm, but it may also be active during tasks such as sight-reading, and in score reading in the absence of playing (Parsons 2001), as well as in the recognition of melody and the processing of musical syntax (e.g., detecting inappropriate chord progressions [Maess et al. 2001]).

The subjects of the study of Broca's area carried out by Sluming were male musicians in a major British orchestra with an age range of twenty-six to sixty-six years (Sluming et al. 2002) and were compared with an age-matched control group of non-musicians. Most other investigations of brain morphology in musicians have focused on students or young professionals, generally less than thirty years of age, so the Sluming study provided an interesting opportunity to examine the effect of musical performance on aspects of brain morphology and function throughout the entire period of a typical career. For musicians under the age of fifty, the degree of enhancement of Broca's area appeared to increase with the number of years of playing. Overall, the control group showed an age-related decline in total brain volume as well as in the volume of gray matter within Broca's area; however, neither of these changes were seen in the musicians. The subjects of the study were given some cognitive tests: one of basic reasoning ability, which provided a general assessment of cognitive function, and one of spatial ability, which therefore tested a cognitive function thought to be related to sight or score-reading skill. On the general reasoning test, the musicians and the control group performed similarly, both showing an age-related decline in performance. In the test of spatial ability, though the performance of the controls declined here also, the performance of the musicians actually improved with age. It is well established that constant practice of a challenging intellectual task can help to maintain particular mental abilities and, over a period of time, stimulate cortical volume increases in adults. One notable example of this is seen in London taxi drivers, who must memorize a vast amount of geographical information as a prerequisite for obtaining their cab license. This is known as "The Knowledge" and it takes several years to acquire. Most drivers do not start on this momentous task until their late teens, and many are considerably older. It has been found that gaining The Knowledge is associated with an increase in the volume of an area of the cortex known as the hippocampus (Maguire et al. 2000), which is responsible for laying down associative memory, including the memory of spatial locations.

LEARNING TO PLAY MUSIC

Developing the skills to play a musical instrument involves a variety of learning tasks. First it is necessary to learn how to produce the sound and finger the notes. For a first instrument, this generally runs in parallel with learning to read musical notation, and the two tasks must be brought seamlessly together so that seeing a note or group of notes on the stave automatically leads the fingers to make the correct movement. The motor behavior is gradually refined, typically over a period of many years, to allow an increase in the speed of execution and the level of control so that the sound generated meets the expectations of the player and audience. Very high levels of control are required not only for accurate rendition of the music, but also to enable it to be played with expression—a rather intangible but generally instantly recognizable element of performance that is realized by subtle manipulation of timing and dynamics. Today, near perfection in the accuracy of execution is expected by audiences spoiled by exposure to recorded music, though most probably never realize the extent of physical practice that is required not only to achieve the required standard, but also to maintain it. In addition, as it is also expected that, for soloists at least, even long pieces will be performed without the score, it must be reliably committed to memory. Many aspects of the way in which these faculties are developed are still beyond the scope of current research, but we will consider some of the more mechanistic aspects of skill acquisition in order to see whether our present perceptions of the underlying biology can provide any insight into how this is achieved.

The Mechanism of Motor Learning

The studies that are of most relevance to understanding how the technical ability to play an instrument or a new piece of music is acquired are based on learning simple patterns of finger movement. Though these resemble patterns used in the playing of keyboard and other instruments, they do not match them exactly. In these studies, the motor skills of musicians and nonmusicians are compared. As the exercises have a degree of novelty for both groups, what is being examined are not changes associated with the specific skills demanded by a particular instrument, but the general mechanisms that underlie the greater levels of motor performance that musicians develop. Several investigations use a task that requires that the pads of different fingers be brought into contact with the pad of the thumb in a particular sequence. The subjects are asked to do this as rapidly and as accurately as possible and without looking at the fingers. The results suggest that we learn to carry out such patterns of movement in several stages (Karni et al. 1995, 1998). An initial period of fast learning takes place over a period of minutes, during which there is a significant improvement in performance; however, this is followed by a subsequent period of consolidation lasting six to eight hours that occurs in the absence of the activity. Thus, when the task is repeated (e.g., the next day) there is a further improvement in performance beyond the final level achieved at the end of the first practice session. Though a gradual and continuous improvement in performance is seen in the period following training that occurs during waking hours, consolidation of motor learning appears to be dependent on sleep (Walker et al. 2003). This results in an improvement in both the speed and accuracy of the learned task (e.g., a finger-tapping sequence), which in the hours following sleep remains at a plateau in the absence of further training on the following day. If additional days and nights are allowed to elapse without further training, performance continues to improve gradually. Though sleep has been implicated in the consolidation of several forms of memory, the crucial phase of sleep involved appears to vary depending on the learning task. In the case of motor learning this is what is called phase 2 sleep, while for visual discriminative tasks it is the slow wave and rapid eye movement periods that are critical (Stickgold and Walker 2005).

During the next few weeks, daily practice sessions produce additional improvement, but the increments in improvement become progressively smaller until an upper level of proficiency is reached. To break through this ceiling requires a considerable increase in effort. Some notions of the mechanisms underlying these processes have been gleaned from imaging brain activity during this type of learning. When the task is carried out for the first time, activity is seen in the primary motor cortex of the hemisphere that controls the hand making the movements (i.e., the one on the opposite side). When first repeated, the activity in the cortex is at first reduced. This is due to an effect called habituation, which is a common phenomenon in the nervous system. However, when the finger sequence has been repeated a certain critical number of times (in this case, a few dozen times), the signal in the cortex becomes larger, and it stays larger during the training sessions on subsequent days. During this stage it is thought that new connections are made between the nerve cells, resulting in a modification of the motor map in the cortex (Kleim et al. 2004). Of course, the primary motor cortex is not the only part of the brain that is active during motor learning. Activity is also seen in other areas such as the premotor and supplementary motor cortex, as well as in the basal ganglia and the cerebellum (Hund-Georgiadis and von Cramon 1999). This occurs particularly during the early phases of motor skill activation and declines as greater competence is achieved (fig. 8-3).

Interestingly, it has been shown that the activity in the cortex during the initial stages of the finger-tapping task differs between pianists and nonmusicians. In pianists there is much less activity in the supplementary motor and premotor areas, and greater activity in the primary motor cortex (Haslinger et al. 2004). It is as if right from the outset, the pianists are showing a pattern of activity that the nonmusicians take some time to achieve, which presumably reflects their previous intensive training in the control of fine finger movement. The supplementary motor cortex is thought to be involved in the control of sequential movements performed in the absence of visual feedback. It is more active when the task is complex; the reduced activity in this region in the pianists therefore implies that the task is less demanding for them. Comparisons of cortical activity between professional and amateur violinists playing the same piece of music reveal a similar phenomenon (Lotze et al. 2003).

The learned movements used in instrumental performance are highly stereotyped. The trajectories of points on the body surface can be accurately measured in two and three dimensions using video analysis. Studies of violin players have revealed that the size and timing of the trajectories of the fingers of the left hand (in a task requiring minimal overall hand displacement) are almost identical when the same note sequence is repeated several times. The same is true of the bow and the right arm in violinists and cellists (Baader, Kazennikov, and Wiesendanger 2005; Turner-Stokes and Reid 1999; Wiesendanger, Baader, and Kazennikov 2006). Nevertheless, the synchronization between the fingering and bowing is not absolutely precise. Even in expert players there is an average discrepancy of around 50 milliseconds between finger placement and bow contact. However, there is a lag between the initial contact of the bow with the string and the onset of the vibration (also typically around 50 milliseconds), and it appears that the synchronization of the left and right hands is determined by the sound that is heard and not by sensory feedback from the movements themselves. The size of the acceptable error in synchrony therefore depends on how accurately the auditory system can determine the beginning of the note (Baader, Kazennikov, and Wiesendanger 2005). In the cello, left-hand excursions during playing can be of considerable magnitude, and their accuracy has been investigated in players of various standards who were asked to make movements of different speeds along the fingerboard in order to play particular notes (Chen, Woollacott, and Pologe 2006). In studies of movement accuracy, it is generally found that the greater the velocity of the movement and the force used, the greater the error observed in the final position reached. Among the cellists, however, neither the distance covered by the hand nor its velocity affected the average accuracy of finger placement. This is probably an effect of the high level of training in left-hand movement that cellists undergo. The accuracy of finger positioning was greatest for the more proficient cellists but was also correlated with the accuracy of their pitch perception. However, the variability in finger placement was not associated with either the level of expertise or pitch perception, which suggests an underlying limitation set by the motor system and its proprioceptive sensory feedback. Surprisingly, all of the cellists in this study tended to play a little sharp, something that has also been noted among wind players (Morrison 2000), but the reason for this is unknown.

Though the left side of the brain controls the right hand and vice versa, there is some evidence that training of the nondominant hand may also cause activation of cortical regions on the same side. This suggests that training one hand may improve the performance of the other through communication between the two hemispheres (Hund-Georgiadis and von Cramon 1999). Such transference has not been observed in all studies, however, and remains controversial, but as we shall see later, occupational focal dystonia in one hand can quickly appear in the other if it is used to carry out tasks formerly assigned to the dystonic one. If, as has been proposed, this type of dystonia is a maladaptive effect of overtraining, its transference to the other hand would be consistent with a bilateral effect of training on the sensorimotor cortex.

Mental Rehearsal

For many professional musicians, mental rehearsal is an integral part of their preparation for performance. It is strongly promoted by some teachers and its use by famous piano soloists such as Horowitz and Rubinstein is a matter of record. In neurobiological terms, mental rehearsal and preparation can be seen to encompass several distinct elements. First, there is the interpretation of the score in terms of an internal representation of sound (i.e., mentally hearing the music when reading the score). Second, there is the committing of the score to memory, which includes not only the notation on the stave, but also the marks of expression. The memory of the score can then be used to support a virtual rehearsal of the movements required to perform it. Another form of mental rehearsal is to read the score and mentally rehearse the performance movements. In its most advanced stages, this may even be used to explore various options for expressive interpretation. For this to be possible, the brain must create an internal image not only of the movements but also of the precise effect they will have on the sound produced. Though they are combined holistically, each of these tasks requires a different set of mental skills, and we will first consider the mental rehearsal of playing movements. It goes without saying that this needs a complete familiarity with and mastery of the instrument and is therefore an option open only to advanced players (Lotze et al. 2003). This form of physical imagery is not unique to musicians; it is widely used in sports that involve complex stereotyped movements. High jumpers can often be seen mentally practicing before a crucial jump, and the complex and precision movements of divers also benefit from this type of rehearsal. The effectiveness of mental practice in improving aspects of the dynamics of movement, such as the accuracy of the movement trajectory, has been verified experimentally (Yaguez et al. 1998). In one study, the effect of mental rehearsal was compared with physical practice of the same simple musical passage (Pascual-Leone 2001). The subjects practiced for two hours daily over five days, and the effect on brain activation and the accuracy of performance was monitored. Though the section of the primary motor cortex that drives the muscles of the hand remained silent in the group carrying out only mental rehearsal, the size of the areas that would have been controlling the muscles moving the fingers increased, while the threshold for their activation was reduced. This was accompanied by a demonstrable improvement in motor performance, though it was not as great as the one achieved by physical practice. However, at the end of the study, a single session of physical practice in the mental rehearsal group was sufficient for them to reach parity of performance with the physical rehearsal group. This result is in general agreement with those of other less physiologically rigorous experiments that suggest that while mental practice is better than no practice, it is not as good as actual practice (Gabrielsson 1999). However, mental practice can be done in the absence of the instrument, and as part of an overall scheme of rehearsal may, by reducing the amount of physical playing, potentially reduce the risk of overuse injury (see chapter 3).

Clearly, one source of information missing in mental rehearsal is feedback from the sensory endings in the fingers and their joints and muscles. The less experienced the player, the more important this feedback will be; however, in experienced players in whom the movements of the fingers have become automatic, its importance may be reduced. There is also, of course, a lack of auditory feedback as there is no tangible output from the virtual activity. The effect of its absence on performance accuracy has been investigated in experienced pianists playing on a silent keyboard (Finney and Palmer 2003). For substantial excerpts of previously learned pieces (e.g., music by Bach, Beethoven, and Rachmaninov), there was no significant difference in error rate between playing with or without sound. In simple sight-reading tests, however, though the absence of auditory feedback had no effect on performance from the score, it did have a deleterious effect on the accuracy of repeating the music from memory. For those interested in developing and optimizing the skills of mental rehearsal, practical information can be found in Connolly and Williamon (2004).

Outside the primary motor region, many of the same cortical areas that are normally active during playing are also active to a lesser extent during virtual practice (fig. 8-

3) (Lotze et al. 2003; Langheim et al. 2002; Meister et al. 2004). Functional imaging studies have revealed activity in premotor and supplementary motor areas that are thought to be involved in the generation of complex motor activity. The premotor area is active when we silently "sing" a melody to ourselves, though not when the melody is simply recalled. Perhaps surprisingly, there was no activity in the primary auditory area during these experiments, despite the fact that virtual rehearsal generally requires a vivid mental realization of the sound associated with the virtual "movements." This is in contrast to imagining a scene, which does produce activity in cortical visual areas. However, when the rehearsal involved real hand movements, activity was present in the right primary auditory cortex and left auditory association cortex, even if the hand was not in contact with the instrument and no sound was produced (Lotze et al. 2003). This suggests that some link exists between the primary motor cortex and the auditory cortex (Bangert and Altenmuller 2003). The right primary auditory area is the main region of the cortex involved in the perception of pitch, harmony, and timbre, and the level of its activity during silent practice with actual finger movements is greater in professional musicians than in the amateurs. A link in the opposite direction between the primary auditory and primary motor cortices has also been demonstrated. A study of advanced piano students demonstrated that listening to a piece of keyboard music with which they were already familiar caused involuntary activity in the primary motor cortex even though the finger muscles were not activated (Haueisen and Knosche 2001). Activity in the motor cortex occurred in the region controlling a finger just before the note it would have played was sounded and so mirrored the activity that would have been required for playing. No such response was seen in a control group of similarly experienced singers who were not pianists. This type of connection would undoubtedly support the ability to play music by ear.

As mentioned previously, one component of mental rehearsal is familiarization with the score. A number of studies have investigated the relative effectiveness of different score-learning strategies based either on playing the music through, examining the score without playing it, or using a combination of both approaches (see Gabrielsson 1999). Unfortunately, differences in methodology make it difficult to draw general conclusions from the results (Gabrielsson 1999). The studies had a variety of different aims, and their design was not compatible with what is now known of the time scale of and requirements for motor learning. Differences in the level of experience of the subjects were also not taken into consideration. This is an important factor because the way in which the score will be analyzed will depend on this (see below) as will the degree to which certain note sequences are familiar to the individual through playing technical studies and other repertoire. In addition, we have already gained some inkling of the differences in brain development and activation patterns that may be present as a result of different lifetime experiences of music.

Physical Practice

In the initial stages of learning a new piece, reading through the score may be used to gain a clear idea of the notes and expression marks in the absence of the distraction of the physical challenges of playing. This may take the form of studying the overall structure of the piece and/or a careful examination of single phrases or their component note sequences. The latter in particular should increase the probability of playing the notes accurately at the first attempt and, in so doing, establishing the correct motor program from the outset. If we relate this to what we already know of motor learning, this should be of considerable advantage because the correct sequence of finger movements will need to be repeated many times to generate the initial increase in cortical responsiveness that underlies the first stage of motor learning. If several variants are played initially, this will at the very least slow the consolidation of the correct motor sequence and at worst lead to the firm establishment of an incorrect variant that may persist for some time as a learned alternative to the correct sequence (especially if the incorrect sequence is easier to perform). The importance of the initial stages of learning is borne out by observations of how high-level performers actually practice. In one study it was found that different short segments of an eight-bar sequence were repeated more than 150 times by a pianist in the first practice session and 50 times in the second session (e.g., fig. 8-5) (Chaffin and Lemieux 2004). The fact that it was not singled out for special treatment on any subsequent session suggests that it had been effectively mastered, demonstrating the efficacy of this highly focused approach to motor learning. In a study of brass and woodwind students, it was found that structured, supervised practice involving this type of approach was more effective than free practice where they were left to their own devices and tended not to use such strategies (Barry 1992). One way of ensuring accuracy right from the start is to play the notes slowly. It has, however, been suggested that in keyboard instruments, which require complex bimanual coordination of several voices, the motor activity used for slow playing is fundamentally different from that used for fast playing (see Gabrielsson 1999). It has been proposed that in such circumstances it would be necessary to adjust the technique of the slow playing used when initially learning the music to compensate for this, or to develop early on the facility to play short segments at close to final speed. However, this problem has yet to be examined more objectively from a physiological standpoint.

Memorizing Music

Until the middle of the nineteenth century, it was unusual for soloists to perform extensively from memory; the ability of musicians such as Franz Liszt and Clara Schumann to do this was regarded as something of a phenomenon. Now most teachers put considerable emphasis on the importance of learning the score by heart, and it is regarded as unusual if a soloist plays directly from the music. From the viewpoint of the biology of performance, freeing the brain from the requirement of reading the score will not only eliminate a considerable cognitive load, but also allow the attention to be focused entirely on the sound being produced, which will undoubtedly be an advantage in refining the performance. Of course, even when reading from the score, many segments will already effectively have been committed to memory, as it is impossible to play fluently otherwise. In many cases there is simply not time to read all the notes when playing at the correct tempo, and the written music is used simply as a cue to bring forth memory of blocks of motor activity whose performance has been refined through extensive practice.

Learning a piece of music by heart involves several types of memory. We must learn the written score, as well as retaining an auditory memory of how it sounds and a motor memory of how it is played. Though the written score is the original source of information, it is for the instrumentalist merely the first stage en route to constructing and learning the motor program. As we have seen, the motor memory is constructed largely by carrying out the activity repeatedly, but becoming familiar with the written score is a more abstract task—the learning of a pattern—and is done in different regions of the brain. At the most fundamental level, the motor memory is created from extensively practiced note sequences based on elements of scales, arpeggios, and chordal progressions (Halpern and Bower 1982). Grouping together a series of such operations that are then remembered as a unit is called "chunking" and makes the memory task easier as there are many fewer chunks to remember than notes. Similarly, learning the score is more efficient if it is perceived to be composed of recognizable musical elements. Music, like language, has a grammar based on scales and progressions, and within this context many patterns are identifiable and predictable. Experienced players who are familiar with musical syntax can use this to simplify the learning task, while less experienced players must create the motor pattern by reading the score by rote in a more literal fashion (Aiello 2001). To use a linguistic analogy, it is easier to remember the phrase "the dog was a golden retriever" than "golden the was retriever dog." Furthermore, the anomaly in the phrase "the dig was a golden retriever" is immediately apparent while less so in "golden the was retriever dig." The memory processes that are used to create a performance in the absence of the score can therefore operate at a variety of levels. Some recent studies have investigated this through statistical analysis of practice strategies, in one case of an individual professional pianist and in another, of groups of pianists of different standards (Chaffin and Imreh 1997, 2002; Aiello 2001).

On the most basic level, a performance can be created by learning a piece of music as a sequential series of chunks. This requires relatively little knowledge of the structure of the music and is often used by inexperienced musicians; however, it is a risky strategy. Each new phrase is required to trigger the memory of the next and as the sequence increases in length, it becomes progressively harder to do this. If there is a break in the sequence due to a lapse in memory, the whole structure may fall. The only recourse in such circumstances is to start the section again and risk another breakdown at the same or a different point in the memory train, which may now be even more likely due to the stress of the previous failure. However, if the structure of the music is analyzed, it can be broken down into a series of elements, which are progressively divided into smaller and smaller units according to a hierarchical scheme. The hierarchy provides a context in which the "chunks" can be reassembled during playing (fig. 8-5). As well as making it easier to memorize, this approach allows a musician to recover from a memory lapse by rejoining the music at the beginning of the next structural element. The bars at the beginning and end of each element become important memory retrieval cues that require greater attention during learning than the bars following. If musicians who have learned pieces in this way are shown isolated bars from the piece, the cue bars are recognized more quickly and more accurately than bars falling within segments, and this is reflected in the pattern of electrical activity they evoke in the brain (Williamon and Egner 2004).

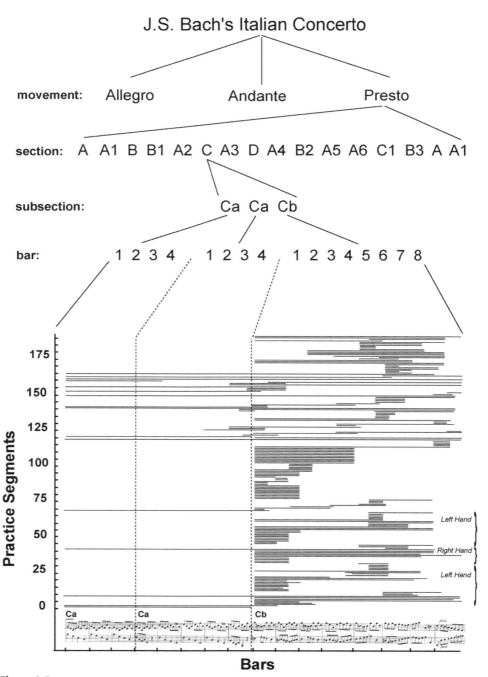

Figure 8-5

Figure 8-5. The upper part of the figure shows the hierarchical structure of the Presto of Bach's Italian Concerto, illustrating the sequential way in which the memory of the piece is unpacked by a pianist playing from memory. Particular attention needs to be given to transitional boundaries between subsections and to the reappearance of similar, but not identical, musical elements (e.g., A1, A2 . . . A6). The lower part of the figure is a record of how a pianist went about preparing and memorizing one section of the piece through intense "deliberate" practice. Each line indicates a segment of music played continuously, and the practice session runs from bottom to top. This session concentrated on a particular section of the movement (Cb); most playing episodes start from its beginning. A sequence of episodes in which the playing is progressively extended further into the section is repeated several times. This is interspersed with practice of short note sequences that pose technical problems. As the session progresses, the sections played start to concentrate on the transitions between adjacent segments and are designed to stitch them together to form a mental image of this part of the movement. Reproduced with permission from Chaffin and Imreh (1997).

An insight into how this works in practice is provided in a study by Chaffin and Imreh (1997, 2002), who recorded and analyzed rehearsal sessions during which a piece of keyboard music (the Presto from Bach's Italian Concerto) was learned by a professional player (Imreh). The results are illuminated by the player's subjective comments on the process. One of the first tasks required in the playing of any piece is to solve the motor problems posed by difficult note sequences, in this case the fingerings. The music in question involves many sequences that, though basically similar, are often subtly different. After some experimentation, the fingering solutions ultimately used were not always the simplest, but the ones that could most consistently be applied to similar phrases. In other words, the resolution of the motor difficulties was viewed in the context of the higher-level problems of memorization. When the fingerings had been converted to automatic motor memories, it was then possible to turn the attention to discrete structural segments of the music, and then to link these together into progressively longer sections. As we would expect from what has been said previously, starts and stops during rehearsal occurred most frequently at cue bars on the boundaries between musical segments.

Figure 8-5 shows the structure of the movement studied by Imreh. The initial theme (A) is repeated in a number of guises throughout the piece, interspersed with other repeated sections (B, C, and D). On the one hand, this gives it a clear structure but on the other, the final bar of theme A does not always signal a switch to theme B; what follows varies depending on where in the piece it occurs. This sets a particular challenge for the memorization, which is reflected in the amount of time devoted to the practice of key bars around these transitions (fig. 8-5). Imreh commented, "A lot of my later practice . . . was practicing throwing those switches. My fingers played the notes just fine. The practice I needed was in my head. As I approached a switching point I would automatically think about where I was and which way to throw the switch." (Chaffin and Imreh 2002). The analogy of "throwing a switch" underlines the fact that motor sequences of the chunks had by this stage become fully automatic.

The emergence of the types of memory skills seen in expert musicians can be observed by examining patterns of practice and levels of achievement seen in individuals at different stages of musical training. Williamon and Valentine (2002) compared pianists grouped into four levels of experience at an early stage in their musical careers, graded according to the scheme of the Associate Board of the Royal School of Music. These represented grades 1–2 (level 1), grades 3–4 (level 2), grades 5–6 (level 3), and grades 7–8 (level 4). Each group was asked to learn and memorize a piece of music of appropriate difficulty. All had some awareness of how the structure of the pieces could be divided into segments, either through guidance from teachers or through their own objective or intuitive understanding. In all groups but level 1, starts and stops during practice sessions tended to coincide with structural boundaries in the music as the familiarity with it increased, but this was particularly marked at the higher levels of proficiency. Starts and stops at difficult bars declined in all groups but level 1 with increasing practice, presumably reflecting the progressive integration of these sections into the rest of the piece as the technical problems were overcome. It therefore seems that the same hierarchical memory retrieval systems seen in expert performers are being employed, in at least a basic form, by all but the least experienced players. From a pedagogical point of view, it is apparent that an ability to understand the underlying musical structure of a piece develops naturally with experience. These results also suggest that the development of these memory retrieval strategies can be encouraged even at an early stage of musical training, which in view of the complexity of the hierarchical schemata required for the memorizing of typical recital pieces may have considerable long-term advantages for the student.

High levels of practical musical expertise are not easily won. By the age of twenty, a proficient pianist is likely to have accumulated in the order of ten thousand hours of practice, and even achieving a standard equivalent to grade 8 typically requires around a third of this (Sloboda et al. 1996), at least for a first instrument. However, it is not the time spent in practice alone that is significant, but also its quality. For maximum benefit the practice must also be "deliberate," that is to say, rather than simply playing through the music, it must be highly structured with the attention focused on improving a particular aspect of performance. We have already encountered this notion in our consideration of motor learning, in which attention is a key factor (Noppeney et al. 1999), as well as in the advantages of supervised practice (Barry 1992). Needless to say, this requires considerable effort and mental concentration, and in view of the fact that the benefits may take some time to become evident, the demands of the practice sessions must be sustainable over a prolonged period from both a mental and a motivational point of view. Consequently, sessions of deliberate practice tend to last only between one hour and ninety minutes. In one study, the amount of effort required appeared to be reflected in the greater incidence of daytime napping in elite musicians. They also tended to play more in the morning when presumably they were most fresh (Ericsson, Krampe, and Tesch-Romer 1993). In addition, the highest achievers not only concentrated more on deliberate practice but were more consistent in their practice schedules.

Comparisons between players of different standards have consistently revealed that the more experienced practice in longer sessions. In many studies, of course, age tends to increase in parallel with expertise, but the increase in session length does not appear to be simply a consequence of greater patience and determination. The improved physical stamina that age brings may be a factor; however, it may also be that once the more mundane problems of basic technique have been mastered, the challenges that open up in terms of interpretation and memorization provide many different focuses of attention, making practice more varied and interesting (Williamon and Valentine 2000).

OCCUPATIONAL FOCAL DYSTONIA

Established instrumental musicians in midcareer sometimes develop a painless but unaccountable inability to control the hand. This often starts as a feeling of heaviness in the fingers but becomes progressively more debilitating so that ultimately the player may only have to pick up or sit at the instrument to find the fingers involuntarily taking up a hyperflexed or hyperextended posture that makes playing impossible. These are the symptoms of occupational focal dystonia.

Dystonia refers to abnormal involuntary and uncontrollable muscle contractions that are most often seen in the hand or in muscles of the neck or face. Though it is usually painless initially, the extreme contraction that may ultimately develop in sets of antagonistic muscles can cause considerable discomfort. The excessive and inappropriate muscle activity may generate abnormal postures of the upper limb or body, a twisting of joints such as the wrist or neck, rhythmic movements, or tremor. Dystonia is said to be focal when it affects only a single muscle or a small group of muscles, and this is generally task specific, appearing particularly during skilled movements that have been practiced habitually over a long period of time, for example, as part of one's occupation. In musicians, though it may be triggered just by holding or touching the instrument, it may not affect a similar movement used to pick up and use a tool or a piece of cutlery. The symptoms tend to come on gradually and in the initial stages may be apparent to the player only as a subjective feeling of difficulty, a heaviness in the arm, or a resistance to movement in the fingers. At first the consequences may not be obvious to the listener, and the condition sometimes takes years to develop fully; in other cases the dystonia may become debilitating in a matter of months (Tubiana 2000).

Occupational focal dystonias have a long history, and a brief but informative account of this can be found in Hochberg, Harris, and Blattert (1990). The first probable description of focal dystonia in Western medicine was written in the early eighteenth century by the father of occupational health studies, Bernardini Ramazzini. He describes an intense fatigue and a loss of power in the right hand of a notary brought on by writing. When the notary tried to solve the problem by using the other hand, it soon became affected as well. This type of dystonia was well known in the nineteenth century and was given the name scrivener's palsy (widely known as writer's cramp). An account by Solly in 1864 as quoted by Hochberg, Harris, and Blattert (1990) describes its essential features: "It comes on insidiously, the first indication often being only a painful feeling in the thumb or forefinger of the writing hand accompanied by some stiffness. . . . The loss of power is not sudden as in a paralytic stroke; nor is it a complete paralysis of any group of muscles. The paralyzed scrivener, though he cannot write, can amuse himself in his garden, can shoot, and cut his meat like a Christian at the dinner table; indeed he can do anything he likes, except earn his daily bread as a scribbler." This was only one of many work-related dystonias (or occupational neuroses as they were sometimes known) that were described at this time. These covered more than fifty occupations, but musicians were said to be second only to writers in their vulnerability to it (Fry 1986). Its origins have long remained obscure, but in recent years the study of affected musicians with modern brain scanning techniques has done much to increase our understanding of focal dystonia.

Because focal dystonia has been widely discussed in recent literature on musicians' health, instrumentalists with an interest in arts medicine may have an exaggerated idea of how common it is. The incidence can be difficult to determine from reports from well-known clinics specializing in musicians' health problems because these attract difficult cases that have not received effective diagnosis or treatment elsewhere. As dystonia is frequently misdiagnosed in the first place, its sufferers are likely to be overrepresented among their patients. Therefore, though their reports would appear to suggest that 5 to 15 percent of musicians with motor problems have focal dystonia, the figure is undoubtedly much lower. The best evidence of its incidence among professional musicians suggests that this is in the order of 1 in 200 to 1 in 500 (Lim, Altenmuller, and Bradshaw 2001), which is around ten times that seen in the general population (Pullman and Hristova 2005; Wynn Parry and Tubiana 1998). Several studies have collated information on the characteristics of focal dystonia among musicians, and a comprehensive review of the more important reports can be found in Lim, Altenmuller, and Bradshaw (2001), who also assess current theories of its origin. However, for a shorter and more accessible overview, readers are directed to Jabusch and Altenmuller (2006) which can be freely downloaded from the journal website http://www.ac-psych.org/. Focal dystonia most commonly appears in the fourth decade of life (Lim, Altenmuller, and Bradshaw 2001; Hochberg and Hochberg 2000; Wynn Parry and Tubiana 1998), though it is certainly not unknown at an earlier age (Jankovic and Shale 1989). This means that it generally affects musicians in midcareer, when they already have a sound and long-established technique. In contrast to their younger colleagues, they are unlikely to be pushing hard to develop a professional level of proficiency or to be competing vigorously to gain their first foothold in the musical world. There is a distinct but unexplained gender bias in the expression of dystonia. Different studies suggest that men are two to six times more likely to be affected (Jabusch and Altenmuller 2006). Most of those affected have problems with coordination of the hand, and there is a high incidence of dystonia among pianists and guitarists, though the hands of other string players and of woodwind and brass players can also be affected. In addition, focal dystonia of the embouchure (see chapter 6) is not uncommon in wind players (Frucht et al. 2001).

Symptoms of Focal Dystonia in Musicians

The onset of dystonia is usually gradual and painless. Among keyboard players there is initially a loss of facility in passages that may have been executed without problems for decades (Hochberg and Hochberg 2000; Tubiana 2000). In rapid passages, particularly those containing arpeggios, some of the fingers may appear to lag behind the others in an unexplainable way. Problems may also be experienced with playing octaves. In string players, difficulties may be found with double stopping as well as passage work, in which a finger or fingers become slow to lift. As the condition progresses, the affected fingers often assume a more flexed posture so that the edge of the nail strikes the piano key or it becomes difficult to raise the finger from between the strings. Finally, the fingers may become completely curled under the palm so that the outer surface of the fingernail instead of the pad strikes the key (Candia et al. 2002). In other cases, the recalcitrant fingers instead become involuntarily extended and cannot be brought down to touch the key or string. The later stages of dystonia are sometimes characterized by a fierce simultaneous contraction of antagonistic flexor and extensor muscles of the digits, which causes fatigue and pain. Interestingly, in patients who play more than one instrument, the dystonia may affect the playing of only one. Activities such as typing, which one might think would share many similarities with keyboard playing, may also be unaffected (Wynn Parry and Tubiana 1998). The typical site of the dystonia varies depending on the instrument. Wynn Parry and Tubiana report that in pianists, it is the right hand that is most usually dystonic (70 percent), in which case the most commonly affected fingers are those closest to the little finger. When the left hand is involved, the affected digits tend to be on the other side. Among guitarists, it is the index and ring fingers of the right hand that are most likely to become dystonic, while in violinists, three-quarters of cases involve the left hand.

Theories of the Origin of Dystonia

Occupational focal dystonias are often described by the medical profession as idiopathic, meaning of unknown cause. This should not make you immediately lose confidence in your doctor! Many well-known illnesses are idiopathic, and though the science of medicine has progressed greatly over the last century and a half, so has our recognition of the incredible complexity of the physiology of the body and its interactions with its environment. Though the origin of focal dystonia is unclear, our knowledge of its symptoms goes much deeper than the abnormal movements it causes. There are many clues as to what may lie at the root of the problem, but none has yet led to a definitive conclusion. Some researchers have proposed a strong causal link between focal dystonia and repetitive strain injury, and one group has even gone as far as to define a condition known as "repetitive strain–induced focal dystonia" (Byl and McKenzie 2000). This theory is not currently widely accepted for human focal dystonia, as the relationship between dystonia and injury, regardless of how it is caused, is for the most part unclear. While some anecdotal evidence has been put forward to support the idea that a variety of injuries might trigger the appearance of dystonia (Jankovic and Shale 1989), a lack of objectivity in the way that much of the data have been collected, and the absence of any rationale to explain the theory, seriously undermines its credibility. However, there is quite good evidence that nerve compression, particularly when it involves the ulnar nerve, is a risk factor (Charness, Ross, and Shefner 1996). One factor that makes this theory convincing is that in dystonic musicians with demonstrable ulnar nerve pathology, the affected muscles are particularly those controlling the little and ring fingers. The ulnar nerve supplies the small muscles within the hand that act on these fingers as well as the skin that covers them.

Furthermore, treatment to relieve ulnar nerve compression can markedly improve or even eliminate the dystonia, though this may take many months. Unfortunately, in other forms of dystonia of the hand in which the affected muscles are supplied by the radial or median nerves, the same link with nerve compression has not been found.

The observation that dystonic symptoms can be generated in monkeys by inducing them to carry out repetitive, stereotyped hand movements appears highly significant (Byl and Melnick 1997), as it is precisely this type of activity that underlies musical practice and performance. However, the context dependency of the symptoms remains a mystery. Dystonia sometimes appears in musicians following a marked increase in the intensity of practice, a substantial change in technique, or upon switching to a different model of instrument that may make slightly different physical demands than the one used previously. Changes in the physical sensations that these new circumstances generate may also be important. In such circumstances it cannot be ruled out that there has been some unidentified trauma, related perhaps to the change in technique or overintensive practice, but this would be inconsistent with the observation that the onset of dystonia is typically painless. In addition, the average age of onset for overuse injuries among musicians is in the midtwenties, while for dystonia it is in the mid- to late thirties (Tubiana 2000). It is also thought that an obsessive perfectionism or anxiety about performance may be a predisposing factor for the emergence of dystonia (Jabusch and Altenmuller 2006), though this needs to be more rigorously investigated. This may lead the player to carry out repeated but futile attempts to exceed the biomechanical limits of the hand, rather than to explore alternative solutions to problems of fingering.

There is a growing acceptance that focal dystonia is not fundamentally a condition of muscle or peripheral nerve malfunction, but is primarily related to changes in the parts of the brain that control and coordinate movement. We have already seen that the wiring of the brain is not fixed, but can be shaped by experience and that this plasticity can alter the sensory and motor maps within the cortex. Studies of the brain of monkeys and humans with focal dystonia reveal changes in the organization of the area of the primary sensory cortex receiving information from the affected region. In monkeys that develop dystonia after being trained to carry out repetitive hand movements, there is a degradation in the sensory map of the hand. The near-simultaneous stimulation of adjacent fingers during tasks that require close attention to maintain accuracy appears to be the most significant factor underlying these changes. The receptive fields of the nerve cells that map the fingers onto the cortex can be enlarged by a factor of ten to twenty, resulting in considerable overlap between the representation of adjacent fingers and even between the front and back of the hand (Byl and Melnick 1997). Receptive fields may also grow to cover several finger joints. The end result is that the brain can no longer tell what part of the finger, or even which finger, is being touched. Investigations of musicians and nonmusicians with focal dystonia of the hand reveal similar maladaptive changes in the cortical mapping. The finger representations of the dystonic hand are much closer together and either overlap or appear in random order (Bara-Jimenez et al. 1998; Elbert et al. 1998; Byl, McKenzie, and Nagarajan 2000; Butterworth et al. 2003). A study by Elbert et al. (1998) has also suggested that there is some degradation in the sensory maps for the nonaffected hand of dystonic patients, though this is not as marked as that of the affected hand. The notion that the sensory maps in each hemisphere are not entirely independent is supported by observations on readers of Braille, who use several fingers simultaneously to read text. The changes this produces in the cortical representation of these fingers is often reflected in the representation of the other hand, even though it is not used for Braille (Sterr et al. 1998). This may partly explain why dystonia sometimes appears quite rapidly in the previously nonaffected hand when dystonic patients try to use it for tasks previously carried out by the dystonic hand (Lim, Altenmuller, and Bradshaw 2001). In brass players with dystonic embouchures, a distortion has also been reported in the cortical mapping of the lips, with a decrease in the ability to detect gaps between fine gratings applied to the upper, though not the lower, lip (Hirata et al. 2004).

Focal dystonia is of course a disorder of motor control, so if the idea that it is caused by changes in the sensory map is valid, it should theoretically be possible to demonstrate some reconfiguration of the motor cortex. In the normal brain, large-scale changes in the motor map have been demonstrated experimentally, and it is clear that these can take place very rapidly, in fact, over a period of just a few hours (Kandel, Schwartz, and Jessell 2000). In dystonic musicians, however, it has not been possible to detect changes in the motor map of the hand. The reason for this is probably that, as we have already seen, there is not the same precise topographical order in the motor map that exists in its sensory partner. Though there is a region devoted to the hand, the representations of muscles moving individual fingers are not discrete, but are normally intermingled. Contraction of a single muscle is reflected in activity at a number of sites in the hand area of the motor cortex and so any changes wrought by dystonia would be difficult to detect.

Changes in other motor areas of the brain such as the premotor cortex and in the basal ganglia have also been shown in dystonic patients, including musicians (Lim, Altenmuller, and Bradshaw 2001; Lim et al. 2004; Ibanez et al. 1999). For example, during the execution of tasks that induce dystonic symptoms in musicians, activity in the premotor cortex fell below normal levels while that in the primary motor and sensory cortices was increased (Pujol et al. 2000). A similar result has been reported in dystonic nonmusicians (Lim, Altenmuller, and Bradshaw 2001). There are several other types of dystonia, most of which are thought to be caused by impaired function of the basal ganglia. This may be the result of trauma such as direct physical injury or damage due to stroke (loss of blood supply), or to changes in neurotransmitter levels. One component of the basal ganglia known as the putamen contains a body map incorporating both sensory and motor information (Romanelli et al. 2005). A study of one group of patients with focal dystonia of the hand (in this case writer's cramp) clearly demonstrated that this map had become disorganized on the side of the brain controlling the dystonic limb, but not on the other side (Delmaire et al. 2005).

One consequence of the intensive training needed to perfect the rapid and continuous finger movements required by instrumentalists is a reduction in the strength of inhibitory pathways within the motor cortex. In nonmusicians, sensation originating from one muscle in the hand reduces the excitability of cortical areas controlling other hand muscles. The training of hand movements that musicians undergo appears to alter this so that muscles that need to be active simultaneously during playing do not inhibit each other so strongly. In dystonic musicians, this loss of inhibition progresses even further to include muscles that are not usually active together. Thus, in the dystonic musician, a process that may facilitate hand control appears to have progressed too far, resulting in a maladaptive state (Rosenkranz et al. 2005). Patients with writer's cramp, a form of dystonia that has some similarities with musicians' hand dystonia, do not show this change. This may reflect the fact that most writer's cramp patients do not have a history of excessive writing; in other words, the origin of their condition, though still unknown, is not due to overtraining, though it may be linked to overuse.

A similar loss of inhibition is found in the interaction between the hand control areas in the opposite hemispheres of the brain. Activity in the primary motor cortex on one side of the brain normally has an inhibitory effect on the equivalent areas on the opposite side; however, in instrumental musicians the level of this inhibition is reduced (Nordstrom and Butler 2002). The reason it is reduced in normal musicians may be the necessity of coordinating very precisely the action of the fingers on each hand. A similar reduction in inhibition is also seen in dystonic nonmusicians. This again suggests that a training-induced change in brain circuitry, while advantageous in moderation, may contribute to the maladaptive changes that underlie dystonia if unbridled. It may also be another reason why dystonia can develop rapidly in the non-affected hand when it takes over tasks previously performed by the dystonic one. Our best guess about the origin of musicians' focal dystonia is therefore that it is a disorder of the integration of sensory and motor activity underlying musical performance. This emerging perception has given new impetus to attempts to devise effective treatments for the condition.

Predisposing Factors

In view of the uncertainty concerning the origins of focal dystonia, theories concerning possible predisposing factors need to be approached with some caution. There is excellent evidence that some families carry a gene that strongly predisposes them to develop a form of early-onset dystonia, which typically affects teenagers (Lim, Altenmuller, and Bradshaw 2001); however, whether focal dystonia has a significant genetic component has not been studied in detail. One report suggests that a minority of dystonic musicians (perhaps around 10 percent) may have close family members with various forms of focal dystonia (Schmidt et al. 2006). Not all of the affected relatives were musicians, and the condition most commonly manifested itself as writer's cramp. Interestingly, in two cases the relatives were professional pianists who suffered from writer's cramp but had no playing-related symptoms.

There has been some speculation about how psychological factors such as stress or anxiety may contribute either directly or indirectly to the development of focal dystonia. It has been proposed that the resistance of focal dystonias to therapy is related to the integration of the motor programs with the emotional and memory-forming elements of the limbic system (see chapter 10). A link between the physical aspects of playing and emotional responses could be a potent force for fixing motor memories, and might support a connection with performance-related stress (Lim, Altenmuller, and Bradshaw 2001).

The repetitive nature of the hand movements required in instrumental performance, especially when repeated for hours at a time, may lend itself to the generation of dystonia in some individuals. The risk factors listed by some authors read like a standard catalogue of poor biomechanical technique: postural tension, instability in the shoulders and other joints, working at the extreme ends of the range of joint motion, heavy use of alternating flexor and extensor muscle activity, and playing with nerve compression syndromes (Byl and Melnick 1997). An investigation of the structure and joint movement ranges of the hands of musicians with focal dystonia revealed that many may be pushing the biomechanical limits of what their hands are capable of (Wilson, Wagner, and Homberg 1993); however, in the absence of control data from a large population of unaffected musicians, this remains only suggestive and not all of those working in the field of focal dystonia believe that it is related to what in the broadest terms might be called faulty technique (Altenmuller 2003). Nevertheless, it underlines the importance for teachers of taking into consideration the physical limitations of their pupils when trying to optimize their technique. The link reported between ulnar neuropathy and focal dystonia might be explained by the related change in sensory input coupled with the compensatory movements used to overcome the ensuing muscle weakness, which together may disrupt the well-established motor programs controlling highly trained stereotyped movements. However, one is left wondering why there is no obvious link with other nerve compressions.

Treatments

Until recently there has been no treatment for focal dystonia that significantly restores the ability to play the instrument at a high level. A small number of recent reports do describe a possible way forward, but their development is at an early stage and they have been so far tried on only a small number of individuals. One must therefore remain cautious about how great an impact they will ultimately make on treatment and rehabilitation. We will first consider the traditional approaches to the treatment of occupational focal dystonia.

Treatment of any medical condition is dependent on three factors: 1) an accurate diagnosis, 2) understanding the cause, and 3) having a procedure or a drug that is effective in correcting the problem. In the past, treatments for occupational focal dystonia have had limited effectiveness because of difficulties with each of these three factors. The first step is, of course, an accurate diagnosis. In one survey of musicians with focal dystonia, several had undergone what appeared to have been inappropriate surgery (Hochberg, Harris, and Blattert 1990). Among another group of 189 patients, 40 percent had been wrongly diagnosed initially (Altenmuller 2003). Altenmuller also stresses that practitioners working with dystonic musicians should discuss the possible treatments realistically with their patients without raising false hopes of rapid recovery and should suggest a pragmatic approach to treatment based on a number of possible therapies. These should take into account the particular situation of the individual and the physical requirements of his or her instrument. Given the possible importance of psychological factors, emotional support is important and the patient should be encouraged to find some way of coming to terms with the limitations imposed by the dystonia and discouraged from indulging in useless therapies.

The term "dystonia" refers to a set of symptoms and not to a single condition, so the several types of dystonia (of which occupational focal dystonia is but one) do not necessarily have the same underlying cause, though they may share some common features. A number of drug treatments are used for dystonias, but most have been developed for other conditions. Finding one that has some beneficial effect remains largely a question of trial and error. Furthermore, the effectiveness of any drug in a particular patient may decline over time. Many of the drugs used are powerful ones that act by interfering with different classes of neurotransmitters (the chemicals used by neurons to communicate with each other; see chapter 7). Unfortunately, these transmitters have many different roles in the nervous system other than the control of movement, so drug treatments often have significant side effects. Furthermore, some may have only a palliative effect on the condition, and while they may reduce symptoms such as the discomfort of chronic muscle contractions, they do not provide a cure (Hochberg, Harris, and Blattert 1990). The major classes of drugs used are as follows:

1. Benzodiazepines and drugs such as baclofen. These act on receptors for the inhibitory neurotransmitter GABA to reduce nerve cell activity within the nervous system. They can be used to induce muscle relaxation by making motor neurons less active. The major side effect of the benzodiazepines is drowsiness.
2. Anticholinergic drugs, which block the neurotransmitter used by the motor neurons. This neurotransmitter is also found in many brain neurons, and it is these that are targeted by the drugs used to treat dystonia. The drug usually employed is trihexyphenidyl (Artane). The rationale for its use is that it damps down circuits in the brain that become overactive when levels of the transmitter dopamine (see below) are reduced. Whether dopamine levels do change significantly in focal dystonia is unclear, but Artane does relieve symptoms in some patients, though it cannot be tolerated for long periods. Side effects can include confusion, hallucinations, drowsiness, memory loss, and dry mouth, among others.
3. Drugs that mimic the effects of dopamine, a neurotransmitter involved in nerve cells within the motor pathways of the central nervous system (e.g., their loss is the cause of Parkinson's disease). Some forms of dystonia can be controlled by these drugs, though side effects may include slowing of movements and depression. They are usually less effective than anticholinergics for focal dystonia.

The chronic muscle contraction caused by dystonias can also be treated by the injection of botulinum toxin directly into the muscles affected. This drug is probably most familiar to the general public under the name of Botox, which is used cosmetically to paralyze muscles that wrinkle the skin of the face. The dosage must be carefully controlled so that it only weakens rather than paralyzes the affected muscles; however, the problem for dystonic musicians is that it is difficult to regulate this sufficiently to preserve the high degree of control required for playing. It is most effective when used on the small muscles that lie within the hand, as there is less chance of affecting the movement of adjacent fingers than when the injections are made into the large muscles of the forearm. However, many of the intrinsic muscles of the hand are involved in the rapid lateral movements of the fingers, which are used constantly by woodwind, string, and keyboard players. For woodwind players, for example, this is particularly crucial where the little fingers must depress several keys, but it is also important for the thumb and the other fingers. Therefore, for these players, Botox injection into hand muscles may be inappropriate (Altenmuller 2003). Finally, even where Botox is used successfully, patients may ultimately develop antibodies that will block its effects.

The discovery of the changes in cortical mapping that are associated with occupational focal dystonia has led to the development of a variety of new treatments based not on drugs but on physical retraining aimed at reversing these trends. The most puzzling aspect of dystonia is that although it is possible to modify sensory and motor maps in the brain very rapidly, it is extremely difficult to reverse the changes associated with focal dystonia. This problem has remained stubbornly resistant to investigation. At the moment there is no consensus on the optimum approach to take; it is also not clear what the limits to recovery will be. The techniques tried so far are based on sensory reeducation of the hand, either alone or together with motor exercises. The tasks used for sensory retraining are designed to require mental attentiveness, as this appears important for the remolding of sensory maps in the cortex. One approach uses Braille reading for sensory retraining without any motor training (Zeuner et al. 2002). The subjects of this study were nonmusicians who exhibited some form of writer's cramp. They had an initial training period of eight weeks, after which some continued with daily practice for up to six months. Spatial acuity (the ability of the fingers to distinguish closely positioned bars) improved significantly, suggesting that some reconfiguration of the sensory map was achieved. Those who persevered with the regimen showed considerable improvement in writing, but those who stopped reverted quite quickly to their dystonic state. In a second study, subjects who suffered from a variety of occupational dystonias were trained using a much heavier schedule involving a range of sensory discriminative tasks that required the tactile identification of objects and patterns by the hands and fingers. This was accompanied by a program aimed at reducing the aberrant motor activity of dystonia and improving general fitness and posture (Byl and McKenzie 2000). Improvements in sensory discrimination and motor accuracy were again evident, and though movements remained slower than normal, most of the subjects were able to return to work. However, none required the high degree of control needed by professional musicians.

There has been only a single study directed at applying retraining techniques to musicians, who are probably one of the most challenging groups in terms of rehabilitation. It used an approach called sensory-motor retuning (SMR) (Candia et al. 2002, 2003; Taub, Uswatte, and Elbert 2002). This study involved six pianists, two guitarists, two flutists, and an oboist, all suffering from dystonia of the hand. In each case, the main finger or fingers that were being used to compensate for the dystonic one were identified and held immobile with splints, leaving the dystonic finger to cope on its own in a series of highly structured exercises involving sequential movements of this and the other free fingers at a series of different tempos. After these exercises, the subjects played first simple and then more complex pieces with the hand unconstrained, during which they generally noticed considerable relief from their symptoms.

Initially the periods of free practice were short, lasting only fifteen to thirty seconds, but were gradually increased to fifteen minutes. It should be noted that SMR differs from constraint-induced movement therapy (CIMT), which is sometimes used for the rehabilitation of stroke victims. In CIMT the compensating part of the body is immobilized for prolonged periods so that the patient is forced to use the affected part for all tasks. In SMR, by contrast, the exercises carried out during immobilization are structured, with the aim of reeducating the affected joints to maintain nondystonic angles, while between training sessions, free-playing sessions are encouraged so that the newly reinforced finger postures are incorporated into the context of normal playing.

During a period of up to a year of sensory motor retraining, the dystonic finger was required to perform repetitive movements demanding coordination of different muscles for an hour or more each day. Many of the subjects showed signs of improvement even after an initial eight days of intensive training, though maintaining and extending this further required that the exercises be continued regularly for many months. There was a significant improvement among the pianists and guitarists who persisted with the training, and some reached a level close to normality. Subjectively, these participants felt that the results were a clear improvement on progress they had made with anticholinergic drugs or Botox injections, and of course there were no side effects from retraining. Objective analysis also demonstrated normalized finger movement. There were also indications of a normalization of the sensory mapping of the fingers within the brain (Candia et al. 2003). Unfortunately, for reasons that are unclear, the therapy produced no improvement in wind players with hand dystonia, and there is no obvious way that such an approach might be extended to embouchure dystonia; nevertheless, SMR therapy is a promising treatment that warrants further trials involving much larger numbers of affected musicians.

Another approach to reducing dystonic hand movements in musicians is limb immobilization (Priori et al. 2001; Pesenti, Barbieri, and Priori 2004), in which a splint is used to completely prevent any movement of the wrist and hand on the affected side for a period of four to five weeks. Because immobilization leads to a reduction in the cortical representation of the affected limb, the rationale behind the treatment is that it will reduce the overlap between the fingers in the cortical map of the hand. Such a long period of immobilization leads to considerable loss of muscle strength, which takes several weeks to be restored, but the treatment was reported to produce considerable long-term improvement in four of seven musicians who took part. It appeared to be most effective in those whose dystonia was of most recent onset. However, the treatment needs a more detailed evaluation, and so far no cortical mapping studies have been done to confirm that the desired changes are actually taking place as a result of treatment.

In conclusion, it can be seen that new ideas about the origin of focal hand dystonia have led to the exploration of new therapies based on a rational understanding of the condition. Though there is some way to go before the causes of this form of dystonia are fully understood, and though further work will be needed to establish the best strategies for rehabilitation, the possibility that effective treatments will ultimately be developed to replace the largely palliative therapies that are currently available looks increasingly hopeful.

REFERENCES

Aiello, R. 2001. Playing the piano by heart. From behavior to cognition. *Ann NY Acad Sci* 930:389–93.

Altenmuller, E. 2003. Focal dystonia: Advances in brain imaging and understanding of fine motor control in musicians. *Hand Clin* 19 (3):xi, 523–38.

Amunts, K., G. Schlaug, L. Jancke, H. Steinmetz, A. Schleicher, A. Dabringhaus, and K. Zilles. 1997. Motor cortex and hand motor skills: Structural compliance in the human brain. *Hum Brain Mapp* 5:206–15.

Amunts, K., G. Schlaug, A. Schleicher, H. Steinmetz, A. Dabringhaus, P. E. Roland, and K. Zilles. 1996. Asymmetry in the human motor cortex and handedness. *Neuroimage* 4 (3 Pt 1):216–22.

Baader, A. P., O. Kazennikov, and M. Wiesendanger. 2005. Coordination of bowing and fingering in violin playing. *Brain Res Cogn Brain Res* 23 (2–3):436–43.

Bangert, M., and E. O. Altenmuller. 2003. Mapping perception to action in piano practice: A longitudinal DC-EEG study. *BMC Neurosci* 4 (1):26.

Bangert, M., and G. Schlaug. 2006. Specialization of the specialized in features of external human brain morphology. *Eur J Neurosci* 24 (6):1832–34.

Bara-Jimenez, W., M. J. Catalan, M. Hallett, and C. Gerloff. 1998. Abnormal somatosensory homunculus in dystonia of the hand. *Ann Neurol* 44 (5):828–31.

Barry, N. H. 1992. The effects of practise strategies, individual differences in cognitive style, and gender upon technical accuracy and musicality of student instrumental performance. *Psychol Music* 20:112–23.

Bengtsson, S. L., Z. Nagy, S. Skare, L. Forsman, H. Forssberg, and F. Ullen. 2005. Extensive piano practicing has regionally specific effects on white matter development. *Nat Neurosci* 8 (9):1148–50.

Butterworth, S., S. Francis, E. Kelly, F. McGlone, R. Bowtell, and G. V. Sawle. 2003. Abnormal cortical sensory activation in dystonia: An fMRI study. *Mov Disord* 18 (6):673–82.

Byl, N. N., and A. McKenzie. 2000. Treatment effectiveness for patients with a history of repetitive hand use and focal hand dystonia: A planned, prospective follow-up study. *J Hand Ther* 13 (4):289–301.

Byl, N. N., A. McKenzie, and S. S. Nagarajan. 2000. Differences in somatosensory hand organization in a healthy flutist and a flutist with focal hand dystonia: A case report. *J Hand Ther* 13 (4):302–9.

Byl, N. N., and M. Melnick. 1997. The neural consequences of repetition: Clinical implications of a learning hypothesis. *J Hand Ther* 10 (2):160–74.

Candia, V., T. Schafer, E. Taub, H. Rau, E. Altenmuller, B. Rockstroh, and T. Elbert. 2002. Sensory motor retuning: A behavioral treatment for focal hand dystonia of pianists and guitarists. *Arch Phys Med Rehabil* 83 (10):1342–48.

Candia, V., C. Wienbruch, T. Elbert, B. Rockstroh, and W. Ray. 2003. Effective behavioral treatment of focal hand dystonia in musicians alters somatosensory cortical organization. *Proc Natl Acad Sci USA* 100 (13):7942–46.

Chaffin, R., and G. Imreh. 1997. "Pulling teeth and torture": Musical theory and problem solving. *Thinking and Reasoning* 3 (4):315–36.

———. 2002. Practicing perfection: Piano performance as expert memory. *Psychol Sci* 13 (4):342–49.

Chaffin, R., and A. F. Lemieux. 2004. General perspectives on achieving musical excellence. In *Musical excellence: Strategies and techniques to enhance performance*, ed. A. Williamon. Oxford: Oxford University Press.

Charness, M. E., M. H. Ross, and J. M. Shefner. 1996. Ulnar neuropathy and dystonic flexion of the fourth and fifth digits: Clinical correlation in musicians. *Muscle Nerve* 19 (4):431–37.

Chen, J., M. Woollacott, and S. Pologe. 2006. Accuracy and underlying mechanisms of shifting movements in cellists. *Exp Brain Res* 174 (3):467–76.

Connolly, C., and A. Williamon. 2004. Mental skills training. In *Musical excellence: Strategies and techniques to enhance performance*, ed. A. Williamon. Oxford: Oxford University Press.

Delmaire, C., A. Krainik, S. Tezenas du Montcel, E. Gerardin, S. Meunier, J. F. Mangin, S. Sangla, L. Garnero, M. Vidailhet, and S. Lehericy. 2005. Disorganized somatotopy in the putamen of patients with focal hand dystonia. *Neurology* 64 (8):1391–96.

Elbert, T., V. Candia, E. Altenmuller, H. Rau, A. Sterr, B. Rockstroh, C. Pantev, and E. Taub. 1998. Alteration of digital representations in somatosensory cortex in focal hand dystonia. *Neuroreport* 9 (16):3571–75.

Elbert, T., C. Pantev, C. Wienbruch, B. Rockstroh, and E. Taub. 1995. Increased cortical representation of the fingers of the left hand in string players. *Science* 270 (5234):305–7.

Ericsson, K. A., R. T. Krampe, and C. Tesch-Romer. 1993. The role of deliberate practice in the acquisition of expert performance. *Psychological Review* 100 (3):363–406.

Finney, S. A., and C. Palmer. 2003. Auditory feedback and memory for music performance: Sound evidence for an encoding effect. *Mem Cognit* 31 (1):51–64.

Frucht, S. J., S. Fahn, P. E. Greene, C. O'Brien, M. Gelb, D. D. Truong, J. Welsh, S. Factor, and B. Ford. 2001. The natural history of embouchure dystonia. *Mov Disord* 16 (5):899–906.

Fry, H. J. 1986. Overuse syndrome in musicians—100 years ago. An historical review. *Med J Aust* 145 (11–12):620–25.

Gabrielsson, A. 1999. The performance of music. In *The psychology of music*, ed. D. Deutsch. San Diego: Academic Press.

Gaser, C., and G. Schlaug. 2003. Brain structures differ between musicians and non-musicians. *J Neurosci* 23 (27):9240–45.

Graziano, M. S., C. S. Taylor, T. Moore, and D. F. Cooke. 2002. The cortical control of movement revisited. *Neuron* 36 (3):349–62.

Halpern, A. R., and G. H. Bower. 1982. Musical expertise and melodic structure in memory for musical notation. *Am J Psychol* 95:31–50.

Hashimoto, I., A. Suzuki, T. Kimura, Y. Iguchi, M. Tanosaki, R. Takino, Y. Haruta, and M. Taira. 2004. Is there training-dependent reorganization of digit representations in area 3b of string players? *Clin Neurophysiol* 115 (2):435–47.

Haslinger, B., P. Erhard, E. Altenmuller, A. Hennenlotter, M. Schwaiger, H. Grafin Von Einsiedel, E. Rummeny, B. Conrad, and A. O. Ceballos-Baumann. 2004. Reduced recruitment of motor association areas during bimanual coordination in concert pianists. *Hum Brain Mapp* 22 (3):206–15.

Hassler, M. 2000. Music medicine. A neurobiological approach. *Neuroendocrinol Lett* 21 (2):101–6.

Haueisen, J., and T. R. Knosche. 2001. Involuntary motor activity in pianists evoked by music perception. *J Cogn Neurosci* 13 (6):786–92.

Hirata, Y., M. Schulz, E. Altenmuller, T. Elbert, and C. Pantev. 2004. Sensory mapping of lip representation in brass musicians with embouchure dystonia. *Neuroreport* 15 (5):815–18.

Hochberg, F. H., S. U. Harris, and T. R. Blattert. 1990. Occupational hand cramps: Professional disorders of motor control. *Hand Clin* 6 (3):417–28.

Hochberg, F. H., and N. S. Hochberg. 2000. Occupational cramps/focal dystonias. In *Medical problems of the instrumental musician*, ed. R. Tubiana and P. C. Amadio. London: Martin Dunitz.

Hund-Georgiadis, M., and D. Y. von Cramon. 1999. Motor-learning-related changes in piano players and non-musicians revealed by functional magnetic-resonance signals. *Exp Brain Res* 125 (4):417–25.

Hutchinson, S., L. H. Lee, N. Gaab, and G. Schlaug. 2003. Cerebellar volume of musicians. *Cereb Cortex* 13 (9):943–49.

Ibanez, V., N. Sadato, B. Karp, M. P. Deiber, and M. Hallett. 1999. Deficient activation of the motor cortical network in patients with writer's cramp. *Neurology* 53 (1):96–105.

Jabusch, H. C., and D. Altenmuller. 2006. Focal dystonia in musicians: From phenomenology to therapy. *Adv Cog Psychol* 2 (2–3):207–20.

Jancke, L., G. Schlaug, and H. Steinmetz. 1997. Hand skill asymmetry in professional musicians. *Brain Cogn* 34 (3):424–32.

Jankovic, J., and H. Shale. 1989. Dystonia in musicians. *Semin Neurol* 9 (2):131–35.

Kandel, E. R., J. H. Schwartz, and T. M. Jessell. 2000. *Principles of Neural Science*. 4th ed. New York: McGraw-Hill, Health Professions Division.

Karni, A., G. Meyer, P. Jezzard, M. M. Adams, R. Turner, and L. G. Ungerleider. 1995. Functional MRI evidence for adult motor cortex plasticity during motor skill learning. *Nature* 377 (6545):155–58.

Karni, A., G. Meyer, C. Rey-Hipolito, P. Jezzard, M. M. Adams, R. Turner, and L. G. Ungerleider. 1998. The acquisition of skilled motor performance: Fast and slow experience-driven changes in primary motor cortex. *Proc Natl Acad Sci USA* 95 (3):861–68.

Kleim, J. A., T. M. Hogg, P. M. VandenBerg, N. R. Cooper, R. Bruneau, and M. Remple. 2004. Cortical synaptogenesis and motor map reorganization occur during late, but not early, phase of motor skill learning. *J Neurosci* 24 (3):628–33.

Langheim, F. J., J. H. Callicott, V. S. Mattay, J. H. Duyn, and D. R. Weinberger. 2002. Cortical systems associated with covert music rehearsal. *Neuroimage* 16 (4):901–8.

Lee, D. J., Y. Chen, and G. Schlaug. 2003. Corpus callosum: Musician and gender effects. *Neuroreport* 14 (2):205–9.

Lim, V. K., E. Altenmuller, and J. L. Bradshaw. 2001. Focal dystonia: Current theories. *Hum Mov Sci* 20 (6):875–914.

Lim, V. K., J. L. Bradshaw, M. E. Nicholls, and E. Altenmuller. 2004. Abnormal sensorimotor processing in pianists with focal dystonia. *Adv Neurol* 94:267–73.

Lotze, M., G. Scheler, H. R. Tan, C. Braun, and N. Birbaumer. 2003. The musician's brain: Functional imaging of amateurs and professionals during performance and imagery. *Neuroimage* 20 (3):1817–29.

Luders, E., C. Gaser, L. Jancke, and G. Schlaug. 2004. A voxel-based approach to gray matter asymmetries. *Neuroimage* 22:656–664.

Maess, B., S. Koelsch, T. C. Gunter, and A. D. Friederici. 2001. Musical syntax is processed in Broca's area: An MEG study. *Nat Neurosci* 4 (5):540–45.

Maguire, E. A., D. G. Gadian, I. S. Johnsrude, C. D. Good, J. Ashburner, R. S. Frackowiak, and C. D. Frith. 2000. Navigation-related structural change in the hippocampi of taxi drivers. *Proc Natl Acad Sci USA* 97 (8):4398–4403.

Meister, I. G., T. Krings, H. Foltys, B. Boroojerdi, M. Muller, R. Topper, and A. Thron. 2004. Playing piano in the mind—an fMRI study on music imagery and performance in pianists. *Cogn Brain Res* 19 (3):219–28.

Morrison, S. 2000. Effect of melodic context, tuning behaviors, and experience on intonation accuracy of wind players. *J Res Music Educ* 48:39–51.

Noppeney, U., T. D. Waberski, R. Gobbele, and H. Buchner. 1999. Spatial attention modulates the cortical somatosensory representation of the digits in humans. *Neuroreport* 10 (15):3137–41.

Nordstrom, M. A., and S. L. Butler. 2002. Reduced intracortical inhibition and facilitation of corticospinal neurons in musicians. *Exp Brain Res* 144 (3):336–42.

Ozturk, A. H., B. Tascioglu, M. Aktekin, Z. Kurtoglu, and I. Erden. 2002. Morphometric comparison of the human corpus callosum in professional musicians and non-musicians by using in vivo magnetic resonance imaging. *J Neuroradiol* 29 (1):29–34.

Parsons, L. M. 2001. Exploring the functional neuroanatomy of music performance, perception, and comprehension. *Ann NY Acad Sci* 930:211–31.

———. 2003. Rethinking the lesser brain. *Sci Am* 289 (2):40–47.

Pascual-Leone, A. 2001. The brain that plays music and is changed by it. *Ann NY Acad Sci* 930:315–29.

Pesenti, A., S. Barbieri, and A. Priori. 2004. Limb immobilization for occupational dystonia: A possible alternative treatment for selected patients. *Adv Neurol* 94:247–54.

Priori, A., A. Pesenti, A. Cappellari, G. Scarlato, and S. Barbieri. 2001. Limb immobilization for the treatment of focal occupational dystonia. *Neurology* 57 (3):405–9.

Pujol, J., J. Roset-Llobet, D. Rosines-Cubells, J. Deus, B. Narberhaus, J. Valls-Sole, A. Capdevila, and A. Pascual-Leone. 2000. Brain cortical activation during guitar-induced hand dystonia studied by functional MRI. *Neuroimage* 12 (3):257–67.

Pullman, S. L., and A. H. Hristova. 2005. Musician's dystonia. *Neurology* 64 (2):186–87.

Ridding, M. C., B. Brouwer, and M. A. Nordstrom. 2000. Reduced interhemispheric inhibition in musicians. *Exp Brain Res* 133 (2):249–53.

Romanelli, P., V. Esposito, D. W. Schaal, and G. Heit. 2005. Somatotopy in the basal ganglia: Experimental and clinical evidence for segregated sensorimotor channels. *Brain Res Brain Res Rev* 48 (1):112–28.

Rosenkranz, K., A. Williamon, K. Butler, C. Cordivari, A. J. Lees, and J. C. Rothwell. 2005. Pathophysiological differences between musician's dystonia and writer's cramp. *Brain* 128 (Pt 4):918–31.

Schlaug, G. 2001. The brain of musicians. A model for functional and structural adaptation. *Ann NY Acad Sci* 930:281–99.

———. 2006. Brain structures of musicians: Executive functions and morphological implications. In *Music, motor control and the brain*, ed. E. Altenmuller, M. Wiesendanger, and J. Kesselring. Oxford: Oxford University Press.

Schlaug, G., L. Jancke, Y. Huang, and H. Steinmetz. 1995. In vivo evidence of structural brain asymmetry in musicians. *Science* 267 (5198):699–701.

Schmidt, A., H. C. Jabusch, E. Altenmuller, J. Hagenah, N. Bruggemann, K. Hedrich, R. Saunders-Pullman, S. B. Bressman, P. L. Kramer, and C. Klein. 2006. Dominantly transmitted focal dystonia in families of patients with musician's cramp. *Neurology* 67 (4):691–93.

Schneider P., M. Scherg, H. G. Dosch, H. J. Specht, A. Gutschalk, and A. Rupp. 2002. Morphology of Heschl's gyrus reflects enhanced activation in the auditory cortex of musicians. *Nat Neurosci* 5:688–694.

Sergent, J., E. Zuck, S. Terriah, and B. MacDonald. 1992. Distributed neural network underlying musical sight-reading and keyboard performance. *Science* 257 (5066):106–9.

Sloboda, J. A., J. W. Davidson, D. G. Howe, and D. G. Moore. 1996. The role of practice in the development of performing musicians. *Brit J Psychol* 87 (2):287–309.

Sluming, V., T. Barrick, M. Howard, E. Cezayirli, A. Mayes, and N. Roberts. 2002. Voxel-based morphometry reveals increased gray matter density in Broca's area in male symphony orchestra musicians. *Neuroimage* 17 (3):1613–22.

Sterr, A., M. M. Muller, T. Elbert, B. Rockstroh, C. Pantev, and E. Taub. 1998. Changed perceptions in Braille readers. *Nature* 391 (6663):134–35.

Stickgold, R., and M. P. Walker. 2005. Memory consolidation and reconsolidation: What is the role of sleep? *Trends Neurosci* 28 (8):408–15.

Taub, E., G. Uswatte, and T. Elbert. 2002. New treatments in neurorehabilitation founded on basic research. *Nat Rev Neurosci* 3 (3):228–36.

Tubiana, R. 2000. Musician's focal dystonia. In *Medical problems of the instrumental musician*, ed. R. Tubiana and P. C. Amadio. London: Martin Dunitz.

Turner-Stokes, L., and K. Reid. 1999. Three-dimensional motion analysis of upper limb movement in the bowing arm of string-playing musicians. *Clin Biomech (Bristol, Avon)* 14 (6):426–33.

Walker, M. P., T. Brakefield, J. Seidman, A. Morgan, J. A. Hobson, and R. Stickgold. 2003. Sleep and the time course of motor skill learning. *Learn Mem* 10 (4):275–84.

Wiesendanger, M., A. P. Baader, and O. Kazennikov. 2006. Fingering and bowing in violinists: A motor control approach. In *Music, motor control and the brain*, ed. E. Altenmuller, M. Wiesendanger, and J. Kesselring. Oxford: Oxford University Press.

Williamon, A., and T. Egner. 2004. Memory structures for encoding and retrieving a piece of music: An ERP investigation. *Brain Res Cogn Brain Res* 22 (1):36–44.

Williamon, A., and E. Valentine. 2000. Quantity and quality of musical practice as predictors of performance quality. *Br J Psychol* 91 (Pt 3):353–76.

———. 2002. The role of retrieval structures in memorizing music. *Cognit Psychol* 44 (1):1–32.

Wilson, F. R., C. Wagner, and V. Homberg. 1993. Biomechanical abnormalities in musicians with occupational cramp/focal dystonia. *J Hand Ther* 6 (4):298–307.

Wynn Parry, C. B., and R. Tubiana. 1998. Dystonia. In *The musician's hand: A clinical guide*, ed. I. Winspur and C. B. Wynn Parry. London: Martin Dunitz.

Yaguez, L., D. Nagel, H. Hoffman, A. G. Canavan, E. Wist, and V. Homberg. 1998. A mental route to motor learning: Improving trajectorial kinematics through imagery training. *Behav Brain Res* 90 (1):95–106.

Zatorre, R. J. 1998. Functional specialization of human auditory cortex for musical processing. *Brain* 121 (10):1817–1818.

Zeuner, K. E., W. Bara-Jimenez, P. S. Noguchi, S. R. Goldstein, J. M. Dambrosia, and M. Hallett. 2002. Sensory training for patients with focal hand dystonia. *Ann Neurol* 51 (5):593–98.

Chapter Nine

Hearing and the Processing of Musical Sound by the Brain

In this chapter we will first consider the physical properties of sound, which are important for an understanding of how the ear responds to and can be damaged by it. We will then consider how sound is detected by the ear and how the information it extracts reaches the brain. Finally, we will examine how music is analyzed by the brain and how some of the effects that it has on us are generated.

THE NATURE OF SOUND

The sensation that we subjectively perceive as sound originates from objects in the environment that vibrate. Most commonly, the effects of these vibrations reach us through the pressure waves that the vibrating objects generate in air, but the auditory system can be stimulated more directly when the vibrating object (e.g., a tuning fork) is applied directly to the bones of the skull, and indeed, some hearing aids work on this principle. In the case of musical instruments, the sound arises from a vibrating string, the vibrations in a column of air within the instrument, or the membrane of a drum and is then conducted through the air to the ears. The properties of the vibrations in the resonating object and those it drives in air are best described initially for a pure tone (a sound of a single frequency). The sounds of natural objects and musical instruments are not like this, but pure tones can be generated electronically using a waveform generator and a loudspeaker. The vibration generating the tone can be represented graphically (fig. 9-1, sound presentation 9-1) as a regular oscillation that is described mathematically as a sine wave representing the displacement of the vibrating object over time. The wave is characterized by its amplitude (which equates to the size of the displacement of the vibrating cone of the speaker, or the loudness of the sound) and its frequency (which represents the number of oscillations per second made by the cone of the speaker), which we may call the pitch of the tone. The vibrations of the speaker cone set up a series of pressure pulses in the surrounding air. As the cone moves forward, it produces an increase in pressure as the molecules of the air are pushed closer together than they would be in the absence of the vibration. As the cone moves

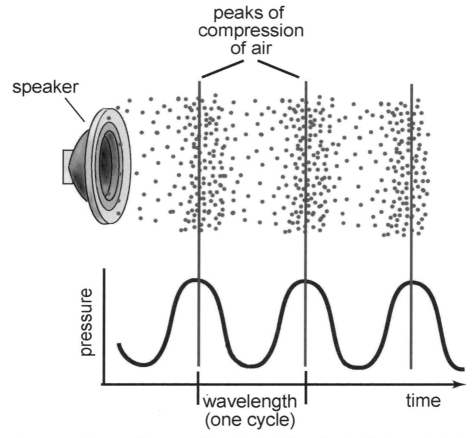

Figure 9-1. When sound is generated by a vibrating body such as the diaphragm of a loud-speaker, the air is compressed, raising its pressure as the diaphragm moves forward, while the pressure falls as it moves back. This can be represented by the waveform at the bottom of the image in which the vertical axis represents air pressure and the horizontal axis, time. The distance between the peaks is the wavelength. Shortening the wavelength is equivalent to increasing the frequency, perceived as a rise in pitch. The greater the amplitude of the waveform, the louder the sound.

backward, the air pressure is reduced, leaving the air molecules farther apart than they would otherwise be (fig. 9-1). These pressure oscillations radiate out from the origin of the sound like the ripples in a still pond that spread from the point at which a stone has hit the water surface and continue for as long as the vibrations persist.

The pressure fluctuations that we perceive as sound can be extremely small. The pressure of air at sea level, which is generated by the weight of the column of gas that extends from there to the edge of the atmosphere, provides a standard measurement that is given the value of 1 atmosphere. It is the same as the pressure that is produced by the weight of 10 cubic meters of water. The quietest sound that can be detected by the auditory system is described as its threshold and is represented by a pressure pulse that is 2×10^{-10} (two ten-billionths) of atmospheric pressure. This arbitrary value is used as the standard sound pressure level (SPL) against which sound intensity or volume is measured. One of the remarkable features of the auditory system is the enormous range of sound pressures that can be detected. The pressure generated by sounds at the top end of the tolerable range (which are perceived as painful) is 10^7 (ten million) times that of the auditory threshold. With this range of pressures, it is not convenient to use a linear scale to describe sound intensities, so a logarithmic scale is used instead. The unit of measure is the decibel (dB), which represents a ratio—in the case of sound pressure this is defined as follows:

sound pressure level (dB SPL) = $20 \log_{10} (P/P_{ref})$,

where P is the pressure of the sound being measured and P_{ref} is the reference sound level that is the human auditory threshold level described above. The standard units in which pressure is measured are called pascals (Pa). The standard value assigned to the auditory threshold is 20×10^{-6} Pa (twenty-millionths of a pascal). However, the main point to bear in mind is that a rise of 20 dB SPL represents a tenfold increase in the sound pressure. For an orchestra, the typical sound levels during performance range from about 40 dB SPL for a pianissimo passage to 90 dB for a fortissimo involving the full orchestra. Players may experience sound pressure levels above this for short periods. Sound levels of over 100 dB are quite commonly reached for electronically amplified music at rock concerts and can rise further to levels that cause temporary or permanent damage to the ear (see below). In the context of its impact on our hearing, the important characteristic of sound is its intensity, which is the amount of energy that is released per unit area. This is expressed in units of watts per square meter (Wm^2). As this is proportional to P^2:

sound intensity (dB) = $10 \log_{10} (I/I_{ref})$,

so a rise of 10 dB represents a tenfold increase, and a 3 dB increase is equivalent to a doubling of intensity. Thus, between the threshold for hearing (0 dB SPL) and the intensity of sound that causes pain (about 140 dB SPL) the intensity of the sound (the amount of energy it carries) increases by a factor of 10^{14} (one hundred trillion). This is a quite extraordinary range of intensities; no other sensory system has to cope with a dynamic range of this magnitude. We will see later some of the mechanisms used by the ear to achieve this feat.

If the sound is represented by a simple sine wave (fig. 9-1), the frequency of the oscillation in sound pressure represents its pitch. The standard unit for the measure of frequency is the hertz (Hz). A frequency of 1 Hz represents a single cycle of the waveform per second. In musical terms, pitch for Western music is now largely standardized, with the A above middle C (A4) providing a reference at 440 Hz. Until the nineteenth century there was no international pitch standard, and in the eighteenth century A4 typically varied between 400 Hz and 450 Hz, a difference of about three semitones. The first attempt at pitch standardization in the 1850s set A4 at 435 Hz, and concert pitch was raised to its present level in the mid-twentieth century. The ten-

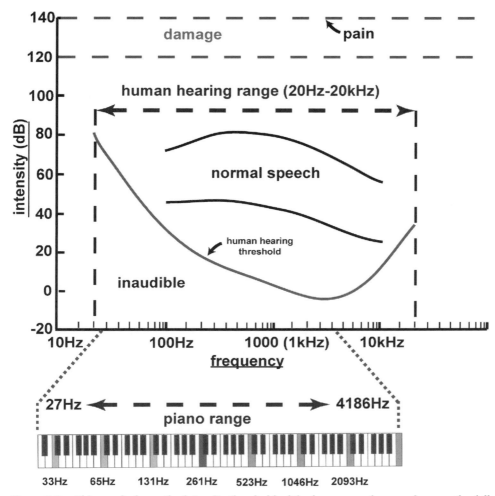

Figure 9-2. This graph shows the intensity threshold of the human ear for sound across the full range of frequencies that it can detect (20–20,000 Hz). The minimum threshold (defined as 0 dB) is found for sounds of about 3,000–4,000 Hz. Above and below this frequency, the threshold rises. For the lowest frequencies detectable by the ear, it reaches 80 dB, which is equivalent to the loudest sound intensity encountered in conversational speech. For reference, the piano keyboard is drawn at the bottom with the frequency of C indicated for each octave. Its range runs from about 27 Hz to 4,000 Hz.

dency for pitch to rise was linked to the need to produce a brilliant sound that would fill large concert halls and was limited mainly by the tensile strength of the E string of the violin. When it became possible to produce strings that would support greater tensions reliably, the pitch could be raised, though this also required structural modifications to the violin so that it could support the increased forces this generated. The change in pitch was perhaps not so welcome to singers, whose instruments cannot be so easily modified!

In humans, the audible frequency range extends from about 20 Hz to 20,000 Hz (20 kilohertz [kHz]), though our ability to discriminate pitch (i.e., to distinguish one note from another) is effectively limited to sounds below 5 kHz. It is important to recognize that the ear is not equally sensitive to all frequencies (fig. 9-2). Its peak sensitivity lies in the range of 3–5 kHz, and the threshold for frequencies between about 300–8,000 Hz lies below 20 dB SPL. This covers the range used in conversational speech. Most significant musical sounds lie below 11 kHz, but fundamental frequencies of the notes on a full concert piano range from 27 Hz (A0) to 4,186 Hz (C8), with middle C (C4) at 261 Hz.

Most of the sounds we hear are not pure sounds of a single frequency but are complex sounds containing many frequencies (sound presentation 9-1). The lowest frequency of the complex sound produced by an instrument is usually the most intense and is called the fundamental. This is overlaid by a series of harmonics. If we consider the vibration of a plucked string, the fundamental (also known as the first harmonic) represents a vibration of the whole length of the string in a smooth curve from one end to the other, with the greatest displacement from the rest position at the point of the string at its midpoint (fig. 9-3). It is quite easy to see this mode of vibration on, for example, a harp string. What is not so apparent is that superimposed on this is a further set of vibrations (harmonics). The second harmonic can be visualized as one in which the midpoint of the string remains at the rest position and the upper and lower segments vibrate at twice the frequency of the fundamental. This creates a note one octave above the fundamental that can be used for effect in many stringed instruments by touching the midpoint of the string during plucking or bowing to suppress the fundamental. The third harmonic is a mode where the string is divided into three vibrating segments and is a fifth above the second harmonic. For the fourth harmonic, the string is divided into four segments giving a pitch a third above the previous harmonic, and so on. When we hear the complex note that results from the sounding of the fundamental and its harmonics, we nevertheless attribute to it a single frequency value that is defined as its pitch. This is usually the frequency of the fundamental, but it may be influenced by the perceived harmonic structure of the note. The perception of pitch is a reflection of how the brain interprets sound; we will see later that the pitch of a note may represent a fundamental frequency that is not actually present! In different instruments or voices, the relative strength of the harmonics in the notes varies, giving each a distinctive sound quality or timbre. For example, among the woodwinds, the clarinet with its cylindrical bore acts like a stopped pipe and generates only the odd harmonics of the fundamental; this is a significant element of its characteristic tone color (Fletcher and Rossing 1998). On the other hand, the oboe, saxophone, and bassoon, because of their conical bore, act as open pipes and so have both odd and even harmonics. For brass instruments, a significant component of their timbre comes from the presence of a mouthpiece and the shape of the bell (Benade 1973). Interestingly, however, much of the information we use to identify the characteristic sound of a particular instrument comes from the transient changes in the harmonics and other extraneous sounds that characterize the onset of the note. If we record a note and cut off the beginning and the end, it becomes almost impossible to identify the instrument

The origin of harmonics in a vibrating string

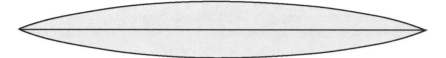

first harmonic mode (fundamental), e.g. 100Hz

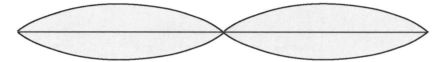

second harmonic mode, e.g. 200Hz

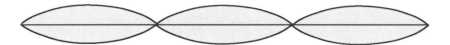

third harmonic mode, e.g. 300Hz

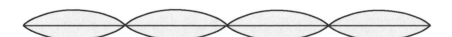

fourth harmonic mode, e.g. 400Hz

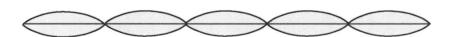

fifth harmonic mode, e.g. 500Hz etc.

Figure 9-3.   The harmonics of a vibrating string. When a string is plucked, a series of frequencies called harmonics or partials are generated. The fundamental frequency (first harmonic) is the result of the vibration seen in the uppermost panel. Superimposed on this are the other modes of vibration shown in the lower panels. These vibrations divide the string into segments of equal length. For the second harmonic the string is divided into two, and the frequency is twice that of the fundamental; for the third harmonic the frequency is three times that of the fundamental, and so on. This type of harmonic series is typical of all real sounds.

that made it. One cannot even say whether the sound comes from a stringed or a wind instrument. This is illustrated in sound presentation 9-1 on the disc accompanying the text. When the onset of the note is restored, the task becomes easy.

The auditory system can be divided into two parts, which we will consider in turn. The first is the ear, which detects the sound and splits it up into its frequency components. This information is then carried to the second part, which lies within the brain; it is here that the frequency components are recombined, analyzed, and interpreted. The brain also compares the information coming from the two ears to create a three-dimensional soundscape, which allows the position of the sound source to be accurately determined, at least for some frequencies.

HEARING AND THE EAR

The Outer and Middle Ear

For descriptive purposes, the ear is usually divided into three parts, the outer, middle, and inner ear (fig. 9-4A). The outer ear is composed of the cartilaginous external ear, which sits on the side of the head, and the auditory canal into which it reflects sound. The external ear is most effective at collecting sound from the front and so has a built-in directionality. Unlike the ears of some other animals such as the cat, our external ears are virtually immobile, though the muscles that move them still exist as rudiments. The auditory canal ends in the eardrum (or tympanic membrane), which separates it from the air-filled middle ear. Like the membrane of a drum, the tympanic membrane must be kept taut if it is to vibrate efficiently in response to sound. On the other side of the tympanic membrane lies the middle ear (fig. 9-4B). The vibrations of the tympanic membrane are communicated to three small bones (or ossicles) that lie in contact with each other within the middle ear cavity. These are called the malleus (hammer), incus (anvil), and stapes (stirrup). The malleus, as its name suggests, is shaped like a hammer with the handle lying in contact with the tympanic membrane. A muscle called the tensor tympanum acts on the handle to keep the tympanic membrane taut. This muscle is supplied by a branch of the trigeminal nerve, which also supplies the large chewing muscles that move the jaw. Vibrations of the tympanic membrane are conducted through the malleus, incus, and stapes to the fluid-filled inner ear, where the structures that detect the vibrations are found. The middle and inner ear lie within one of the bones of the skull (the temporal bone). There are two windows in the bony wall separating the inner ear from the middle ear, one of which is round and the other oval (fig. 9-4B). The stapes ends in a flat disk called the footplate, which sits in the oval window. Because the fluid in the inner ear (which is mainly water) is incompressible, vibrations of the footplate would be unable to set up vibrations in it if it were a sealed chamber. The second window (the round window) is covered with a membrane, and as the footplate pushes into the oval window, this membrane bulges outward. This allows the vibrations to radiate through the fluid. The ear ossicles are not there simply to carry the vibrations across the middle ear chamber; they also concentrate the energy of the sound that is vibrating the eardrum onto the much smaller area of

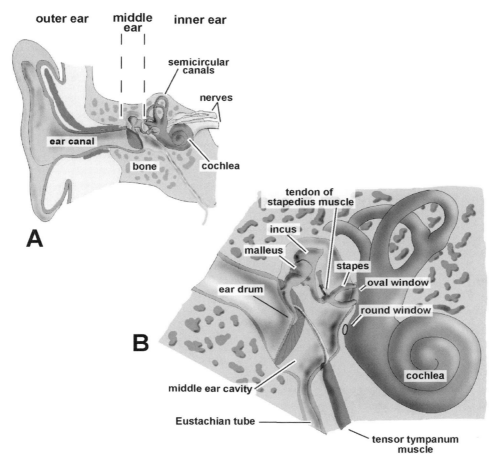

Figure 9-4.   The structure of the ear. A. The ear can be divided into three distinct regions. The outer ear consists of the cartilaginous part on the outside of the head and the auditory canal into which it reflects sound. The canal ends in the tympanic membrane, behind which lies the middle ear. This is an air-filled cavity containing three small bones (ossicles) called the malleus (hammer), incus (anvil), and stapes (stirrup). The middle ear chamber is connected to the back of the throat by the Eustachian tube to allow pressure equalization. The inner ear is made up of a series of convoluted spaces filled with fluid. These are the cochleas, which respond to sound, and the semicircular canals and vestibule, which are involved in balance. B. The middle ear. The tympanic membrane is attached to the "handle" of the malleus and is kept taut by the action of the tensor tympanum muscle. The stapes ends in a broad "footplate" that is pushed into the oval window, a hole in the bone that contains the inner ear. The movement of the stapes can be limited by the stapedius muscle, whose tendon attaches to its head.

the oval window. The ossicles also act as a system of levers, further contributing to this effect so that there is an increase in the force exerted per unit area of about twenty times. This amplification is necessary because the airborne vibrations of the tympanic membrane would otherwise be too weak to drive the vibrations in the fluid of the inner ear; in fact without this mechanism, most (over 99 percent) of the energy would be reflected from the surface of the fluid.

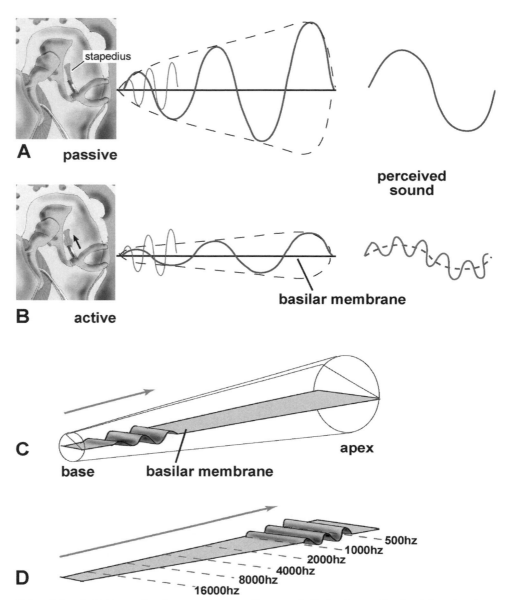

Figure 9-5. A–B. Protecting the ear. The stapedius muscle limits the amplitude of the vibrations of the stapes and so the amount of energy this transfers to the inner ear. It is more effective in blocking low-frequency than high-frequency sound. When a high-pitched and a low-pitched sound are presented together, each sets up a traveling wave that runs along the basilar membrane (solid line). Without the stapedius muscle, the wave produced by the low-frequency sound (dark) can mask that of the high-frequency sound (light), making it impossible to detect. When the stapedius is active, the greater reduction in the low-frequency wave allows the high-frequency sound to emerge. The resultant waveform perceived by the cochlea is shown on the right. C–D. Because the physical properties of the basilar membrane change along its length, waves caused by high-frequency sounds travel only a short distance before being damped, while successively lower frequencies generate waves that travel ever farther. How far the wave runs therefore indicates its frequency. This is the principle of tonotopy, and this is one source of information that can be used by the nervous system to determine the pitch of the sound.

The movement of the stapes is controlled by the stapedius muscle, which is attached to its neck (fig. 9-4B). When we are exposed to very loud sounds, the muscle contracts and so limits the extent to which the stapes can vibrate, which helps to protect the delicate receptor apparatus of the inner ear. The contraction of the muscle is brought about by an involuntary reflex (the stapedius reflex) (fig. 9-5A, B). The stapedius restricts the movement of the chain of ossicles, with the result that they transmit high frequencies more efficiently than low frequencies. When the stapedius is active, the chain of ossicles therefore acts as a filter, making it easier to detect a high-frequency sound against a low-frequency background. The muscle becomes active just before we speak or sing. During speech the sound of one's own voice is transmitted to the ears not only through the air, but also through the tissues of the neck and head, which most effectively transmit low-frequency vibrations. This is one reason why our voice sounds very different when we listen to it in a recording. The volume of the voice is also normally set at a level that will carry the sound at a comfortable volume to a listener who typically is much farther away from us than the distance between our mouth and our own ears, and so it is appropriate to activate the reflex to reduce the sensitivity of our hearing during speech. The stapedius muscle is supplied by the facial nerve, which also supplies the small muscles in the face that are used to generate facial expression or to control the embouchure. This nerve is sometimes damaged in a condition known as facial nerve palsy (Bell's palsy), which causes paralysis of the facial muscles (see chapter 6). One symptom of facial nerve palsy is an intolerance of loud noise, which is a direct consequence of the paralysis of the stapedius muscle.

Like all gases, air changes its volume depending on its pressure. The air in the middle ear is no exception. We experience changes in atmospheric pressure constantly as weather systems pass over or if we climb a hill or a mountain. During flying or scuba diving, the pressure changes can be both rapid and dramatic. The cabin of a commercial passenger aircraft is pressurized because at the cruising height for a typical long-haul flight (a mile or more higher than Mount Everest), we would rapidly become unconscious due to low oxygen pressure. However, the cabin pressure is usually set at a level equivalent to about 6,000 feet above sea level, which is why we still have to make adjustments during takeoff. If the pressure in the middle ear is not the same as the outside air, the eardrum will bulge inward or outward. At best this is uncomfortable, but as the pressure difference increases, it rapidly becomes painful and the eardrum will ultimately rupture. Though this would normally heal spontaneously over a couple of months, hearing would be affected until the process is complete. There must therefore be a link between the middle ear and the outside air to allow pressure equalization; this duct, which links the middle ear to the back of the throat, is the Eustachian or auditory tube (fig. 9-4B). For part of its length it travels through bone, but the end of the tube is made of cartilage. Most of the time this section is closed, but part of the muscle layer lining the inside of the throat is attached to it and during swallowing, the contraction of the muscle opens the tube briefly. This is why swallowing or any activity that promotes it (e.g., sucking on a sweet) is encouraged by cabin staff during takeoff. The eardrum may also rupture following an explosion, where the increase in air pressure occurs too rapidly for pressure equalization to take place via the eustachian tube.

The Inner Ear

The inner ear is composed of a convoluted chamber lying within the temporal bone of the skull. Because of the mazelike complexity of its passageways, it is known as the labyrinth. One part of the inner ear contains the sensory apparatus that monitors the orientation and acceleration of the head, information that the brain uses to help us maintain our balance. This system does not concern us here. The other part, where sound is detected, is called the cochlea (fig. 9-6). This is a spiral of two and three-quarter turns with a central bony core, and a cast of it would look rather like a snail shell; indeed, the name cochlea is derived from the Latin word for "shell." The base of the cochlea opens into a large space called the vestibule, which has the oval window in its wall (fig. 9-4B). A cross-section through the cochlea reveals that it contains three long, narrow, fluid-filled chambers running in parallel up to the tip of the spiral. Each of these spaces is given the name "scala." This comes from the Latin word for "ladder" or "staircase" and has the same origin as the musical scale. The central tube, called the scala media (or cochlear duct), comes to a blind end at the apex of the cochlea. On either side are the scala vestibuli and the scala tympani, which communicate with each other at the tip of the spiral. The floor of the scala media is formed by the basilar membrane (figs. 9-5C, D, 9-6). This is a complex structure whose physical properties are responsible for separating complex sounds into their different frequency components. It is about 3.5 millimeters long and is relatively narrow and stiff at the base of the spiral but broad and floppy at the apex. The vibrations in the fluid cause traveling waves to run along the membrane. To understand what is meant by a traveling wave, lay a piece of rope on the ground and whip one end up and down; a wave will run along the rope to its other end. This is analogous to what happens with the basilar membrane, but how far the wave travels depends on its frequency. High-frequency sounds run well where the membrane is stiff but die out as it becomes floppier toward the tip of the cochlea. The lower the frequency of a sound, the farther it can run along the membrane. As it travels, the wave increases to a peak then abruptly collapses as the propagation fails, so with increasing frequency the peak occurs farther and farther along the basilar membrane. The frequency of a harmonic can therefore be identified by the position of the peak on the membrane. This principle is called tonotopy (*topos* is the Greek word for "place") and has an important influence on the architecture of the auditory pathways linking the cochlea to the brain.

The vibrations of the basilar membrane are detected by the organ of Corti, a long, narrow structure composed of sensory cells (hair cells) and nerve endings that runs along its surface within the scala media (fig. 9-6B). It is named after the microscopist Marchese Corti, who first described its structure in 1851. The flask-shaped hair cells are held upright by specialized support cells (fig. 9-7A). Hair cells are so named because on their upper surface they have three rows of hairlike projections (stereocilia) that project into the fluid of the scala media (figs. 9-6, 9-9A). These lie in contact with a gelatinous flap called the tectorial membrane that cantilevers out from the bony core of the cochlear spiral. When the basilar membrane vibrates, the hair cells move relative to the tectorial membrane and the stereocilia are deflected from side to side.

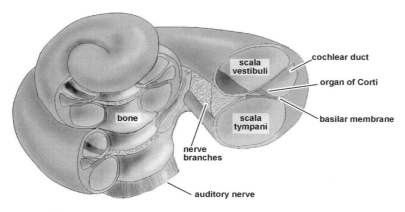

A Cochlea

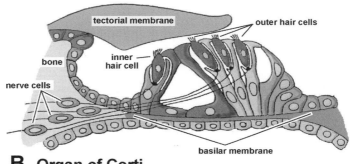

B Organ of Corti

Figure 9-6.   A. The cochlea is a spiral made up of three parallel tubes running around a core of bone that contains the auditory nerve. The three tubes are the scala vestibuli and scala tympani and the cochlear duct (scala media) lying in between. The cells that detect the vibrations caused by sound are found in the organ of Corti, which sits on the basilar membrane forming the floor of the cochlear duct. B. The organ of Corti contains four rows of hair cells, which detect vibrations. When the basilar membrane moves up and down, the "hairs" on the tips of these cells are pushed from side to side by a gelatinous flap called the tectorial (roof) membrane. The hair cells send signals to nerve cells, which carry information to the brain.

The three rows of stereocilia on each hair cell are not the same height. The row nearest the edge of the cell is tallest, the middle row is shorter, and the inner row, shorter still. The tips of adjacent stereocilia in the three rows are connected by fine strands called tip links. When the stereocilia bend in the direction of the tallest row, the distance between the tips increases and the tip links are stretched. When they bend in the opposite direction, the tip links relax. The increase in tension is transmitted to the membrane of the stereocilia, where it causes minute pores or channels in the membrane to open. This allows potassium ions to flow into the hair cells from the fluid in the scala media. As a result, an electrical potential is generated within the hair cell that causes it to release a neurotransmitter (glutamate) to branches of nerve cells that lie in the core of the cochlear spiral. As a result, a series of electrical impulses run along their axons and into the central nervous system. The hair cells are phenomenally sensitive to vibration, and at the threshold for hearing, the deflection of the stereocilia is no greater than the diameter of a single atom.

There are four rows of hair cells, a single inner row that lies closest to the central core of the cochlea, and three outer rows (figs. 9-6, 9-9A). These are ranged on either side of a tunnel that passes along the length of the organ of Corti. The inner and outer hair cells have very different functions. The inner hair cells have abundant connections with nerve cells, and despite being in the minority, they are mainly responsible for detecting the vibrations generated by sound. The outer hair cells have much sparser connections with nerve cells, and their main role is to increase the sensitivity of the organ of Corti. When the outer hair cells are excited by the movement of the basilar membrane, they respond by actively contracting (becoming shorter) as the stereocilia move in one direction, then relaxing (elongating) as they move back in the opposite direction (fig. 9-7B). The length of the cells oscillates in time with the rise and fall of the basilar membrane, and this increases the amplitude of the movement in the same way that a gymnast on a trampoline rises ever higher by jumping in phase with its bounce. The maximum height of the traveling wave is increased by about one hundred times by this mechanism (fig. 9-7C, D). This activity by outer hair cells constitutes what is known as the cochlear amplifier. The vibration it induces in the basilar membrane can cause it to operate like the diaphragm of a loudspeaker so that it can actually generate sound. These are called otoacoustic emissions and are usually too weak to be audible over ambient noise; however, in very quiet surroundings, or if the cochlea has been damaged by loud noise or disease, they may become audible. One famous and well-verified story of otoacoustic emissions concerns a man who noticed that a dog sitting next to him on a sofa appeared to be humming. On further investigation he was able to determine that the sound was coming not from the dog's throat, but from one of its ears!

Tartini Tones

The cochlea is not only sensitive to sounds that exist in the outside world, but can also give the illusion of sounds that do not actually exist. This was first described in the eighteenth century by the violinist and composer Giuseppe Tartini. An analysis of Tartini's theories on this and other matters can be found in Planchart (1960). He found that when two notes are played simultaneously, other notes may also be heard at mathematically related pitches. These are referred to as Tartini or difference tones. They are best achieved with relatively low intensity sounds of about 50–65 dB, a sound level that is comparable to the volume of conversational speech. If the two real sounds have frequencies of f_1 and f_2 (where f_2 is the higher frequency), the Tartini tones will have frequencies of $f_2 - f_1$, $f_2 + f_1$, $2f_1 - f_2$, $2f_2 - f_1$, and so on. An example can be heard in sound presentation 9-2 on the accompanying disc. This is a phenomenon well known to organ builders, who have used it for well over a century to generate what is known as the Acoustic Bass stop. The name is more than a little ironic as the Acoustic Bass stop gives the impression of a set of pipes that do not exist, but instead is an illusion created entirely within the auditory system. For example, combining C3

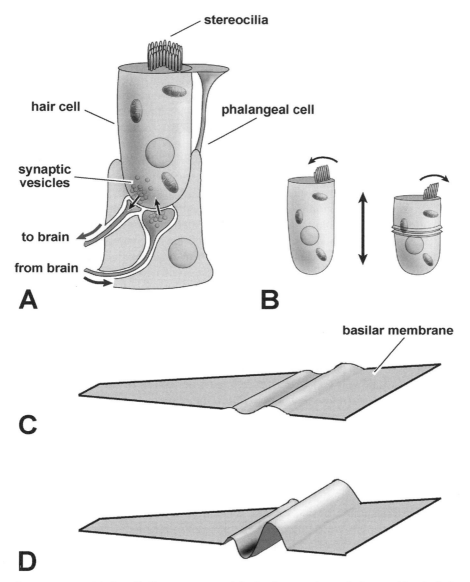

Figure 9-7.   A. A hair cell. The movement of the basilar membrane is detected by the hair cells (see fig. 9-6B). These are supported by phalangeal cells, which have a strutlike extension that helps to hold them upright. The tips of the cells carry three rows of "hairs" (or stereocilia). When these are deflected one way, the hair cells are excited, and when they are moved in the other direction, the cells are inhibited. When excited, their synaptic vesicles release a neurotransmitter that stimulates the branches of the nerve cells that carry the information to the brain. The responsiveness of the hair cells can also be controlled by signals traveling in the opposite direction, from the brain. B–D. The extreme sensitivity of the cochlea is partly due to a mechanism called the cochlear amplifier. When the outer hair cells are activated by the deflections of their stereocilia, they respond by rapidly shortening and lengthening in phase with the vibrations that excited them (B). This increases the amplitude of the traveling wave. C represents diagrammatically the amplitude of the wave in the absence of the cochlear amplifier, and D when the cochlear amplifier is active, though the difference in the amplitude of the wave is much greater in reality.

at 126 Hz, played on a four-foot-long organ pipe, with G3 at 190 Hz on a pipe that is two feet eight inches long, can be used to generate the illusion of C2 at 64 Hz (190 − 126 = 64, i.e., $f_2 − f_1$) without the need to build an eight-foot C2 pipe to produce it. In this example, the fundamentals of the notes played represent the second and third harmonics of the Tartini tone frequency and so when heard together, the three will give the impression of a single pitch, although this will be less rich than that produced by an actual eight-foot pipe. In this example, the ratio of f_2 to f_1 is 1.5, close to the optimum for producing the effect, which is about 1.2. (Further details of the use of Tartini tones in the organ can be found in Bicknell 1999 and Audsley 1965). Outside the arcane world of organ building, the role of Tartini tones in music is a relatively minor one, as they are generally rather weak, though some violinists use them to control the intonation of double-stopped notes (Rasch and Plomp 1999).

It is possible to examine the movement of the basilar membrane as a note of a particular frequency is sounded. If a pure sound of a single frequency is presented, then one peak of vibration is seen on the membrane. If two pure tones are presented, we would intuitively expect to see two peaks; however, if the frequencies of the tones strongly stimulate the same section of the organ of Corti, several additional peaks may appear, each representing the frequency of a Tartini tone. The Tartini tones are thought to originate from the outer hair cells as a consequence of changes in the elasticity of the hair bundles when the tip links flip the potassium channels between their open and closed states (Jaramillo, Markin, and Hudspeth 1993). This disturbs the otherwise linear relationship between the degree of deflection of the stereocilia and the force they generate—a force that acts to return them to the rest position. The response is therefore said to be nonlinear, and the resulting wave on the basilar membrane is called a distortion product. The nonlinear response introduces an instability into the backward and forward movements of the stereocilia, which either directly, or through the contractile mechanisms of the outer hair cells, causes the basilar membrane to vibrate at the new frequencies. This generates traveling waves that run along the basilar membrane in exactly the same way that those generated by external sounds do. They are therefore interpreted by the nervous system as sound even though they have no reality in the external world. Blocking the potassium channels eliminates the Tartini tone responses but has no effect on the vibrations generated by the two real tones used to create them. Nevertheless, the vibrations of the basilar membrane that underlie Tartini tones can sometimes give rise to real sounds in the form of otoacoustic emissions. While the Tartini tones important in music are usually at a frequency equal to $f_2 − f_1$, a strong otoacoustic emission can, with suitable equipment, be generated at a frequency of $2f_1 − f_2$. This is known as a distortion product otoacoustic emission (DPOAE). These can be used clinically to investigate the health of the inner ear (particularly the functional integrity of the outer hair cells) and are useful in patients such as infants who are unable to give a clear voluntary response.

Control of Hair Cell Activity by the Central Nervous System

Microscopic examination of the synaptic contacts at the base of the hair cells reveals that they not only send information to the brain, but also receive it. This allows the brain to exert a degree of feedback control over hair cell responsiveness (Brown 1999). The contacts (fig. 9-7A) are found mainly on the outer hair cells that lie within the sections of the organ of Corti that are responsive to mid- to high-frequency sound. The nerve cells responsible lie in a region of the brain stem called the superior olivary complex, and they effectively turn down the volume control on the cochlear amplifier. This is probably a protective mechanism to prevent damage to the hair cells by high-intensity sounds, as the nerve cells are most active when such conditions are experienced. When two sounds of different frequencies occur simultaneously, the vibrations of the basilar membrane created by one can by various means obscure those generated by the other. The feedback from the brain onto the outer hair cells can also reduce this interference by toning down the response to the louder frequency.

The superior olivary nucleus is also capable of influencing the signals carrying pitch information from the inner hair cells. It does this not by direct connections with the hair cells, but by acting on the neurons within the cochlea that receive signals from them. Because of the technical difficulties of studying such connections, much less is known about this system; however, it appears to embody two types of feedback control. One of these would have a blanket effect across a large proportion of the auditory range, while the other would be capable of the selective control of narrow frequency bands (Warr and Boche 2003). Though there is currently no direct evidence for this, such a system might help us to concentrate on sound frequencies characteristic of a particular instrument against the background of an orchestra, or on one particular voice in a room full of people. However, if it does play such a role in selective attention, this feedback is probably only part of the mechanism involved, as the most complex analysis of sound (e.g., the recognition of the harmonic structure characteristic of the sound of a particular instrument or voice) is only possible within the cortex.

PROBLEMS AFFECTING THE EAR

Hearing impairment is clearly a great worry for musicians. Most hearing problems originate from the ear and not from the processing of sound by the nervous system. There are two major categories of hearing loss—conductive deafness and nerve deafness. Conductive deafness occurs as a result of damage to or changes in the properties of the eardrum or ear ossicles. The small moving parts in the middle ear are extremely vulnerable and may be affected by many diseases or sources of physical damage. Though several remarkable surgical procedures are now available to treat some of these conditions and offer an improvement, they generally cannot completely restore the level of hearing to its original state. By contrast, neural deafness is caused by damage to the hair cells, the auditory nerve, or the auditory pathways in the brain and is irreversible.

Problems Affecting the Eardrum

Anything that interferes with the vibration of the tympanic membrane will reduce the keenness of hearing. Getting water in the ear after swimming is an example that most of us are familiar with. This quickly resolves itself as the water evaporates, but a buildup of earwax can cause similar symptoms. The wax is secreted by glands in the external ear canal. Its purpose is to protect the skin lining the canal from moisture and to discourage fungal or bacterial growth. The idea that because of its bitter taste (take my word for it!) this wax acts as a deterrent to insect invasion of the ear canal is still perpetuated in some medical textbooks, but there appears to be no objective evidence to back it up. The notion relies on the insect world having similar tastes to ours, and a moment's reflection will make it clear that this is often not the case. In a blocked ear, the wax may become hard, but it can be softened by putting a few drops of light vegetable oil into it for a few days before washing it out with a large syringe (without a needle!) containing warm water. The movement of the tympanic membrane and of the ear ossicles can also be impeded by mucus, which may build up inside the middle ear as a result of an ear infection (e.g., otitis media). This is most common in children, in whom it is often known as glue ear, but is sometimes experienced by adults. If the mucus cannot drain effectively through the Eustachian tube, a grommet (a small rubber tube) may be inserted through the eardrum for this purpose. The grommet ultimately drops out and the hole heals spontaneously without further treatment.

Problems Affecting the Ear Ossicles

The free movement of the ear ossicles can be impeded by abnormal bone growth in a condition known as otosclerosis. It is usually the stapes that is most affected, losing its ability to move freely in the oval window. Otosclerosis can have a genetic component and may therefore run in families, though the hearing may not be noticeably affected in all individuals who have it. It is twice as common in women than in men, and the symptoms (hearing loss sometimes accompanied by dizziness and tinnitus [see below]) may become more noticeable during pregnancy or at menopause. It is now frequently treated by surgery to replace the damaged stapes with an artificial one made of Teflon.

Drug-Induced Hearing Loss

Some commonly used prescription drugs may cause tinnitus or damage hair cells in the cochlea (leading to deafness) or vestibular system (involved in balance) of the ear. These include some classes of antibiotics (particularly, but not exclusively a group called aminoglycosides), the antimalarial drug chloroquine, some nonsteroidal anti-inflammatory drugs (including aspirin in high doses), and certain drugs used for treating fluid retention. The effects are usually dependent on the dose and length of time over which the drug is taken. Some of the symptoms of drug toxicity may be reversible (e.g., tinnitus).

Tinnitus

The word *tinnitus* literally means a ringing sound, and though this is a common symptom, the term is used to cover a wide variety of sounds (clicking, high-pitched whistling, rhythmic or intermittent roaring, etc.) that do not originate from the outside world. It is quite often associated with a hypersensitivity to sound (hyperacusis).

Though it can be a symptom of a wide variety of auditory problems including deafness, most of us would notice mild tinnituslike symptoms if we were to be placed in a soundproof room or if our perception of external sounds was reduced because the movement of the tympanic membrane or ossicles was limited by earwax, glue ear, or otosclerosis. This is because some forms of tinnitus represent real sounds that occur in the head. These may result from the flow of blood through vessels in and around the ear, spasms of the muscles of the middle ear, or movement of the jaw joint. The presence of this type of sound can sometimes be confirmed by a doctor using a stethoscope. In other circumstances, tinnitus may be an auditory illusion created by damaged hair cells (e.g., following exposure to loud noise) or by tumors in the ear or central nervous system. Because it has so many possible causes, tinnitus requires careful investigation; however, in many cases an obvious cause cannot be established. Where there is a clear organic cause this can be addressed directly. Treatment may be as simple as removing earwax or changing long-term medication. More rarely, delicate surgery on blood vessels in the ear or treatment of tumors may be required. In most cases, however, the approach taken is to help the patient cope with the symptoms. Masking the tinnitus by listening to music or by generating sound in the ear canal may be effective in reducing its annoyance. A more recent development is tinnitus retraining therapy, which encourages the brain to become used to the tinnitus to the extent that it can be ignored. This is called habituation and is an important mechanism by which the nervous system disregards much of the sensory input it receives so that it does not become overloaded with information of little significance. For example, in an office near a busy road, we quickly cease to be aware of the traffic noise when working, just as we cease to notice the contact of our clothes with the skin, though a new stimulus such as a light touch on the hand will be recognized immediately.

As tinnitus is a common condition, it is not surprising that many famous musicians (including Beethoven and Schumann) have suffered from it; however, it is perhaps most dramatically exemplified by Smetana. In the mid-1870s he became deaf, probably as a result of syphilis, and complained of a piercing whistling sound in his ears. In his autobiographical first string quartet, "From My Life," he illustrates this in the final Vivace movement by having a high E played continuously for several bars (224–230) by the first violin (fig. 9-8). Lasting as it does for only a few bars, this must rank as a remarkably restrained evocation of his symptoms (though in the preceding section, the E an octave below struggles to establish itself over a more tumultuous background). Many quartets today play the high E with such a fine sense of musicality that it loses much of its sinister nature and hardly does justice to the distress it caused Smetana. The extract from this movement, recorded specially for the accompanying disc by the Mavron Quartet, presents a more dramatic evocation of the sound that blighted the last few years of Smetana's life.

Menière's Disease

Menière's disease is caused by a swelling of the part of the ear involved in balance. This produces the symptoms of dizziness or vertigo, sometimes associated with unusual movements of the eyes, which use information from this part of the ear to

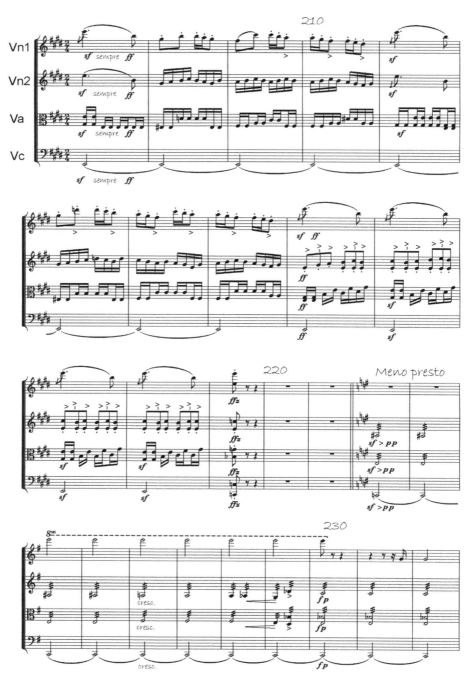

Figure 9-8. Tinnitus (a ringing, whistling, or growling noise originating within the ear) has been experienced by many composers. Smetana illustrates this musically in the final movement of his string quartet "From My Life." In the meno presto, a persistent high E over a rumbling, monotonous bass briefly (and with commendable restraint) represents what the phenomenon sounds like. The accompanying disc contains a recording of part of this movement made by the Mavron Quartet.

compensate for movement. Nausea and sweating may be experienced. Disturbances in hearing also frequently occur, including loss of sensitivity to low frequencies in the affected ear and tinnitus. The immediate cause is unknown but it can be triggered by middle ear, respiratory, or viral infections, head trauma, adverse reactions to prescription drugs, alcohol, or stress.

Age-Related Hearing Loss (Presbycusis)

As we age we tend to experience a progressive loss of hearing, starting quite young with the highest frequencies of the auditory range. If you remember the squeaks of echolocating of bats in your youth and wonder why they now appear to have fallen silent, this is the reason. Age-related hearing loss affecting less extreme parts of the range generally first becomes noticeable at around the age of fifty. By age sixty-five, approximately 25 percent of people will experience it to some degree and by seventy-five to eighty, 40–50 percent are affected. The reasons for age-related hearing loss are unclear, though there appears to be a genetic predisposition for it in some families. One suggestion is that it is the result of the accumulated effects of a lifetime's exposure to noise; however, there is no clear evidence for or against this. It is, however, probably a mistake to consider it to be a single, well-defined condition, as a whole range of problems (e.g., otosclerosis described above, exposure to loud noise) may contribute to its onset. There is no cure, though specific problems such as otosclerosis may be amenable to treatment.

Noise-Induced Hearing Loss

Perhaps of greatest relevance to musicians is the possible risk of noise-induced hearing loss. Protective mechanisms such as the stapedius reflex are effective in defending the ear against sounds only up to a certain level. When these defenses are overwhelmed, physical damage to the hair cells occurs, ultimately destroying the stereocilia and killing the hair cells (fig. 9-9). While this was once considered to be due directly to physical forces acting on the stereocilia (e.g., their forceful impact with the tectorial membrane), it now appears that its major cause is an overloading of the metabolic pathways of the hair cells. An excellent account of current thinking on the origin of noise-induced hearing loss can be found in Henderson et al. (2006). A detailed examination of the sound-abused ear reveals that the damage is not solely confined to the hair cells, but can involve the other classes of cell within the organ of Corti that help to maintain a stable environment for them. Exposure to high-intensity sound has the additional consequence of reducing the blood flow to the cochlea during the period when the hair cells are at their most active and therefore have their highest demand for oxygen and nutrients. One consequence of the active state of the hair cells is that there is a buildup of molecules called reactive oxygen species that oxidize and damage cellular components such as the lipids that form the cell membrane. This initially has a disruptive effect on the structure of the stereocilia, breaking the tip links that are necessary for their responsiveness and making them lose contact with the grooves in the tectorial membrane into which they are normally inserted. It is the outer hair

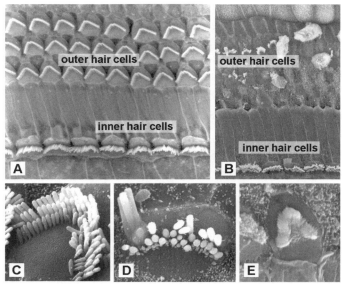

Figure 9-9. This figure shows high-magnification images of normal and damaged hair cells in the organ of Corti obtained using a scanning electron microscope. A. A view looking down onto the tips of hair cells in the normal cochlea reveals the "hairs" (stereocilia) that detect movement of the basilar membrane during hearing. Three rows of outer hair cells and one row of inner hair cells are clearly visible. B. Prolonged exposure to very loud noise or to certain drugs damages the "hairs," especially those of the outer hair cells, as shown in this photograph. This destroys the cochlear amplifier and greatly reduces hearing sensitivity. Photographs C–E show progressively more severe damage to the "hairs." In C they are only slightly distorted while in D, most have lost their tips and only a small tuft on the left appears normal. In E, all that remains of the "hairs" is a fused mass that will be totally unresponsive to sound. (Reproduced with permission from R. V. Harrison, Auditory Science Laboratory of the Hospital for Sick Children, Toronto, Canada).

cells that are most affected because their metabolism must support the energetically demanding cellular contractions that underlie the cochlear amplifier. Any impairment of their activity results in marked reduction in hearing sensitivity. The effects are at first reversible, causing what is known as a temporary threshold shift in hearing. After being at a loud concert, we may feel our hearing is muffled in the following hours or even days, and this can make speech comprehension difficult. It may also be accompanied by other symptoms such as tinnitus. If the damage is not too severe, the hair cells gradually recover. The stereocilia may return to normal and insert once more into the pits on the tectorial membrane, and hearing sensitivity is restored. However, prolonged exposure to intense noise results in a permanent threshold shift (a loss of hearing sensitivity) as a result of the death of the hair cells. Unfortunately, these never regenerate in humans, though in some animals such as birds this does occur. The outer hair cells at the basal (high frequency) end of the cochlea are the first to be affected, but ultimately the damage spreads to the other regions of the cochlea and may affect the inner hair cells as well.

The damage caused by high-intensity sound is frequency specific because the region of the basilar membrane showing the greatest amplitude of vibration is dependent on frequency. Before the advent of occupational health legislation that made ear protection mandatory, sound-induced deafness was a major hazard among industrial workers. It was often known as "boilermaker's deafness" and was particularly serious if it affected the frequency range most used in speech (500–4,000 Hz). Noise-induced hearing loss is frequently first observed between 3,000 and 6,000 Hz. This loss at the upper end of the main speech range makes consonants difficult to distinguish. Though industrially induced hearing loss is now rarely seen in the West, the rise of the personal stereo has caused a new wave of noise-induced deafness. Because music usually covers most of the audible frequency range, the effects are much less selective than those of industrial deafness. In addition, the gradual onset of deafness may go undetected, and the natural reaction is to progressively increase the volume in the headset to compensate for it, which ultimately exacerbates the problem.

Music-induced deafness among rock musicians, who use electrical amplification to very high levels (often peaking at over 120 dB), is unsurprising, though they may be more able to take preventive action by moving about the stage (e.g., to position themselves out of the main line of fire of the speakers), and be quite content to wear visible ear protection. A general awareness that classical musicians (particularly those working in orchestras) may also be exposed to damaging levels of sound has been slower to gain acceptance, though it is unlikely to come as a surprise to the musicians themselves! It is not only the absolute intensity of ambient noise that needs to be taken into consideration, but also how efficiently different frequencies are transmitted by the ear canal, that is, its resonance characteristics. The intrinsic resonance of the ear canal lies between 2 and 4 kHz, with a peak at around 3 kHz. The enhancement of these frequencies due to ear canal resonance ranges from less than 10 dB to nearly 30 dB. This can result in a peak in intensity within the ear at around 3 kHz even though the intensity envelope of the sound, as measured externally, is actually falling at this frequency (Henoch and Chesky 1999). Audiograms of patients with noise-induced hearing loss generally first show a reduction in sensitivity in this region. The degree to which sound exposure for a particular musical note is increased by ear canal resonance varies from instrument to instrument, as it depends not only on the intensity of the fundamental frequency, but also on the strength of the harmonics. For example, the intensity spectrum for both G4 (392 Hz) on the trumpet and G5 (783 Hz) on the oboe peak at about 3–3.5 kHz, as G7 at 3,136 Hz is a strongly projected harmonic of these notes in each case.

A useful review of current literature on hearing loss in musicians, providing a critical assessment of the problems that exist with much of this literature, can be found in Behar, Wong, and Kunov (2006). Though many studies have sought evidence for music-related hearing loss in classical musicians (Sataloff 1991; Palin 1994), no clear picture has so far emerged. There are a number of possible reasons for this. First, the numbers of musicians examined in each study are often small, and different studies use different methodologies, making it hard to pool their data. In order to correlate the quality of hearing with the levels of noise players experience during performance, it is first necessary to measure the intensity of the sound the orchestra creates. However, there has been no attempt to standardize the points at which sound intensity is measured on the stage in different studies, nor the type or volume of music being performed when the measurements are taken. The structure of the concert hall or recital room will also be a significant factor. Ambient sound levels are higher if the player is sitting close to a wall, which reflects the sound. Measurements of hearing sensitivity in players are also not necessarily made at the same frequencies by different investigators. Further difficulties arise when it comes to interpreting the results obtained. Two players of the same instrument and of similar age, sitting side by side in the orchestra, may have quite different hearing thresholds, but it is difficult to determine whether this is due to differences in their professional experience or to other factors. There are many additional considerations that need to be taken into account in the analysis. For example, unless the same group of musicians is tested at regular intervals, it is necessary to find a control population for comparison, but who should be used? Should it be those with the best hearing found within a population, that is, those who have always lived in a quiet environment, or should the control group come from a noisier urban environment more typical of that inhabited by the musicians? Then, what level of loss should be regarded as indicative of impairment? For some clinicians, at least, an increase in threshold of 20 dB at a given frequency is regarded as clinically significant. This represents a tenfold loss of sensitivity, and though this may seem a major impairment, it must be viewed in the context of the extreme sensitivity of the auditory system. When measuring hearing thresholds, care must also be taken to allow some time to elapse (usually forty minutes to one hour) after exposure to significant noise levels before any auditory tests are carried out, as, if the noise is of sufficient intensity, it may cause a temporary threshold shift. This lasts longer with increasing sound intensity or length of exposure. As a consequence of these and other sources of variability, similar results from different studies have been used to justify quite opposite conclusions. Nonetheless, the evidence that sound levels experienced during playing can, over time, cause damage to hearing is accumulating. Sound intensities above 90 dB may by generated within the orchestra over a significant proportion of playing time for certain pieces, and peak intensities in excess of 110 dB are sometimes experienced. Off the concert platform, playing in small, bare practice rooms with a reverberant acoustic may be flattering to the tone but will also maximize the intensity of the sound. In many cases, the greatest sound intensity experienced by the musician comes from his or her own instrument. Brass and upper woodwind players seem to produce the highest sound levels. In the case of trumpet players, the increase in bore size of many modern instruments is actually designed to raise the volume of sound produced. Interestingly, violinists often show an asymmetry in the hearing thresholds between the two ears, the left ear being less sensitive, presumably because its greater proximity to the belly of the instrument means that it experiences greater sound intensities.

Orchestras are now beginning to take sound exposure to their members seriously. The Association of British Orchestras recently initiated a project entitled "A Sound Ear" to look into the question. This has been made particularly timely by legislation from the European Union (directive 86/188) governing noise in the workplace, which seeks to reduce exposure levels to a time-weighted average of 87 dB over a week of five days of eight hours each, while the National Institute for Occupational Safety and Health (U.S.) guidelines set the acceptable level at 85 dB. Every 3 dB increase in sound intensity represents a doubling of the energy it contains and a halving of the acceptable exposure time. So taking 87 dB as the starting value, exposure at 90 dB should be limited to four hours, at 93 dB to two hours, and so on. Consequently, if you are attending a rock concert where the sound reaches 110 dB, you have less than two minutes before you exceed the recommended exposure time!

How acceptable levels can be maintained in orchestras performing with only acoustic instruments is less clear, both to the music industry and the legislators. A further related EU directive (2003/10/EC) states that "the particular characteristics of the music and entertainment sectors require practical guidance for the effective application of the provisions laid down by this directive" and goes on to say that there will be a transitional period to work this out. One way in which individual players (and indeed concertgoers) can reduce the intensity of sound they perceive is to use earplugs. The crude variety that simply block the external ear canal do not offer a practical solution because they do not reduce all frequencies to the same extent. High frequencies are blocked most effectively, so the sound reaching the cochlea appears muffled and distorted and does not accurately represent the ambient sound. This is obviously not satisfactory in a musical context. Earplugs specially tailored for the needs of musicians have been designed to reduce most frequencies in the audible spectrum to the same degree, so wearing them is equivalent to turning down the volume on a stereo. The best of the earplugs have to be custom-made to fit the ear canal of the individual wearer and so they are not cheap. On the other hand, given the importance of protecting the ears for musicians, this is probably a price worth paying. They can be designed to reduce the sound intensity to differing degrees up to about 25 dB. In some instruments such as the clarinet, there is significant conduction of sound from the instrument to the ear through the bone of the skull due to the contact between the teeth and the mouthpiece. In such circumstances, the wearing of earplugs may lead the player to experience a buzzing noise due to bone conduction by this route, which may interfere with their perception of the tone of the instrument (Hart et al. 1987).

The intensity of sound on the stage or in the pit obviously depends to some extent on the proximity of other instruments, particularly the brass. One measure used to reduce sound exposure to other players is to deploy screens behind the chair to create a sound shadow. These are in use by some orchestras; however, they are only effective if they are sufficiently close to the head (about 15–20 centimeters) and lose their efficacy if, for example, the player sits forward in the seat (Wright Reid 1999). Stage layout can also be used to shield players from the sound of others. Moving players farther apart will help, as does raising loud instruments like the brass above the rank of seats in front, though the difference in height required to make a significant difference (0.5–1.0 meters) may not always be achievable. In the pit, of course, the situation is worse as players are generally closer together, all on the same level and in an enclosed space whose walls may reflect the sound. Clearly varying the repertoire so that particularly loud pieces are mixed with quieter ones in performance and rehearsal also helps to avoid discomfort among players. In addition, the conductor needs to be aware of the state of his or her hearing. If an older conductor has a decreased sensitivity to high frequencies and is unaware of it, he or she may ask for more from instruments playing in this range. The result is not only potentially damaging for the hearing of the players, but will of course not produce for the audience the balance of sound being sought by the conductor.

Beethoven's Deafness

The most celebrated case of deafness in musical history is, of course, that of Beethoven. Remarkably, his body not only underwent a postmortem, but a copy of the report is still in existence. In a rather macabre twist, although his ear ossicles and the region of the skull containing the inner ear were retained for further examination, they were later "lost or stolen"! The autopsy clearly supports his own accounts of serious gastrointestinal problems including chronic diarrhea, vomiting, colic, and jaundice. The immediate cause of his death appears to have been liver failure. This may have been associated with inflammatory bowel disease, a condition that could explain many of his other symptoms. The question of the origin of Beethoven's deafness is rather less clear. He describes its onset as being accompanied by continual whistling and buzzing (i.e., tinnitus) and of first losing the ability to hear high frequencies. The tinnitus started in about 1796 at the age of twenty-six, and he had lost much of his hearing by 1801. In cases of major historical figures, there is always a tendency to read too much into the little contemporary information still in existence. From a musical standpoint, it is the distressing nature of the symptoms that is most significant. One conservative suggestion is that the deterioration in his hearing may have been a combination of nerve deafness and otosclerosis probably unrelated to his other health problems (Kubba and Young 1996).

HEARING AND THE BRAIN

How the Nervous System Codes Sound

The nerve cells that send auditory signals to the brain lie in the bony core of the cochlea. Like most other nerve cells, these carry information as pulses of electrical activity called action potentials. This is a digital signaling system and so it is very robust and resistant to degradation as it transmits information through numerous relay stations, all the way up to the cortex. Two major strategies are used by the auditory system to code sound frequency. The first is action potential frequency, and the second is tonotopy (i.e., the relative position of the lines carrying signals representing different frequencies). Even under the most favorable circumstances, action potentials cannot be generated at frequencies above about 1,000 Hz and so they cannot code directly the sound frequency across much of the auditory range. On the other hand, the tonotopic map on the basilar membrane is unable to distinguish between sounds with frequencies at the lower end of the range. The two systems are therefore complementary. For the lower octaves of the auditory range, action potential frequency in single nerve cells

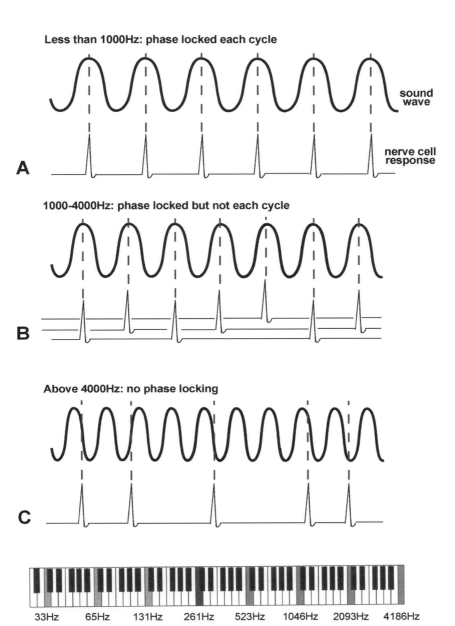

Figure 9-10. This figure shows two ways in which nerve cells of the auditory system code sound frequency. A. At low frequencies, single nerve cells can accurately convey frequency information. Each nerve cell can fire a digital signal (an action potential) at the same point on each cycle of the sound wave; that is, the signal is phase-locked. B. From 1,000 to 4,000 Hz, single nerve cells cannot fire action potentials fast enough to keep up; however, they still fire phase-locked potentials on some cycles. By pooling the information from many nerve cells supplying the same region of the basilar membrane, the brain can still determine the pitch of the sound from the combined action potential frequency. C. Above 4,000 Hz, the nerve cells still fire occasional action potentials, but these are no longer phase-locked. Under these circumstances, the sound frequency can only be determined by knowing the region of the basilar membrane from which the signal originates (i.e., by using the principle of tonotopy).

matches sound frequency (fig. 9-10A), as long as each nerve cell fires an action potential in phase with the sound pressure oscillation. These phase-locked action potentials
are evenly spaced in time, and the sound frequency is a function of the time interval
between them. The upper theoretical limit for this type of signaling represents fundamental frequencies of notes of around C6 (two octaves above middle C). However,
even for lower notes, we need information about their harmonic structure in order to
appreciate the timbre of the sound, which gives each instrument or voice its distinctive character. Between about 1,000 Hz and 4,000 Hz, it is still possible to use action
potential frequency as an indicator of the pitch of the fundamental if information from
many nerve cells that are stimulated by the same region of the basilar membrane is
pooled. Each nerve cell need not fire an action potential for every oscillation, but as
long as they are all phase-locked to the same place on the waveform, their collective
output can still be used to determine frequency directly (fig. 9-10B). Above 4 kHz, the
nerve cells lose their ability to phase-lock and instead fire randomly when stimulated
(fig. 9-10C). In this range, frequency can only be coded by tonotopy—the position
on the basilar membrane from which the signal is coming. It is therefore vital that
this order is retained within the bundle of axons that carry the signal to the brain and
that it is maintained through the many relay stations on the way. How this is ensured
is unknown, but the axon bundle forms a ribbon with the lowest-frequency fibers at
one edge and highest-frequency fibers at the other. Though it is possible to detect frequency tuning above 5 kHz in nerve cells in various parts of the auditory system, we
cannot subjectively attribute pitch to the sound, so this change from frequency coding
to tonotopy appears to have important perceptual consequences. The highest note on
the piano (C8 at 4,186 Hz) is close to this boundary where tonotopy takes over (fig.
9-2). In addition to frequency, the intensity of the sound must also be conveyed to
the brain. This is encoded both by the number of action potentials generated and the
number of nerve cells activated, that is, the total number of action potentials generated
in a particular frequency channel of the auditory pathway.

The auditory information from the cochlea runs to the brain along the vestibulocochlear nerve (the eighth cranial nerve) and passes through many relays within the
brain stem on the way to the auditory cortex (fig. 9-11). As it is passed from one to
another, the way in which the sound is coded changes. One of these relay stations is
the superior olivary nucleus, which we have encountered before when discussing its
role in the feedback control of hair cell activity. It is also involved in the signal processing that makes it possible to identify the position of a sound source in space (see
below). Another important relay station lies in the roof of the midbrain (the inferior
colliculus). Here there is a map of auditory space that is linked to a similar map of
visual space in a nearby region (the superior colliculus). When we suddenly become
aware of a new sound, we may turn quickly toward it to look to the place from which
it appears to be coming. This is a hardwired reflex response that is controlled by
these midbrain auditory centers. The maximum frequency of the action potentials in
individual nerve cells is less in the inferior colliculus and cortex than in nerve cells
that leave the cochlea, so even coding for relatively low sound frequencies becomes
tonotopic at these upper levels (Fujioka et al. 2003).

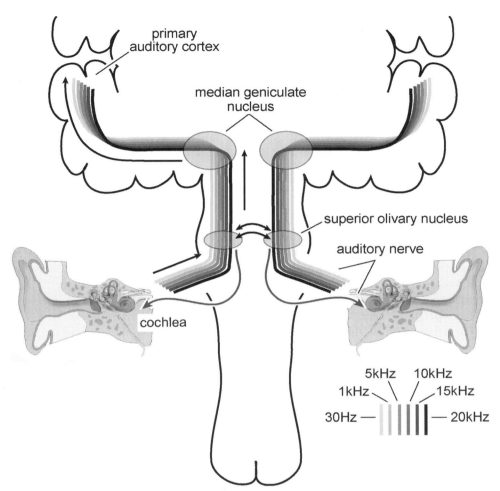

Figure 9-11. The pathway by which information from the cochlea is carried to the auditory cortex. The different shaded lines represent nerve fibers coding different sound frequencies. The tonotopic order of these lines must be preserved throughout the entire pathway if the auditory cortex is to decipher the frequency carried by each. By comparing the information reaching the two ears, nerve cells in the superior olivary nucleus determine the direction from which a sound is coming. With this information the inferior colliculi can create a map of the soundscape. The superior olivary nucleus also feeds back onto the outer hair cells to control the sensitivity of the cochlear amplifier.

Pitch and Missing Fundamentals

When presented with a complex sound, whether derived from a single instrument, a number of instruments playing a chord, or from something more mundane like a car engine, we can usually attribute to it a single pitch. This impression is created by an analysis of the harmonic structure of the sound by the brain, and the pitch attributed to the sound is generally that of its fundamental frequency. With practice it is possible to resolve some of the harmonics separately, but overriding the pitch perception mechanism requires an effort of will and is a skill that must be consciously developed by musicians. Combining sound from different sources to create the impression of a single pitch is important in pipe organs. A given note can be generated by an open pipe or by a stopped pipe (one whose open end is blocked) of half the length. For reasons of cost and design, using shorter pipes is often more convenient, especially for low stops. One problem with stopped pipes is that the sound generated contains only the odd harmonics of the fundamental; the even ones are missing. As a result, the Tartini tone generated by the odd harmonics has the pitch of the second harmonic (i.e., an octave above the fundamental). However, if an open pipe with a pitch an octave higher is played simultaneously, it provides not only the missing harmonics but also Tartini tones, which support the fundamental frequency, so that together the two stops simulate an open pipe at the same pitch as the stopped one.

The mental process that allows us to attribute pitch to a complex sound can sometimes be fooled into creating the sensation of a fundamental frequency that is not actually present in the sound spectrum—the so-called missing fundamental illusion. For example, if a series of pure tones at 300, 400, 500, 600, and 700 Hz are presented simultaneously, the perceived pitch is 100 Hz. This is logical, as these frequencies are equivalent to the lower partials (excluding the second harmonic at 200 Hz) of a note at 100 Hz (sound presentation 9-3A). The perceived pitch is most strongly influenced by frequencies that fall into what is known as the dominance region of our hearing range where the ear is most sensitive, that is, between about 500 and 2,000 Hz (C5–C7). At higher frequencies the missing fundamental illusion fails. When a series of tones at 1,000, 2,000, 3,000, 4,000, 5,000, and 6,000 Hz are presented together, the combined pitch is perceived as 1,000 Hz, but if the lowest two harmonics are dropped, the pitch becomes dominated by that of the lowest remaining tone at 3,000 Hz (sound presentation 9-3B).

So what is the mechanism of the missing fundamental illusion? If we return to the example of the pure tones presented at 300, 400, 500, 600, and 700 Hz, one way in which the pitch of 100 Hz could be derived by the nervous system would be from the presence of the regular periodicity generated in the complex waveform produced when these frequencies are combined, as this exhibits regular fluctuations at 10-millisecond intervals. This is the cycle interval (or period) of the 100 Hz missing fundamental. We have seen already that the nervous system can code frequency information by summing activity in different nerve cells all stimulated by the same part of the cochlea. An extension of this type of analysis could generate the perceived frequency here (Yost 2000). However, this is not the whole story. If we now consider the series 850, 1,050, 1,250, 1,450, and 1,650 Hz, this has a periodicity of 200 Hz even though all of the notes are also high harmonics of 50 Hz. The perceived pitch appears close to, but not exactly

200 Hz (sound presentation 9-3C). Instead it lies at 208.3 Hz, which represents the fundamental pitch whose harmonics would most closely match the tones presented; in other words, it represents a "best fit" solution. Other studies, however, have cast doubt on a mechanism of pitch perception based purely on periodicity. If, instead of a small number of pure tones, the sound presented has many intermediate frequencies of varying intensity across the same range, but which tend to be of greatest amplitude at 500, 750, 1,000, 1,250, 1,500, and 1,750 Hz, the periodicity of the combined waveform will be completely lost, yet the perceived pitch remains at 250 Hz (Yost 2000).

In view of what has been said so far about the role of tonotopy in coding the frequency of a pure sound, it is perhaps surprising that recent studies have suggested that it can contribute to the perception of pitch (Penagos, Melcher, and Oxenham 2004). It appears to be particularly significant for the low-frequency components of complex sound because, as the higher harmonics become closer and closer together, the corresponding peaks of the traveling waves on the basilar membrane cannot be clearly distinguished from one another. As the individual waves interfere, the resulting complex does show a periodicity related to the fundamental frequency, though in itself this does not appear to make a major contribution to pitch recognition. The origin of pitch perception is clearly an area that requires further investigation. However it is achieved, the perception of pitch by the brain requires a sophisticated mechanism for pattern recognition. For notes of low pitch, the illusion of the missing fundamental can be created with as little as two pure tones representing its harmonics. It can even be achieved when the two tones are presented to different ears. This demonstrates unequivocally that the illusion is created not in the ear, but in the central nervous system (Rasch and Plomp 1999).

The obvious question that arises from our consideration of pitch is what is the significance for hearing in general, and music in particular, of the way in which complex sounds are analyzed by the brain? If each sound frequency was treated separately by the brain, the soundscape would be incredibly complex and difficult to interpret. The ability to attribute a single pitch (and therefore source) to harmonically related clusters of frequencies greatly simplifies the auditory world and allows us to interpret it in a logical way. The relative strengths of the harmonics in complex sounds gives them a distinctive timbre, which further helps us to identify their source. From a musical point of view, a group of instruments playing in an ensemble can present an impression of a sound of a single pitch when they contribute to a chord (albeit colored by the particular harmonics they contribute). However, the flexibility of the analysis carried out by the nervous system allows this to be realized without prejudicing our ability at other times to follow several melodic lines created simultaneously by the same instruments. In addition, the illusion of the missing fundamental is vitally important in a number of circumstances. As with difference tones, the devious minds of organ builders have again found that it can contribute to the Acoustic Bass stop. Indeed, for some notes in this stop, a low difference tone may also represent a missing fundamental and so the cochlear and the mental illusion reinforce one another. However, the missing fundamental illusion has a much broader significance for instruments with a low frequency range in their register. A reexamination of figure 9-2 will remind you that the threshold for hearing varies considerably with frequency. As sound frequency descends from 100 to 30 Hz, this rises from about 40 to 80 dB. As this frequency range represents the bottom two octaves of the piano (A0–G2), we are not dealing with unfamiliar territory. For these notes, eliminating the fundamental frequency and the next couple of harmonics makes almost no difference to the perceived pitch or to the timbre. The implication is that the perception of pitch in this range is almost entirely dependent on the missing fundamental illusion, particularly if the notes are not loud. It also explains why the acoustic bass can work so well on the organ. The lowest notes on the organ descend even farther than those of the piano. A thirty-two-foot open pipe produces a fundamental frequency of only 16 Hz, which is actually below the threshold for complex sounds, lying as it does at around 30 Hz for human hearing (Pressnitzer, Patterson, and Krumbholz 2001). In the small number of acoustic organs that have this stop, the bottom few notes on the thirty-two-foot rank may actually all play the same pipe (Bicknell 1999)! This gives a suitably gratifying rumble of subjectively indeterminate pitch, as the harmonic structure of the notes generated by the wooden pipes in this rank is weak. The perceived pitch can then be dictated by other stops representing the upper harmonics for the required notes. The missing fundamental illusion is also important in an orchestral context. The average spectral peak of the sound produced by the orchestra lies at about 500 Hz (C5), from which it rapidly declines. For instrumental or vocal soloists, and indeed for solo passages from orchestral players, the missing fundamental illusion will make a significant contribution to our ability to follow their melodic line against a loud orchestral accompaniment.

At the lowest end of the range of the pipe organ, the appreciation of sound at or below the auditory range may be accentuated by the effects of vibration on sensory endings throughout the body and not just in the ear. When of reasonable large amplitude, the low-frequency vibrations generated within the organ will be conducted through the walls and floor of the building as well as through the air. These can be detected by vibration sensors in the skin and joints, or even those associated with structures inside the chest or abdomen. Obviously such sensations can really only be experienced in a live venue such as a church or concert hall and are hard to reproduce in recording, no matter how tolerant the neighbors may be!

Analysis of Sound by the Brain

The auditory pathways that originate in the cochlea finally terminate in the region of the forebrain called the primary auditory cortex. This lies in the temporal lobe and forms the central two-thirds of a ridge on its upper surface known as Heschl's gyrus (fig. 9-12). Within the primary auditory cortex, the frequency of sound is mapped in an orderly tonotopic fashion. From here this raw auditory information is sent out into a belt of secondary auditory cortex that includes the region known as the planum temporale, which lies behind and above Heschl's gyrus. It has been proposed that information on pitch and timing of sound is processed here before being distributed to other areas of the temporal and frontal lobes for higher-level analysis (Griffiths 2001; Griffiths and Warren 2002). The processing of different aspects of auditory information is modular. Analysis of the temporal aspects of sound, such as meter and rhythm, and melodic aspects involving pitch contour, phrasing, and harmony are to a

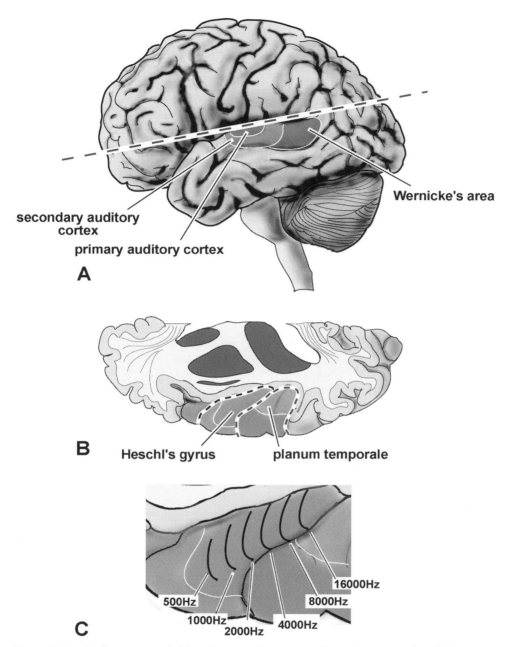

Figure 9-12.   Auditory cortex. A. The primary auditory cortex lies on the upper edge of the temporal lobe. This is surrounded by the secondary auditory cortex, where higher-level auditory processing takes place. One region of the secondary auditory cortex is Wernicke's area (left hemisphere
only), which is involved in language processing. B. A horizontal section through the brain along the
plane marked by the dashed line in A. This reveals more of the upper surface of the temporal lobe,
which is obscured by the overhanging regions of the frontal and parietal cortices. The primary
auditory cortex takes up much of a region known as Heschl's gyrus. Behind this lies the planum
temporale of which Wernicke's area forms a part. C. This shows a schematic representation of the
sound frequency maps in the primary auditory cortex; however, it is now thought that the primary
and secondary auditory cortices may contain several distinct maps of this type.

considerable degree carried out in different places. This can be dramatically revealed following damage to discrete areas of the cortex. For example, a patient may be able to discriminate between different tones in simple tests, yet not be able to distinguish tonal and atonal music. The principle of modular processing of different parameters of sensory information is well established in other systems. In vision, for example, color, movement, and form are processed in different areas of the cortex.

The primary auditory cortex, like the cortex in general, is a thin sheet of gray matter made up of an array of columns that run vertically through the sheet. Within each column the nerve cells respond to the same type of information. In many regions of the primary auditory cortex, each column responds to a particular frequency. A commonly presented but rather simplistic view of its organization is that the columns are arranged in an orderly fashion to form a single tonotopic frequency map, with those toward the anterior and lateral edge responding to low frequencies and those lying more posteriorly and medially, to high frequencies (fig. 9-12C). In fact there appear to be several such maps (perhaps as many as seven) within the primary and adjacent secondary areas of the auditory cortex (Kaas, Hackett, and Tramo 1999; Talavage et al. 2004). Information on the loudness of the sound is also coded here, as some of the nerve cells respond best to their preferred frequency when it is at a particular intensity. In addition, some rows of columns are excited most strongly by sound that comes from both ears, while others respond best to sound from one ear and are inhibited when it comes from both (Schreiner and Winer 2007). There has been considerable debate as to whether the primary auditory cortex responds predominantly to individual sound frequencies or to the overall pitch of complex sounds, or indeed both (Pierce 1999). Studies that record the electrical activity of single neurons often suggest that primary auditory maps are based on frequency, whereas those that monitor the simultaneous activity of many neurons suggest that these assemblies code for pitch. However, it has recently been demonstrated that some auditory neurons respond not only to a pure tone of a given frequency but also to a harmonic series that represents the same frequency as a missing fundamental. They do not, however, respond to the individual pure tones that make up such a series (Bendor and Wang 2005) and so they can be regarded as being pitch sensitive. Evidence is beginning to emerge that while the tonotopic maps in the primary auditory cortex are based on frequency, neurons that respond to pitch are present in the adjacent areas of the secondary cortex that lie more anteriorly or laterally on the upper surface of the temporal lobe (Bendor and Wang 2005, 2006; Penagos, Melcher, and Oxenham 2004).

Neurons in the primary auditory cortex carry information not only on frequency but also on the temporal aspects of the sound. This is processed in the secondary auditory cortex and elsewhere in the brain to provide information on rhythm and meter (the pattern of stresses in a rhythmic beat that allows us to distinguish a waltz from a march). Both the left and right primary auditory cortices respond to musical sounds, but while there appears to be a right-sided bias for frequency information, the temporal component is more bilaterally represented (Evers et al. 1999). Indeed, some studies even suggest slightly greater activity on the left side for this type of information (Jamison et al. 2006), though, like many aspects of the analysis of auditory processing, this remains a matter of debate (Zatorre, Chen, and Penhune 2007).

The development of modern imaging techniques that enables us to measure various aspects of neuronal activity in the intact living brain has led to a proliferation of studies into how musical sound and language are analyzed; however, many aspects of this remain highly controversial. This stems partly from the difficulty of designing experiments that effectively isolate particular parameters of musical sound. For example, without rhythm, a melody loses much of its character to become simply a series of intervals, and this may not be analyzed in the same way or in the same region of the brain as an intact melody. Rhythm is easier to isolate in the absence of pitch or melody, but is closely linked to meter, which may be seen as a higher-order property of rhythm analysis, interpreted by a different network. Furthermore, though the new technology provides unprecedented opportunities, the complexity of the brain circuitry makes sensible interpretation of data very challenging. A single region may be involved in a range of tasks, and establishing the common denominator can be extremely difficult. We have seen from the previous chapter the many other problems that beset the unwary when carrying out such studies, but these methods nonetheless offer unprecedented opportunities for studying this area.

One theory of the way that auditory processing is carried out in the cortex postulates that this is done along two processing streams. One reason for this notion is that a simple way of explaining how the visual system operates is based on a similar idea, which suggests that there is a ventral stream concerned with processing information about object identity (what) and a dorsal stream concerned with object position (where). The first auditory stream is said to run anteriorly along the upper and lateral surfaces of the temporal lobe, through the secondary auditory regions including the planum polare, which lies toward the anterior end of the lobe (fig. 9-13A). This stream is also said to encompass some areas in the ventral regions of the frontal lobes. It is proposed that, like the ventral stream in the visual system, this is concerned with identity (what). As the equivalent visual stream also extends into the temporal lobe, this theory has the advantage of providing a potential mechanism for bringing together the visual and auditory aspects of object recognition. The proposed second stream runs dorsally and medially through the parietal lobe and into the dorsal regions of the frontal lobe. Here the analogy with the "where" stream of the visual system is rather less helpful. The most obvious role of this stream is to link auditory and motor activity, and it appears to underpin rhythm perception (fig. 9-13B). It has been suggested that the planum temporale may form a central node for the distribution of information along the two streams. One hypothesis is that by matching the harmonic structure and temporal patterning of incoming complex sounds with previously remembered templates, the planum temporale can then distribute the information appropriately to other cortical areas for higher-level processing (Griffiths and Warren 2002). In this regard, it is interesting to note that in European musicians the planum temporale has been shown to be more active when hearing culturally familiar (Western) music than culturally unfamiliar (Chinese) music (Nan et al. 2008). On the left side of the brain, the planum temporale includes Wernicke's area, which is crucial for linguistic comprehension, and it has a strong projection to a region in the left frontal lobe called Broca's area, which is associated with verbal fluency and intonation. As we will see, Broca's area is also active when the brain is analyzing music.

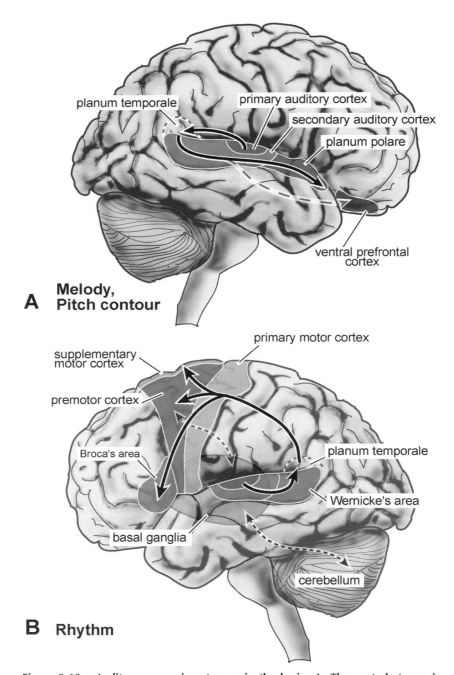

Figure 9-13. Auditory processing streams in the brain. A. The ventral stream is thought to process pitch contour, melody, and timbre. Auditory information runs from the primary auditory cortex to the planum temporale, then along the upper surface of the temporal lobe to the planum polare. A tributary of this stream runs into the prefrontal lobes and may be concerned with melodic memory, among other things. B. The dorsal stream is strongly implicated in processing rhythm. This recruits the motor network of the brain, including areas of the cortex involved in movement control as well as the basal ganglia and cerebellum.

The recognition of melody is based on the identification of pitch changes over time. There is accumulating evidence that this involves the posterior regions of the secondary auditory cortex, including the planum temporale (Patterson et al. 2002; Liegeois-Chauvel et al. 1998; Peretz and Zatorre 2005). As the analysis extends to the perception of melody, activity appears to spread along the superior temporal gyrus to the planum polare (fig. 9-13A). This therefore suggests a hierarchical sequence of processing along the ventral stream. Several distinct processes may be involved. Determination of the overall contour of the melody (disregarding interval size), may use a mechanism that would also be useful for analyzing speech inflection. Musical analysis would also require matching pitch relations regardless of absolute frequency (i.e., recognizing the similarities between transposed melodies) or key violations of individual notes in the sequence. Most of the tasks used to obtain these results involve memory to compare whether two presented melodies are the same or different. As a result, regions of the brain implicated in associative and working memory are also implicated, for example, the hippocampus (temporal lobes) and inferior frontal lobes (Peretz and Zatorre 2005; Watanabe, Yagishita, and Kikyo 2008). Given that timbre is likely to be a significant component in sound source recognition, one might expect that it would also be processed in the ventral processing stream. Cortical responses related to timbre have so far received relatively little attention, but both its perception and its mental imaging lead to activity in and around the superior temporal gyrus and on the border between Heschl's gyrus and the planum temporale (Halpern et al. 2004; Menon et al. 2002). Attending to harmonic discrepancies activates similar regions on the ventral stream, down into the planum polare (particularly in the left temporal lobe) in addition to the frontal cortex in the region of Broca's area and its equivalent on the right side (Passynkova, Sander, and Scheich 2005; Parsons 2001). A similar pattern (with the additional involvement of motor areas) was noted during vocal repetition of a melody or a vocal harmonization task, though in this study the activations were bilateral (Brown et al. 2004).

When we listen to rhythmic music we often find our feet tapping or our head nodding to the beat or may experience a strong urge to dance. If this observation appears self-evident, compare it to the complete lack of response we experience when watching rhythmic movement in the absence of sound. It is only through the auditory system that the urge for movement is generated. It will therefore come as no surprise to learn that the motor areas of the brain play a central role, not only in the production of rhythmic movement, but also in the perception of auditory rhythms (fig. 9-13A). Our response to rhythm does not rely simply on an interpretation of incoming signals, but also on an ability to predict how the rhythm will continue. Without this, our dancing, foot tapping, and indeed music making would lag behind the beat. This implicates the brain circuitry involved in the temporal patterning of sequential movements and is consistent with the observation of activity in the basal ganglia, the cerebellum, and the supplementary motor cortex in response to auditory rhythms (Limb et al. 2006; Grahn and Brett 2007). This is present even in the absence of overt movement, during which the primary motor cortex remains silent. It has been proposed that while the basal ganglia and supplementary motor area play a key role in the timing of motor activity over periods of several seconds, the cerebellum is responsible for the precise synchronization movement in the subsecond range (Zatorre, Chen, and Penhune 2007). In basal ganglion diseases such as parkinsonism, in which motor sequences break down, leading to a slowing or freezing of movement, music or the beat of a metronome can be an effective means of starting it up again and can help the individual with the condition to maintain a regular walking cadence (Suteerawattananon et al. 2004; Zatorre, Chen, and Penhune 2007; Sacks 2007). Rhythm also evokes activity within the frontal premotor cortex including Broca's area, which lies in its ventral region. However, as the rhythms (either perceived or produced) become progressively more complex, the dorsal parts of the premotor cortex are increasingly recruited (Zatorre, Chen, and Penhune 2007). The basic pattern of activity described so far appears equally applicable to both musicians and nonmusicians, though musicians show additional foci of activity in the prefrontal cortex, which may indicate a greater involvement of working memory (the neural equivalent of computer RAM) in the analysis of the temporal structure of rhythm (Chen, Penhune, and Zatorre 2008). The perception of meter appears to have a different origin, requiring the involvement of the anterior superior temporal gyrus (the upper surface of the temporal lobe some distance in front of the primary auditory cortex) (Grahn and Brett 2007; Liegeois-Chauvel et al. 1998).

The history of our understanding of the role of Broca's area in speech and in the analysis of musical sound is instructive in demonstrating how the properties of a given brain region may fit it for a range of different functions. It should also be seen as a warning against applying simplistic functional labels to particular regions of the brain, something that is all too tempting with functional imaging. Broca's area lies on the left inferior region of the frontal lobe and was first described by Pierre Paul Broca in 1861, following examination of the brains of two of his patients who had lost the ability to speak. The brains are still in existence and have recently been scanned to reveal that the lesions extend considerably beyond what is now known as Broca's area (Dronkers et al. 2007). In the 1990s, animal experiments revealed that Broca's area and its equivalent on the right side of the brain contain what are known as "mirror neurons." These respond both when we perform an action and when we watch the same action being performed by another. It was subsequently discovered that some mirror neurons also respond to the sounds that are generated during such actions (Kohler et al. 2002). Though for ethical reasons the properties of single neurons in Broca's area cannot be studied directly in humans, circumstantial evidence strongly supports the likelihood that some mirror neurons within our own brains also have this property (Gazzola, Aziz-Zadeh, and Keysers 2006). This may help to explain the long-established association of Broca's area with speech (Zatorre, Chen, and Penhune 2007; Gazzola, Aziz-Zadeh, and Keysers 2006). Neurons in Broca's area respond when sounds are created using movements of the hand or the mouth, and the level of activity has been shown to be higher in musicians than in nonmusicians (Bangert et al. 2006). A similar response is seen in the equivalent region on the right side of the brain, though it is not as intense. Though it doesn't itself contain mirror neurons, the secondary auditory cortex in the middle temporal gyrus may also be involved in this system. Functional imaging studies now suggest that Broca's area contributes to the processing of several aspects of musical syntax including harmonic structure, melody, rhythm, and timbre (Brown and Martinez 2007; Koelsch 2006), though its precise role in these activities has yet to be explained.

Consonance and Dissonance

Certain combinations of pure or complex tones are perceived as more harmonious than others. In general pairs of notes, those whose fundamentals are related by simple ratios appear to us more consonant than those with more complex ratios. Examples of consonant intervals are the octave (ratio 2:1), the perfect fifth (2:3), and the perfect fourth (4:3), while the minor second (16:15) and the tritone (45:32) are dissonant intervals (Tramo et al. 2001). Several explanations have been put forward for this. One is that consonant combinations of complex sounds tend to have harmonics that are common or are numerically related. For the perfect fifth, for example, half of the harmonics of the upper note coincide with harmonics of the lower one (Burns 1999). This is reflected in a regular periodicity of the combined waveform and in the response of the population of neurons in the auditory nerve that respond to the sound thus generated. It is the same phenomenon discussed above in the context of the perception of missing fundamentals, and indeed these will be generated by consonant note combinations. For dissonant intervals, not only are any periodicities much weaker, but they would be indicative of fundamentals that are not related to the notes being played (Tramo et al. 2001). A second theory of consonance is that the circuitry of the auditory system is designed to look for harmonic relationships. Again this is the system that assigns a single pitch to complex sounds. Any mismatch of the harmonic components that does not allow the fitting of a pitch to the set of frequencies presented is therefore very noticeable. At the very least, the perceived pitch clashes with some of the harmonics so that they stand out as noticeably alien components. When subjects are presented with a series of chords that include unexpected dissonances, activity is seen in the region in front of the primary auditory cortex (the anterior superior temporal gyrus), the planum temporale, and the region of the frontal lobe in and around Broca's area and its equivalent on the right hemisphere (Koelsch 2006; Maess et al. 2001; Parsons 2001; Passynkova, Sander, and Scheich 2005).

Cortical Plasticity in the Auditory System

From previous chapters on the sensory and motor areas of the cortex, the idea that the brain is molded by experience will be a familiar one. This is equally true of the auditory cortex. In a study of Heschl's gyrus using brain imaging techniques, the region occupied by the primary auditory cortex in amateur and professional musicians was found to be more than twice as large than that in nonmusicians (Schneider et al. 2002; Gaser and Schlaug 2003; Luders et al. 2004). In professional musicians it is also larger than in amateurs. The auditory cortex of musicians shows a greater response to the sound of their own instrument than to the sound of other instruments (both of which are complex sounds composed of a fundamental frequency and many harmonics), as well as to pure tones of a single frequency. There is a general trend for the magnitude of the signal generated to the sound of the player's own instrument to be greatest in those who started playing before the age of about eight (Pantev et al. 1998, 2003).

The left and right side of the brain are not symmetrical in terms of function. For example, linguistic skills are usually located mainly on the left side, close to the auditory areas. The auditory cortex itself also shows asymmetry. It appears from some studies that perception of pitch is primarily located on the right side but that the temporal pattern of the sound is analyzed mainly on the left side (Liegeois-Chauvel et al. 2001; Zatorre 2001). It has also been suggested that a right-sided bias for analysis of harmony and melody may be greater in females (Evers et al. 1999). It has been proposed that the reason that analysis of language lies on the left is that it is mainly the temporal changes in the sound that are important for interpreting speech. On a slightly longer time scale, the inflections found in speech that carry nonverbal grammatical information have some similarities with melodic phrases. When amateur musicians and nonmusicians are set difficult tasks requiring analysis of the harmonic and melodic structure of a piece of music, the regions of the brain involved in interpreting music on both sides of the brain are used in relatively equal measure. In highly trained professional musicians, there is greater activity on the left side of the brain than on the right, implying that the information is being processed in a different way (Altenmuller 2001; Ohnishi et al. 2001; Evers et al. 1999). This is probably more marked in those whose formal musical training started early, as the brain is more able to alter its internal connections in childhood. The types of changes seen here are not unique to musicians. It is known, for example, that in those who are brought up to be bilingual from birth, the region of the cortex that controls the muscles used in speech is identical for both languages; however, when a second, fluently spoken language is learned later in life, the areas controlling speech in the two languages are separate (Kim et al. 1997).

Perfect Pitch

Pitch and interval discrimination are important abilities that musicians must develop. The majority have what is called good relative pitch, which is to say that when presented with a note, they can sing on demand another that is separated from it by a particular musical interval (e.g., a minor third or a fifth), or on hearing a named note, they can name the pitch of another that is played soon after. This is based on short-term memory of the first note, which can be erased with a burst of white noise, a silent interval of a minute or less, or a brief distracting acoustic or nonacoustic task. Perfect or absolute pitch is less common and is the ability to name the precise pitch of a single note played in the absence of any reference cues. An individual with perfect pitch can therefore typically name up to seventy notes or "varieties of pitch," whereas most ordinary mortals can recognize only six to eight ranges of pitch without reference points (Zatorre 2001, 2003). It should be noted, however, that those with perfect pitch are not more accurate at identifying pitch deviations than those without absolute pitch; their unusual abilities are confined to pitch labeling only and do not extend to pitch perception (Levitin and Rogers 2005). The problem of pitch recognition is similar to that posed by colors. Our computer monitor may be capable of producing several million shades, but we can accurately label little more than the seven spectral colors we define in the rainbow. We have all had futile arguments over such common intermediate shades as turquoise, or had the embarrassment of guessing a paint shade in a home improvement store, only to discover when we get the paint tin home that it is nothing like the color on the wall. The limitations of the analogy are also instructive. One of the requirements for developing an absolute hue perception comparable to absolute pitch would be the presence of a system for naming discrete shade intervals across the continuum of the visible spectrum. However, the musical intervals of the scale have a greater internal structure, as they are formed from a repeated series of steps related to the harmonics of a particular note. In modern tuning, the interval of the octave is absolutely precise and even small deviations from this are easily detected by the beats between two notes. The common property that we perceive in notes one or more octaves apart is described by the word "chroma" but ironically, despite the name, such a precise scale cannot be devised for color.

To acquire perfect pitch it is necessary both to have the innate ability and to be exposed at an early age to an environment in which notes and their names are presented simultaneously. Interestingly, and for reasons that are currently unknown, this appears to be easier for the white notes on the piano than the black ones (Pierce 1999). Most musicians with perfect pitch start their musical education before the age of seven and during their early learning period have not had their absolute judgment of pitch clouded by consciously learning relative pitch. Many adults have struggled long and hard in an attempt to develop perfect pitch, with an almost total lack of success. What we are seeing here is an example of a phenomenon well known in brain development called a critical period. Though the brain remains able throughout life to change its wiring patterns in response to the demands made upon it by changing conditions, the degree to which this is possible declines with age. Many circuits can be radically altered only during a short critical period of a few months or years in early life. For example, if a child has a squint (a walleye), this should be corrected before the age of six, otherwise the circuitry for binocular vision, which requires both eyes to point in the same direction, will not develop. The ability to develop perfect pitch may also depend on genetic factors (see below), as it is seen more often in children of the same parents than would be expected by chance and is more common in some ethnic groups than others, notably in people of Asian origin (Zatorre 2001). It does not, however, appear to be due to the inheritance of a single gene.

Perfect pitch is associated with an increase in the asymmetry of the planum temporale, the area of association auditory cortex that lies behind Heschl's gyrus. This was demonstrated in a comparison of brain structure between thirty musicians, some of whom had perfect pitch, and thirty nonmusicians. In the nonmusicians, and the musicians without perfect pitch, the left planum temporale was 22 to 26 percent larger than the one on the right. However, the greatest asymmetry was seen in male musicians with perfect pitch, in whom the left planum temporale was nearly 80 percent larger than on the right side (Schlaug et al. 1995; Luders et al. 2004). This was not due to its being larger in absolute terms, but because the right planum temporale was actually smaller than normal in this group (Schlaug et al. 1995; Keenan et al. 2001). In female musicians, by contrast, there was no increase in the size of the left planum temporale associated with perfect pitch (Luders et al. 2004). Interestingly, studies of brain function suggest that perfect pitch may be related to the absence of a process that refreshes short-term working memory of pitch change. In those who only have relative pitch, this process is required to establish the interval relationships between different notes.

Perfect pitch is only absolutely "in tune" if the reference pitch the brain acquires correlates with international concert pitch. It has been said of those who have it that "perfect pitch" is the pitch of their mother's piano, so parents who aspire to raise musical geniuses should not skimp on paying for the tuner! While it may have many advantages, perfect pitch also has its drawbacks. A solo singer who persists in maintaining concert pitch when the choir goes flat may not be asked back. Much has also been made of the fact that the reference pitch of individuals with perfect pitch may not remain constant throughout life. Many (but not all) individuals with this ability have reported that their perception of pitch changes with age, sometimes by several half-steps in one direction or another (Pierce 1999). If the musician has definite feelings about the character of different keys, this can be disturbing. Suggestions based on anecdotal evidence that absolute pitch changes during pregnancy or the menstrual cycle have not been supported by more objective testing; however, it does appear to be true that in both males and females, pitch can drift up and down over a range of 10–20 Hz over a period of a few months.

Tone Deafness and Amusia

President Ulysses S. Grant once explained to a reporter that he knew two tunes: one of them was "Yankee Doodle" and the other wasn't. He suffered from tone deafness (congenital amusia) and was not simply unmoved by music but found it positively irritating (Munte 2002). Tone deafness may be quite common; one survey of six hundred students found an incidence of 10 percent (Shuter-Dyson 1999), but a more generally accepted figure is that it affects 4–5 percent of the population. There is some evidence that it may have a genetic component in at least a proportion of those affected (Peretz and Hyde 2003). Those who are tone deaf find it impossible to recognize or hum a melody, to sing in tune (or even to recognize that they are not doing so), regardless of whether they have had musical training in childhood. It is found in people of all mental abilities and does not preclude good verbal skills in one or more languages. In many people with congenital amusia (though not all), the ability to perceive rhythm is unaffected. Even small children can normally recognize dissonance, and the lack of this ability in those who are tone deaf seems to reflect a difficulty in identifying small deviations in pitch and in relating tones to musical scales (Peretz and Hyde 2003; Foxton et al. 2004). Strangely, this difficulty is only experienced in the context of music. The perception of inflection in language, such as the rising tone at the end of a question in English and other Indo-European languages, is essential for interpreting the precise meaning of spoken phrases. In languages such as Mandarin, inflection is even more important in giving meaning to words. These tasks, however, pose no problem to those who are tone deaf. The reason resides partly in the relative sizes of the pitch excursions in language and music. While recognition of melodic lines requires identification of pitch increments as small as one-twelfth or less of an octave, linguistic inflections typically extend over half an octave or more, so a deficit in pitch perception of sufficient magnitude to interfere with the interpretation of music (typically one or more tones) will generally have little consequence for the nonverbal elements of spoken language

(Peretz 2002). However, that is not the whole story, as pitch changes in the range typical of speech are more easily detected when delivered as words than when not (Ayotte, Peretz, and Hyde 2002). Comparisons of the brains of normal subjects and individuals with congenital amusia using magnetic resonance imaging analysis have revealed anatomical anomalies associated with tone deafness. There is a thickening of the gray matter in the right superior temporal gyrus and both thicker gray matter and reduced white matter in the right inferior frontal gyrus (Hyde et al. 2006, 2007). This is thought to be due to malformation of the cortex during development. The superior temporal gyrus is strongly implicated in the fine pitch discrimination and sequential pitch analysis that underpins the perception of melody, while the inferior frontal gyrus is thought to be involved in melodic pitch encoding and memory.

Musical disability that arises as the result of brain damage or disease is a quite different phenomenon. This is usually referred to as acquired amusia, a name that covers a number of disorders, not only of the central processes underlying music recognition and interpretation but also of the reading, composition, and performance of music. When it produces symptoms similar to tone deafness, the areas affected are generally the primary and secondary auditory cortices on the superior temporal gyrus. One composer who developed amusia of a different type in later life was Ravel. He ceased to compose in his midfifties, and his amusia was a symptom of a degenerative age-related disease that today would probably be labeled frontotemporal dementia (Sacks 2007). Though he retained some memory of his own compositions, he became unable to sight-read or name notes and also found it difficult to copy music either from a manuscript or from dictation (Marin and Perry 1999). Oliver Sacks has even suggested that the monotonous repetition and lack of development that characterizes *Bolero* may have been an early indication of the onset of his condition.

The degree to which case studies of individuals who have suffered localized damage to the cortex can dramatically illustrate how musical information is processed is well demonstrated in a series of studies by Peretz (2002). She describes one young woman who underwent several operations to repair ruptured blood vessels in the brain, which resulted in a loss of part of the auditory cortex on both sides of the brain together with regions of the adjacent frontal cortex on the right side. It is a testament to the ability of the brain to compensate for damage that she not only retained her linguistic abilities but also suffered no loss of intellect or general memory function; however, she was no longer able to recognize or memorize music or sing a tune. Though not a musician, she was brought up in a musical family and music had been an important part of her life before surgery. She is described as suffering from amusia without aphasia (aphasia is the loss of the ability to produce or understand speech). A mirror image of this deficit was seen in the case of the Russian composer Shebalin. He suffered two strokes (loss of blood supply to part of the brain), which affected a large area of the left half of the cortex. Though he lost the ability to speak, during the remaining four years of his life he nevertheless composed a symphony, four quartets, two sonatas, eleven songs, and more than a dozen chorales. Shostakovich, who was a contemporary, considered that this music was indistinguishable in quality from that composed before his illness. Shebalin's deficit was therefore aphasia without amusia.

Auditory Synesthesia

For a small number of people, hearing music generates strong involuntary sensations normally associated with senses other than hearing. For example, particular notes or keys may appear to assume specific colors. This is just one form of a wider phenomenon called synesthesia, in which stimulation of one sense produces illusions belonging to another. In its other manifestations, numbers may be associated with colors, or touching certain objects may induce the sensation of a particular taste. Though there has been some controversy in the past about whether this is a real phenomenon and not simply a learned response, or perhaps a drug-induced state or even a form of fakery, the evidence has become increasingly cogent (Ramachandran and Hubbard 2003). The fact that it appears to have a genetic component (i.e., it runs in families) helps to support this view. Because it was apparently experienced by some well-known composers, synesthesia triggered by music has some historical significance. Messiaen, Rimsky-Korsakoff, and Scriabin were all apparently synesthetes. The latter two, who were friends, could not agree on the colors associated with particular keys but with characteristic robustness, Scriabin came up with a theory to explain Rimsky-Korsakoff's "mistaken" perceptions. Scriabin's synesthesia led him to experiment with the color organ, an instrument that presented colored light as an accompaniment to music and for which he wrote the orchestral piece *Prometheus, the Poem of Fire.*

The origin of synesthesia is unknown, though it is thought to be a product of the way in which the brain is wired. When we think of a place, an object, an animal, or a person, we bring together stored information from many of our senses to create a holistic impression in our mind. Information from any one sense may trigger the same complete memory. An important design principle of the brain is therefore to bring different sensory streams together. The difference with synesthesia is that the associations either are with abstractions (e.g., linking tonality with color) or involve matching sensations that cannot be generated by the same object. This suggests that its roots lie in atypical connections between brain regions that deal with abstracted sensory information. On theoretical grounds, a particular region of the cortex that lies above and behind the planum temporale has been proposed as a site for synesthetic associations; however, there is as yet no direct evidence to support this.

Sound Localization

One major task of the auditory system is to calculate the position from which a sound is coming. This has important survival value for all animals and is calculated by the brain from a comparison of the way the same sound appears to each of the two ears. It is only necessary to switch the hi-fi between mono and stereo to appreciate how much information we can gain from this. Two major mechanisms have been proposed for sound localization; these are based on 1) a determination of the difference in the time at which the same sound reaches each ear (the interaural time delay; fig. 9-14A) and 2) the difference in intensity between the sound in each ear (the interaural intensity difference—fig. 9-14B).

Differences in the time at which a sound reaches each ear are extremely small and their detection is a major challenge for the nervous system. If a sound comes from

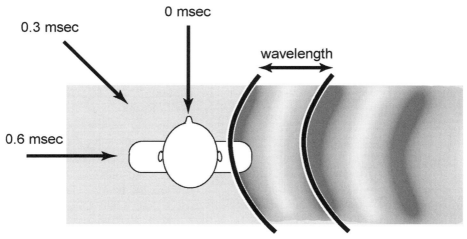

A. Interaural time delay

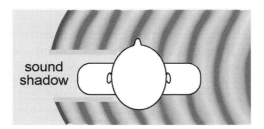

B. Interaural intensity difference

Figure 9-14.   Sound localization. The brain has two ways of working out where a sound is com-ing from. A. The first uses the difference in time between a sound reaching the left and the right ears (interaural time delay). When the sound is coming from directly in front or behind, it reaches both ears simultaneously. The maximum time difference (when the sound is coming from the right or left) is 0.6 milliseconds, and lower delays code for the intervening angles. This method of sound localization only works if the wavelength is greater than the width of the head. For shorter wavelengths (higher frequencies) where distance between the two ears is equivalent to two or more wavelengths, time delay does not give a unique solution for sound direction. Under these circumstances, differences in intensity of the sound reaching the two ears is used (B). The sound shadow created by the head is greatest for sources coming from the right or left and falls to zero for sounds that originate from directly in front or behind.

directly in front or behind the head, it reaches both ears simultaneously, but if it comes from the side, the maximum time difference is only 0.6 milliseconds (six ten-thou-sandths of a second), which is the time sound takes to travel the 20 centimeters or so that separate the ears. Of course in your dog, hamster, or budgerigar this distance is much smaller and the task correspondingly more difficult! The start of a sound is a clear signal whose arrival time can be easily compared. For a continuous sound the situation is more complicated, and the interaural time delay must be measured from the same point on the sound wave (e.g., the peak amplitude) in both ears. If the wavelength is smaller than the distance between the ears, the signal will be ambiguous for continuous sound because it will depend on how many cycles of the waveform lie between the peaks detected in each ear. Sounds of 3,000 Hz and above (top G on the piano) can fit two or more cycles in that distance and so the system that uses interaural time delay starts to generate ambiguous results at about 1,500 Hz, which is an octave below. For higher frequencies, differences in sound intensity must therefore be used for sound source localization. Sounds coming from directly ahead or behind will again be equally loud in both ears, but for those coming from the side, the head creates a sound shadow so that the sound appears quieter in the ear on the opposite side from the source. This mechanism does not work for low frequencies because the longer wavelength sounds can bend around the head, reducing the perceived intensity difference. Interaural time delays and intensity differences do not allow any discrimination of the elevation of the sound source above the horizon. This appears to be achieved by analyzing the distortion of the sound by the external ear, which selectively alters different frequency components depending on the vertical position of the source. Stereophonic effects in the horizontal plane can readily be generated by recording sound from two microphones placed at different positions on the stage, but this cannot be used to produce the illusion of sound sources at different heights.

The accuracy of sound localization in the horizontal plane is quite remarkable, typically in the range of 3°–10°. This can be improved with practice and consequently tends to be better in blind people (Roder et al. 1999). Interestingly, research has shown that conductors have unusually good sound localization abilities. When their performance in sound localization tasks was compared with musicians such as pianists and nonmusicians, all groups performed equally well when the sound sources were more or less directly ahead, but the conductors were much better at localizing sounds from either side. It has been suggested that this superior performance may be developed through learning to use spectral differences in sound coming from different directions. This would involve detecting changes generated both by the filtering properties of the external ear and by the head shadow (Munte et al. 2001). From brain scanning studies, it has been possible to show that the cortical analysis of the spatial organization of the auditory world is carried out in the posterior region of the planum temporale at a position that is quite distinct from the regions that interpret the sequential changes in pitch that underlie melody (Warren and Griffiths 2003). Spatial analysis of the sound world also occurs outside the cortex in the inferior colliculi, which forms part of the roof of the brain stem (fig. 9-11).

Brain Circuitry Underlying Emotional Responses to Music

Music activates not only the parts of the brain that overtly analyze its structure and syntax, but as we all well know from personal experience, it also influences areas that generate emotional responses. Indeed, the main reason we listen to music is for its emotional impact. Of course, our emotional responses to a piece of music may be due as much to the associations it has for us as to its musical structure. One only has to think of the strong reactions that can be generated by the dire music of most national anthems to realize that it is not always the quality of the composition that is the most important factor. To give another example, being Scottish, I find the sound of the bagpipes both stirring and highly evocative and likely to produce feelings of nostalgia, while the same sound once prompted a young relative of mine to complain to her mother that she didn't like "the men playing the Hoovers"! For most composers, however, success depends on their ability to manipulate the emotions of the audience directly through the music. This requires that particular musical elements produce predictable effects on the brain (Peretz, Gagnon, and Bouchard 1998). We may not all be touched by the same pieces, but within the Western musical tradition at least, warlike pieces tend to be strongly rhythmic and sometimes discordant, love songs harmonious and legato, happy music lively and in major keys, and sad pieces slower and in minor ones. Many other sensory stimuli also generate strong emotions, for example, the sight of particular facial expressions, the intonation of the voice, a smell, or a taste; but it has been argued that music differs from these in that it is an abstract phenomenon that does not intrinsically carry signals from our environment that are important for survival (Blood et al. 1999). While this is to some extent true, our responses to the other sensory signals, such as smell, are often as much related to learned associations as to their objective information content. While we may all be repelled by the odor of spoiled food (a response with an obvious survival value), we may as individuals be comforted by familiar odors specific to the environment in which we grew up, odors that to others may appear neutral or even disquieting. In this regard, the response to music is not so different; however, the personal nature of our reactions can make studying them difficult. One attempt to do this compared the reaction of the brain to different degrees of dissonance, which is a quality most listeners can agree upon as being unpleasant. The research revealed consistent differences in the pattern of brain activity induced by consonance and dissonance in regions thought to be involved in emotional responses (Blood et al. 1999). However, music sometimes leads to brief positive responses that are not just mildly pleasant, but positively euphoric. This can induce a physical sensation that may be either visceral or feel like a "shiver down the spine." Both of these types of sensation imply the involvement of the autonomic nervous system (see chapter 10), which engenders responses over which we have no conscious control. The autonomic nervous system supplies the visceral organs and also the blood vessels and glands, including structures in the skin such as sweat glands and the minute muscles that cause the hairs to rise (piloerection). It is probably the action of the piloerector muscles that is responsible for the aforementioned shivers. When music is able to generate such reactions, they are accompanied by detectable increases in heartbeat and breathing rate. This provides an objective verification of the timing and genuineness of the euphoric feelings and so enables them to be correlated with brain activity. The brain regions concerned are the same ones that are activated by other hedonistic stimuli such as food, sex, and drugs of abuse (Blood and Zatorre 2001). They are part of a reward system within the central nervous system that includes structures known to be connected to the autonomic nervous system but is quite distinct from the regions activated by mildly pleasant musical stimuli such as consonance.

In order to appreciate how music achieves its emotional impact on the brain, it is first necessary to understand something of the organization of the circuitry that has

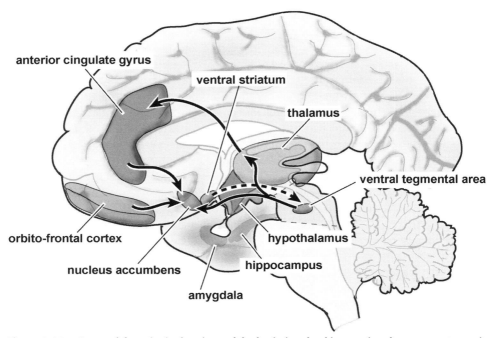

Figure 9-15. Some of the principal regions of the brain involved in emotional responses to music and other stimuli are shown here. These lie mainly in the ventral regions of the brain and include several elements of the limbic system, for example, the cingulate gyrus—particularly its anterior part; the amygdala and hippocampus, which lie at the tip of the temporal lobe; and the ventral prefrontal cortex. The ventral tegmental area of the midbrain contains nerve cells that send their axons forward to the thalamus, hypothalamus, ventral striatum, and nucleus accumbens. Activity in this latter structure is strongly linked to pleasurable emotions. Emotional responses also involve the orbitofrontal cortex, which lies just in front of the nucleus accumbens. The arrows indicate some of the major connections between these regions.

been implicated in pleasurable and unpleasurable sensations. Unfortunately, this is a complex area, not least because it is still incompletely understood, and even the simplified outline presented here may initially appear rather impenetrable. However, as we prize music mainly for its emotional impact, some readers may wish to delve further into this subject, and with a little perseverance this introduction should give them the means to make some sense of the original literature. The parts of the brain discussed below are illustrated in figure 9-15.

The pathways that mediate pleasure originate mainly in the ventral regions of the brain. Some of the centers involved lie in the brain stem, particularly within the midbrain. One key element is a region known as the ventral tegmental area. This lies on the midline of the midbrain and is populated by nerve cells that use dopamine as their neurotransmitter. The axons of these neurons course forward toward the thalamus, hypothalamus, and limbic system (see chapter 7) and are consequently described as mesolimbic fibers (meso = mid). The parts of the limbic system most strongly linked to emotional responses are the amygdala, which contributes the emotional coloring to memory, and the anterior part of the cingulate gyrus, an area of the cortex that sits immediately above the corpus callosum. An important target of the mesolimbic pathway is a structure known as the nucleus accumbens, which sits at the front of the basal ganglion complex. Some studies refer to this general area as the ventral striatum, because the corpus striatum is another name for the components of the basal ganglia that are found here. The nucleus accumbens is linked to the area of the cortex that sits immediately anterior (in front) of it. This is known as the orbitofrontal cortex, as it lies immediately above the part of the skull that forms the roof of the eye socket (or orbit). Though this is not an exhaustive list of the areas that are implicated in positive and negative emotions, it is sufficient to support a general description of the effects of music.

Some insight into the pleasure network of the brain in humans has been gathered from subjective accounts of people who, for various clinical reasons, have had stimulating electrodes implanted in a few of the areas listed in the previous paragraph. From the accounts of these patients it is clear that we need to distinguish between wanting (feeling compelled) to do something and liking (gaining pleasure from) it (Berridge 2003). Stimulation of the mesolimbic dopamine pathway is compulsive, and it has been suggested that activity in these fibers is linked to addiction. Stimulation of the nucleus accumbens, on the other hand, appears to evoke pleasurable sensations. This is dependent on the release of opiatelike chemicals (e.g., enkephalins and endorphins) that act as neurotransmitters (see chapter 1). Activity in the orbitofrontal lobes and in the anterior cingulate gyrus is often associated with pleasure but may also be involved in negative emotions. The physical manifestations of these emotions are largely brought about by the hypothalamus and to some extent by a region of the cortex known as the insula, which lies tucked out of sight behind the temporal lobe. Both of these exert a controlling influence over the autonomic nervous system. Having gained an overview of the effect of pleasurable sensations on the brain, we can now move on to consider the emotional consequences of music.

If we return to the studies of Blood and Zatorre, we can now appreciate their observations that during music that induced the "chills" in their subjects, increased activity was observed in the midbrain, the ventral striatum, the orbitofrontal cortex, and the insula but activity in the amygdala was reduced. The imaging system used here had a rather low spatial resolution, so it was not possible to specifically identify the nucleus accumbens due to its small size. However, similar studies carried out at higher resolution not only confirmed this overall pattern of brain activity but clearly demonstrated the involvement of the nucleus accumbens (Menon and Levitin 2005; Brown, Martinez, and Parsons 2004). When the effects of "happy" and "sad" music were compared, the former activated the ventral striatum and anterior cingulate gyrus, while the latter produced activity in the hippocampus and amygdala (Mitterschiffthaler et al. 2007). The introduction of dissonance into musical stimuli also led to increased activity in the amygdala (Koelsch et al. 2006). This is consistent with its well-known role in the recognition of negative emotion (particularly fear) in the facial expression of others. Its response to the emotional content of music has been further explored through observations on a patient in whom it was completely destroyed on both sides of the brain, while adjacent regions of the temporal cortex involved in music processing were preserved (Gosselin et al. 2007). In comparison to normal control subjects, the ability to label musical extracts correctly as "scary" or "sad" was considerably impaired, while the recognition of music as "happy" or "peaceful" was much more close to normal. This was not due to a failure to extract relevant aspects of musical structure, as the response to tempo and mode remained intact. The reward system evolved to motivate animals to carry out behavior important for survival. Though this is not the case for music, its ability to tap into this system in a nondetrimental way allows it to play a significant role in supporting our emotional well-being.

The "Mozart Effect"

There has been much debate concerning whether music can improve mental performance. In 1993, Rauscher et al. published a short letter in the prestigious scientific journal *Nature* that purported to show that a brief period of listening to Mozart resulted in improved performance in certain tasks forming one element of a battery of standard intelligence tests. This resulted in a considerable degree of fevered press speculation along the lines that listening to the music of Mozart or other socially acceptable classical composers increases intelligence. It is only through the many attempts by other researchers to replicate the effect that the truth has slowly emerged. The claims of the original papers by Rauscher et al. were rather modest (Rauscher, Shaw, and Ky 1993, 1995). A group of college students spent ten minutes listening to a piece of music by Mozart (the first movement [Allegro] of the Sonata for Two Pianos, K. 448) or to taped relaxation instructions, or spent the same length of time sitting in silence. The precise nature of the movement of the Mozart sonata used turns out to be crucial; it is of course fast but also in a major key, with a lively interaction between the two instruments as they pass elements of the melody back and forth. After listening to the music or sitting in silence, the subjects of the study were asked to perform a spatial reasoning test called the Paper Folding and Cutting (PF&C) task. This involves predicting the pattern produced if a piece of paper is folded repeatedly and small sections are then cut out, as might be done to make a symmetrical Christmas snowflake decoration. Interestingly, tasks of this nature should show a gender bias in favor of men (Kimura 1999), but most studies of the Mozart effect do not mention the sex composition of the experimental or control groups. The results obtained by Rauscher suggested that the students who listened to Mozart performed slightly better than the control groups on the PF&C task but that this was short-lived, and neither these nor any subsequent studies have found any evidence of an enhancement in other measures of intelligence or cognitive ability. The idea behind the original experiments was based on some interesting but unproven theories suggesting that higher brain function is dependent on how patterns of activity in small columns of nerve cells within the cortex change over time. The rationale runs as follows: 1) because computer models of these theoretical patterns (which might represent fundamental neural activity) can be used to generate music-like sounds, responses to music early in life may be based on them; 2) Mozart was composing at a very early age, so his music in particular may express features of this patterning particularly strongly; 3) the PF&C task also involves analyzing patterns that change with time and which might, by some unspecified mechanism, be improved by unspecified intrinsic properties of Mozart's music that reflect the relevant mental activity. Needless to say, this is a rather tenuous line of reasoning. Apart from the flaws in the underlying logic, there are problems with the experimental design, as many subsequent researchers who have attempted to replicate the experiments have pointed out. The effect of the music was compared to the effect of silence, which is unstimulating by comparison. Music is an extremely complex stimulus; even pieces of music by the same composer will generate very different emotions depending on their structure. It is vital that such factors are controlled for in experiments that investigate this question. Mozart appears to have been chosen for the reputation he has with a (lamentably perhaps!) small proportion of the general population who mostly share a common cultural background. The fact that he was twenty-five at the time he composed K. 448 in 1781 and that his style had developed very much in keeping with prevailing cultural trends is not recognized by logic backing the theory. Other composers or (heaven forbid) other musical styles were not compared in the original study. It is hard to imagine school boards pushing the music of Led Zeppelin had this been shown to improve performance in the PF&C test! We know nothing of the cultural background or musical tastes of the control group in the original study, which could have significantly influenced their response to the music and hence perhaps their performance in the test. Many studies that have tried to replicate the Mozart effect have failed (Chabris 1999; Steele et al. 1999), though it must be recognized that a significant proportion of them have severe methodological flaws of their own. In several, however, attempts were made to address some of the problems of the original experimental design, for example, by comparing the effect of music by Mozart with that of other classical or nonclassical composers or with listening to a story. The results of some studies suggested that improvement in the PF&C task was related to listening to a preferred sensory experience, whether musical or not (Nantais and Schellenberg 1999) and was related to the mood or degree of arousal that this induced (Thompson, Schellenberg, and Husain 2001; Nantais and Schellenberg 1999). In a telling experiment, a comparison was made between the effects of K. 448 played at the original tempo or at a much slower one, and of a version in a minor key played at a fast or slow tempo. The same conclusion was reached (Husain, Thompson, and Schellenberg 2002).

Given the often frenzied attention that has been (and is still being) given to the "Mozart effect" and its continued promotion in the popular media, it is only fair to give the last word to the only author of the original paper who continued to study it: "The Mozart effect was studied only in adults, lasted only a few minutes, and was found only for spatial-temporal reasoning. Nevertheless the effect has spawned a Mozart industry . . . claiming that listening to classical music can make children 'smarter.' In fact no scientific evidence supports (this) claim. . . . Although the Mozart effect is of scientific interest, its education implications appear to be limited" (Rauscher 2003).

The broader question of whether acquiring practical musical skills, as opposed to passive listening, exerts any educational influence on nonmusical abilities in children is an equally controversial issue. Isolating the effect of musical training, per se, from the stimulation of being in a select group receiving special attention, or the effect of coming from a background that supports involvement in such schemes, is difficult to achieve in an ethical way. A good review of research in this area can be found in

Schellenberg (2006). The best that can be said, once these extraneous factors have been eliminated, is that the benefits appear marginal and may not be long-lasting. Given that an active participation in any form of music making is such a personally enriching experience, the need to justify it on other grounds seems rather to miss the point, particularly if this is linked to a narrow cultural agenda. What is clear is that providing good support for music, of whatever genre, within the educational system, will lead to more practicing musicians within the community, and this should be a worthy objective both for the individual and for society.

Epilepsy

The effect of Mozart's music on brain activity linked to epilepsy has also received some attention. This is rather more amenable to objective study because epilepsy is associated with clearly identifiable patterns of synchronized electrical activity in the brain that can easily be recorded and analyzed statistically. There is evidence from one group that listening to Mozart's K. 448 can reduce the frequency of the electrical activity associated with epileptic seizures (Turner 2004; Hughes 2001, 2002). This piece appears to be more effective than several other pieces of music, including those by other classical composers such as Beethoven; however, the number of patients who have been studied and the number of pieces of music that have been tested are both very small, so much more work is needed to validate the effect. Hughes analyzed the structural features of the music of several composers and, based on the characteristics of K. 448, has made certain predictions about which pieces by Mozart and other composers might be most useful in controlling seizures. For example, he considered that the music of Haydn would be a good candidate, though it might not be quite as effective as that of Mozart. Unfortunately, his hypothesis remains as yet untested.

Interestingly, music can also induce epileptic attacks in some individuals (Kaplan 2003). The nineteenth-century Chinese poet Kung Tzu-chen gives what appears to be an early account of music-induced epilepsy: "Since my remote boyhood I have always been absentminded while hearing the sound of the street vendor's flute. I fall sick when I hear the sound of the flute in the evening sun, although I do not know the reason." The suggestion by some authors that the following Shakespearean quote from *The Merchant of Venice* (act IV, scene 1) also refers to musicogenic epilepsy is perhaps on shakier ground (Wieser et al. 1997):

> Some men there are, love not a gaping pig;
> Some are mad, if they behold a cat;
> And others, when the bagpipe sings i' the nose
> Cannot contain their urine.

Though the ability of flashing lights of certain frequencies is well known to trigger epileptic seizures, there is no evidence that rhythm or any other elements of musical structure consistently have this effect. Instead, the type of music (if any) likely to induce an attack is highly specific to the individual. In most cases, the musical stimulus is of external origin but in some patients an attack can be induced by their own singing. Music of all styles (classical orchestral or opera, religious, folk, jazz, military, dance, music evoking a particular mood or of cultural significance, etc.) has been known to trigger attacks, but the underlying mechanisms remain unknown. Pure tones do not induce seizures, and the crucial aspects of musical stimuli (which may include its emotional impact) suggest that the attack does not arise from activity in the primary auditory cortex, but in regions where higher-order processing of music takes place.

REFERENCES

Altenmuller, E. O. 2001. How many music centers are in the brain? *Ann NY Acad Sci* 930:273–80.

Audsley, G. A. 1965. *The art of organ-building: A comprehensive historical, theoretical, and practical treatise on the tonal appointment and mechanical construction of concert-room, church, and chamber organs.* New York: Dover.

Ayotte, J., I. Peretz, and K. Hyde. 2002. Congenital amusia: A group study of adults afflicted with a music-specific disorder. *Brain* 125 (Pt 2):238–51.

Bangert, M., T. Peschel, G. Schlaug, M. Rotte, D. Drescher, H. Hinrichs, H. J. Heinze, and E. Altenmuller. 2006. Shared networks for auditory and motor processing in professional pianists: Evidence from fMRI conjunction. *Neuroimage* 30 (3):917–26.

Behar, A., W. Wong, and H. Kunov. 2006. Risk of hearing loss in orchestra musicians: Review of the literature. *Med Prob Perform Artists* 21:164–68.

Benade, A. H. 1973. The physics of the brasses. *Sci Am* 229 (July):24–35.

Bendor, D., and X. Wang. 2005. The neuronal representation of pitch in primate auditory cortex. *Nature* 436 (7054):1161–65.

———. 2006. Cortical representations of pitch in monkeys and humans. *Curr Opin Neurobiol* 16 (4):391–99.

Berridge, K. C. 2003. Pleasures of the brain. *Brain Cogn* 52 (1):106–28.

Bicknell, S. 1999. Harmonics and "Cheats," at www.stephenbicknell.org/3.6.01.php (accessed April 23, 2008).

Blood, A. J., and R. J. Zatorre. 2001. Intensely pleasurable responses to music correlate with activity in brain regions implicated in reward and emotion. *Proc Natl Acad Sci USA* 98 (20):11818–23.

Blood, A. J., R. J. Zatorre, P. Bermudez, and A. C. Evans. 1999. Emotional responses to pleasant and unpleasant music correlate with activity in paralimbic brain regions. *Nat Neurosci* 2 (4):382–87.

Brown, M. C. 1999. Audition. In *Fundamental neuroscience*, ed. M. J. Zigmond, F. E. Bloom, S. C. Landis, J. L. Roberts, and L. R. Squire. San Diego: Academic Press.

Brown, S., and M. J. Martinez. 2007. Activation of premotor vocal areas during musical discrimination. *Brain Cogn* 63 (1):59–69.

Brown, S., M. J. Martinez, D. A. Hodges, P. T. Fox, and L. M. Parsons. 2004. The song system of the human brain. *Brain Res Cogn Brain Res* 20 (3):363–75.

Brown, S., M. J. Martinez, and L. M. Parsons. 2004. Passive music listening spontaneously engages limbic and paralimbic systems. *Neuroreport* 15 (13):2033–37.

Burns, E. M. 1999. Intervals, scales and tuning. In *The psychology of music*, ed. D. Deutsch. San Diego: Academic Press.

Chabris, C. F. 1999. Prelude or requiem for the "Mozart effect"? *Nature* 400 (6747):826–27; author reply 827–28.

Chen, J. L., V. B. Penhune, and R. J. Zatorre. 2008. Moving on time: Brain network for auditory-motor synchronization is modulated by rhythm complexity and musical training. *J Cogn Neurosci* 20 (2):226–39.

Dronkers, N. F., O. Plaisant, M. T. Iba-Zizen, and E. A. Cabanis. 2007. Paul Broca's historic cases: High resolution MR imaging of the brains of Leborgne and Lelong. *Brain* 130 (Pt 5):1432–41.

Evers, S., J. Dannert, D. Rodding, G. Rotter, and E. B. Ringelstein. 1999. The cerebral haemodynamics of music perception. A transcranial Doppler sonography study. *Brain* 122 (Pt 1):75–85.

Fletcher, N. H., and T. D. Rossing. 1998. *The physics of musical instruments.* 2nd ed. New York: Springer.

Foxton, J. M., J. L. Dean, R. Gee, I. Peretz, and T. D. Griffiths. 2004. Characterization of deficits in pitch perception underlying "tone deafness." *Brain* 127 (Pt 4):801–10.

Fujioka, T., B. Ross, H. Okamoto, Y. Takeshima, R. Kakigi, and C. Pantev. 2003. Tonotopic representation of missing fundamental complex sounds in the human auditory cortex. *Eur J Neurosci* 18 (2):432–40.

Gaser, C., and G. Schlaug. 2003. Brain structures differ between musicians and non-musicians. *J Neurosci* 23 (27):9240–45.

Gazzola, V., L. Aziz-Zadeh, and C. Keysers. 2006. Empathy and the somatotopic auditory mirror system in humans. *Curr Biol* 16 (18):1824–29.

Gosselin, N., I. Peretz, E. Johnsen, and R. Adolphs. 2007. Amygdala damage impairs emotion recognition from music. *Neuropsychologia* 45 (2):236–44.

Grahn, J. A., and M. Brett. 2007. Rhythm and beat perception in motor areas of the brain. *J Cogn Neurosci* 19 (5):893–906.

Griffiths, T. D. 2001. The neural processing of complex sounds. *Ann NY Acad Sci* 930:133–42.

Griffiths, T. D., and J. D. Warren. 2002. The planum temporale as a computational hub. *Trends Neurosci* 25 (7):348–53.

Halpern, A. R., R. J. Zatorre, M. Bouffard, and J. A. Johnson. 2004. Behavioral and neural correlates of perceived and imagined musical timbre. *Neuropsychologia* 42 (9):1281–92.

Hart, C. W., M. A. Gletman, J. Schubach, and M. Santucci. 1987. The musician and occupational sound hazards. *Med Prob Perform Artists* 2:22–25.

Henderson, D., E. C. Bielefeld, K. C. Harris, and B. H. Hu. 2006. The role of oxidative stress in noise-induced hearing loss. *Ear Hear* 27 (1):1–19.

Henoch, M. A., and K. S. Chesky. 1999. Ear canal resonance as a risk factor in music-induced hearing loss. *Med Prob Perform Artists* 14:103–6.

Hughes, J. R. 2001. The Mozart effect. *J R Soc Med* 94 (6):316.

———. 2002. The Mozart effect: Additional data. *Epilepsy Behav* 3 (2):182–84.

Husain, G., W. F. Thompson, and E. G. Schellenberg. 2002. Effects of music tempo and mode on arousal, mood and spatial abilities. *Music Perception* 20 (2):241–58.

Hyde, K. L., J. P. Lerch, R. J. Zatorre, T. D. Griffiths, A. C. Evans, and I. Peretz. 2007. Cortical thickness in congenital amusia: When less is better than more. *J Neurosci* 27 (47):13028–32.

Hyde, K. L., R. J. Zatorre, T. D. Griffiths, J. P. Lerch, and I. Peretz. 2006. Morphometry of the amusic brain: A two-site study. *Brain* 129 (Pt 10):2562–70.

Jamison, H. L., K. E. Watkins, D. V. Bishop, and P. M. Matthews. 2006. Hemispheric specialization for processing auditory nonspeech stimuli. *Cereb Cortex* 16 (9):1266–75.

Jaramillo, F., V. S. Markin, and A. J. Hudspeth. 1993. Auditory illusions and the single hair cell. *Nature* 364 (6437):527–29.

Kaas, J. H., T. A. Hackett, and M. J. Tramo. 1999. Auditory processing in primate cerebral cortex. *Curr Opin Neurobiol* 9 (2):164–70.

Kaplan, P. W. 2003. Musicogenic epilepsy and epileptic music: A seizure's song. *Epilepsy Behav* 4 (5):464–73.

Keenan, J. P., V. Thangaraj, A. R. Halpern, and G. Schlaug. 2001. Absolute pitch and planum temporale. *Neuroimage* 14 (6):1402–8.

Kim, K. H., N. R. Relkin, K. M. Lee, and J. Hirsch. 1997. Distinct cortical areas associated with native and second languages. *Nature* 388 (6638):171–74.

Kimura, D. 1999. *Sex and cognition.* Cambridge, Mass.: MIT Press.

Koelsch, S. 2006. Significance of Broca's area and ventral premotor cortex for music-syntactic prcessing. *Cortex* 42:518–20.

Koelsch, S., T. Fritz, D. Y. v. Cramon, K. Muller, and A. D. Friederici. 2006. Investigating emotion with music: An fMRI study. *Hum Brain Mapp* 27 (3):239–50.

Kohler, E., C. Keysers, M. A. Umilta, L. Fogassi, V. Gallese, and G. Rizzolatti. 2002. Hearing sounds, understanding actions: Action representation in mirror neurons. *Science* 297 (5582):846–48.

Kubba, A. K., and M. Young. 1996. Ludwig van Beethoven: A medical biography. *Lancet* 347 (8995):167–70.

Levitin, D. J., and S. E. Rogers. 2005. Absolute pitch: Perception, coding, and controversies. *Trends Cogn Sci* 9 (1):26–33.

Liegeois-Chauvel, C., K. Giraud, J. M. Badier, P. Marquis, and P. Chauvel. 2001. Intracerebral evoked potentials in pitch perception reveal a functional asymmetry of the human auditory cortex. *Ann NY Acad Sci* 930:117–32.

Liegeois-Chauvel, C., I. Peretz, M. Babai, V. Laguitton, and P. Chauvel. 1998. Contribution of different cortical areas in the temporal lobes to music processing. *Brain* 121 (Pt 10):1853–67.

Limb, C. J., S. Kemeny, E. B. Ortigoza, S. Rouhani, and A. R. Braun. 2006. Left hemispheric lateralization of brain activity during passive rhythm perception in musicians. *Anat Rec A Discov Mol Cell Evol Biol* 288 (4):382–89.

Luders, E., C. Gaser, L. Jancke, and G. Schlaug. 2004. A voxel-based approach to gray matter asymmetries. *Neuroimage* 22 (2):656–64.

Maess, B., S. Koelsch, T. C. Gunter, and A. D. Friederici. 2001. Musical syntax is processed in Broca's area: An MEG study. *Nat Neurosci* 4 (5):540–45.

Marin, O. S. M., and D. W. Perry. 1999. Neurological aspects of music perception and performance. In *The psychology of music*, ed. D. Deutsch. San Diego: Academic Press.

Menon, V., and D. J. Levitin. 2005. The rewards of music listening: Response and physiological connectivity of the mesolimbic system. *Neuroimage* 28 (1):175–84.

Menon, V., D. J. Levitin, B. K. Smith, A. Lembke, B. D. Krasnow, D. Glazer, G. H. Glover, and S. McAdams. 2002. Neural correlates of timbre change in harmonic sounds. *Neuroimage* 17 (4):1742–54.

Mitterschiffthaler, M. T., C. H. Fu, J. A. Dalton, C. M. Andrew, and S. C. Williams. 2007. A functional MRI study of happy and sad affective states induced by classical music. *Hum Brain Mapp* 28 (11):1150–62.

Munte, T. F. 2002. Brains out of tune. *Nature* 415 (6872):589–90.

Munte, T. F., C. Kohlmetz, W. Nager, and E. Altenmuller. 2001. Neuroperception. Superior auditory spatial tuning in conductors. *Nature* 409 (6820):580.

Nan, Y., T. R. Knosche, S. Zysset, and A. D. Friederici. 2008. Cross-cultural music phrase processing: An fMRI study. *Hum Brain Mapp* 29 (3):312–28.

Nantais, K. M., and E. G. Schellenberg. 1999. The Mozart effect: An artifact of preference. *Psychol Sci* 10:370–73.

Ohnishi, T., H. Matsuda, T. Asada, M. Aruga, M. Hirakata, M. Nishikawa, A. Katoh, and E. Imabayashi. 2001. Functional anatomy of musical perception in musicians. *Cereb Cortex* 11 (8):754–60.

Palin, S. L. 1994. Does classical music damage the hearing of musicians? A review of the literature. *Occup Med (Lond)* 44 (3):130–36.

Pantev, C., R. Oostenveld, A. Engelien, B. Ross, L. E. Roberts, and M. Hoke. 1998. Increased auditory cortical representation in musicians. *Nature* 392 (6678):811–14.

Pantev, C., B. Ross, T. Fujioka, L. J. Trainor, M. Schulte, and M. Schulz. 2003. Music and learning-induced cortical plasticity. *Ann NY Acad Sci* 999:438–50.

Parsons, L. M. 2001. Exploring the functional neuroanatomy of music performance, perception, and comprehension. *Ann NY Acad Sci* 930:211–31.

Passynkova, N., K. Sander, and H. Scheich. 2005. Left auditory cortex specialization for vertical harmonic structure of chords. *Ann NY Acad Sci* 1060:454–56.

Patterson, R. D., S. Uppenkamp, I. S. Johnsrude, and T. D. Griffiths. 2002. The processing of temporal pitch and melody information in auditory cortex. *Neuron* 36 (4):767–76.

Penagos, H., J. R. Melcher, and A. J. Oxenham. 2004. A neural representation of pitch salience in nonprimary human auditory cortex revealed with functional magnetic resonance imaging. *J Neurosci* 24 (30):6810–15.

Peretz, I. 2002. Brain specialization for music. *Neuroscientist* 8 (4):372–80.

Peretz, I., L. Gagnon, and B. Bouchard. 1998. Music and emotion: Perceptual determinants, immediacy, and isolation after brain damage. *Cognition* 68 (2):111–41.

Peretz, I., and K. L. Hyde. 2003. What is specific to music processing? Insights from congenital amusia. *Trends Cogn Sci* 7 (8):362–67.

Peretz, I., and R. J. Zatorre. 2005. Brain organization for music processing. *Annu Rev Psychol* 56:89–114.

Pierce, J. R. 1999. Pitch. In *The psychology of music*, ed. D. Deutsch. San Diego: Academic Press.

Planchart, A. E. 1960. A study of the theories of Giuseppe Tartini. *J Music Theory* 4:32–61.

Pressnitzer, D., R. D. Patterson, and K. Krumbholz. 2001. The lower limit of melodic pitch. *J Acoust Soc Am* 109 (5 Pt 1):2074–84.

Ramachandran, V. S., and E. M. Hubbard. 2003. Hearing colors, tasting shapes. *Sci Am* 288 (5):52–59.

Rasch, R., and R. Plomp. 1999. The perception of musical tones. In *The psychology of music*, ed. D. Deutsch. San Diego: Academic Press.

Rauscher, F. H. 2003. Can music instruction affect children's cognitive development? *ERIC Digest* (September).

Rauscher, F. H., G. L. Shaw, and K. N. Ky. 1993. Music and spatial task performance. *Nature* 365 (6447):611.

———. 1995. Listening to Mozart enhances spatial-temporal reasoning: Towards a neurophysiological basis. *Neurosci Lett* 185 (1):44–47.

Roder, B., W. Teder-Salejarvi, A. Sterr, F. Rosler, S. A. Hillyard, and H. J. Neville. 1999. Improved auditory spatial tuning in blind humans. *Nature* 400 (6740):162–66.

Sacks, O. W. 2007. *Musicophilia: Tales of music and the brain.* New York: Alfred A. Knopf.

Sataloff, R. T. 1991. Hearing loss in musicians. *Am J Otol* 12 (2):122–27.

Schellenberg, E. G. 2006. Exposure to music: The truth about the consequences. In *The child as musician: A handbook of musical development*, ed. G. E. McPherson. Oxford: Oxford University Press.

Schlaug, G., L. Jancke, Y. Huang, and H. Steinmetz. 1995. In vivo evidence of structural brain asymmetry in musicians. *Science* 267 (5198):699–701.

Schneider, P., M. Scherg, H. G. Dosch, H. J. Specht, A. Gutschalk, and A. Rupp. 2002. Morphology of Heschl's gyrus reflects enhanced activation in the auditory cortex of musicians. *Nat Neurosci* 5 (7):688–94.

Schreiner, C. E., and J. A. Winer. 2007. Auditory cortex mapmaking: Principles, projections, and plasticity. *Neuron* 56 (2):356–65.

Shuter-Dyson, R. 1999. Musical ability. In *The psychology of music*, ed. D. Deutsch. San Diego: Academic Press.

Steele, K. M., S. dalla Bella, I. Peretz, T. Dunlop, L. A. Dawe, G. K. Humphrey, R. A. Shannon, J. L. Kirby, Jr., and C. G. Olmstead. 1999. Prelude or requiem for the "Mozart effect"? *Nature* 400 (6747):827–28.

Suteerawattananon, M., G. S. Morris, B. R. Etnyre, J. Jankovic, and E. J. Protas. 2004. Effects of visual and auditory cues on gait in individuals with Parkinson's disease. *J Neurol Sci* 219 (1–2):63–69.

Talavage, T. M., M. I. Sereno, J. R. Melcher, P. J. Ledden, B. R. Rosen, and A. M. Dale. 2004. Tonotopic organization in human auditory cortex revealed by progressions of frequency sensitivity. *J Neurophysiol* 91 (3):1282–96.

Thompson, W. F., E. G. Schellenberg, and G. Husain. 2001. Arousal, mood, and the Mozart effect. *Psychol Sci* 12 (3):248–51.

Tramo, M. J., P. A. Cariani, B. Delgutte, and L. D. Braida. 2001. Neurobiological foundations for the theory of harmony in western tonal music. *Ann NY Acad Sci* 930:92–116.

Turner, R. P. 2004. The acute effect of music on interictal epileptiform discharges. *Epilepsy Behav* 5 (5):662–68.

Warr, W. B., and J. E. Boche. 2003. Diversity of axonal ramifications belonging to single lateral and medial olivocochlear neurons. *Exp Brain Res* 153 (4):499–513.

Warren, J. D., and T. D. Griffiths. 2003. Distinct mechanisms for processing spatial sequences and pitch sequences in the human auditory brain. *J Neurosci* 23 (13):5799–5804.

Watanabe, T., S. Yagishita, and H. Kikyo. 2008. Memory of music: Roles of right hippocampus and left inferior frontal gyrus. *Neuroimage* 39 (1):483–91.

Wieser, H. G., H. Hungerbuhler, A. M. Siegel, and A. Buck. 1997. Musicogenic epilepsy: Review of the literature and case report with ictal single photon emission computed tomography. *Epilepsia* 38 (2):200–207.

Wright Reid, A. 1999. A sound ear, at www.symphony.dk/3info/sound-ear.htm (accessed April 23, 2008).

Yost, William A. 2000. *Fundamentals of hearing: An introduction*. 4th ed. San Diego: Academic Press.

Zatorre, R. J. 2001. Neural specializations for tonal processing. *Ann NY Acad Sci* 930:193–210.

———. 2003. Absolute pitch: A model for understanding the influence of genes and development on neural and cognitive function. *Nat Neurosci* 6 (7):692–95.

Zatorre, R. J., J. L. Chen, and V. B. Penhune. 2007. When the brain plays music: Auditory-motor interactions in music perception and production. *Nat Rev Neurosci* 8 (7):547–58.

Chapter Ten

Performance-Related Stress and Its Management

The stress response is a natural reaction of the body that has evolved to prepare us for extreme physical activity, usually in the face of a major threat from the environment or from the creatures within it. In both animals and humans, this increases the chance of escaping from the danger and as such is vital for survival. In our everyday lives, however, it may be triggered repeatedly by situations that are far from life threatening, and this can interfere with our ability to function normally. This not only has emotional consequences but reduces our control over activities that require precise motor skills. Nowhere is this more evident than in performance-related stress (such as stage fright), which is common among musicians, a group in which it has been studied extensively (for a review see Smith, Maragos, and van Dyke 2000). Performance-related stress can be broken down into two components. The first is known as state anxiety, meaning that it is triggered by particular types of situations. However, the degree to which an individual is susceptible to these situations will depend on his or her psychological makeup. Those who are most vulnerable to it are said to exhibit trait anxiety, that is, they have a predisposition to find the experience of performance threatening rather than challenging or stimulating. Trait anxiety is most common in people who are self-absorbed and have low self-esteem (Kendrick et al. 1982).

Stress can be acute, that is to say, a short-term response to isolated events. However, it can also be a chronic state in which the body is maintained for long periods (days, weeks, or months), and this can have serious consequences for general health. For many people, the origin of stress is in the workplace, where they spend a major proportion of their waking hours. Being at the mercy of an unreasonable or tyrannical boss or conductor will produce stress in most people. Ironically, the behavior of the tyrant may itself stem from a feeling of insecurity at being in the seat of command or from the worries about fulfilling the expectations or demands of superiors. Chronic stress may also be a self-generated symptom of trait anxiety, arising from feelings of inadequacy. The sufferer may feel that his or her performance is not up to standard or that colleagues are critical of his or her abilities, regardless of whether this has any basis in fact.

Though stress is primarily associated in our minds with unpleasant situations, this is by no means always the case. The thrill of anticipation before a first date is brought

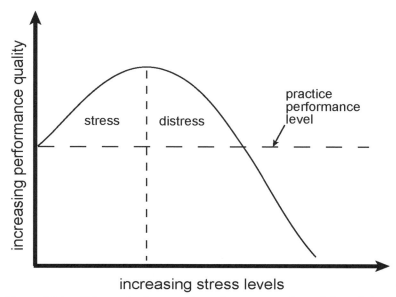

Figure 10-1. This graph gives a schematic representation of the relationship between stress and performance. Low levels of stress increase alertness and prime the body for action, all of which can improve the quality of the performance. As stress levels rise, however, the performer may experience a loss of fine muscle control and experience muscle tremor. A number of other symptoms such as dry mouth, rapid breathing, feelings of nausea, and failure of short-term memory may appear, all of which conspire to reduce the ability to perform effectively.

about by the physical manifestations of the stress response, while the attraction of many rides at fairgrounds or theme parks or of extreme sports comes from the adrenaline rush generated by brief exposure to a more or less controlled stressful situation.

Performance, whether musical or sporting, is likely to benefit from a degree of stress. As we shall see, the stress response prepares the metabolic systems of the body for activity and so is necessary for peak physical performance. If you go onstage feeling too relaxed or lethargic, your performance will remain lackluster, even if it is technically very proficient. For a really excellent performance, not only must all the resources for the physical aspects of playing or singing be at your command, but it is also necessary to be mentally alert or charged. We can therefore imagine a notional relationship between the level of stress and performance quality such as the one shown in figure 10-1. Here quality increases with stress up to a certain level, beyond which it declines as the physical symptoms of stress become increasingly deleterious (Steptoe and Fidler 1987; Everly and Rosenfeld 1981). In this diagram, the section labeled "stress" reflects not simply the physical changes that have been wrought on the body, but how we as individuals respond to this psychologically. As we become more experienced with performance or as we acquire strategies to deal with it, the physical symptoms of performance-related stress may or may not decline, but how we respond to or harness these changes to our advantage certainly does. This chapter will therefore pay particular attention to a range of methods that can be used to manage stress.

THE PHYSICAL SYMPTOMS OF STRESS

We are all familiar with the physical manifestations of acute stress; we experience them during an audition, a job interview, or when we find ourselves in an emotional or physical confrontation or a frightening situation. Our heart rate increases and may become more forceful so that we feel it thumping in our chest. We start to sweat, but because the skin has not yet become heated by the activity of the muscles beneath, this sweat feels cold. We may feel the hair on the scalp or the rest of the skin rising, have the sensation of butterflies in the stomach, and even become nauseous. Breathing becomes rapid and shallow and the mouth dry, and the muscles (including those involved in breathing and controlling the hands) may tremble, making the physical aspects of singing and playing difficult. In addition, the mind may go blank (a failure of working memory) so that music previously safely committed to memory becomes difficult or impossible to recall. If you have a vivid imagination, you may already be feeling uncomfortable just from reading this list! With chronic stress, additional symptoms may arise. One of these is called somatization, which is the appearance of physical symptoms that, while perfectly real to the sufferer, may have no organic basis. These symptoms can include pain (e.g., in the arm, chest, or abdomen), headaches, or fatigue. Somatization is one reason why accurate diagnosis of musicians' ailments (e.g., hand or arm pain) can be difficult and needs to be based on a complete case history and an appreciation of all of the relevant lifestyle factors. Without this, there is a risk that inappropriate and potentially damaging treatment may be advocated. Chronic stress may also lead to a reduction in the effectiveness of the immune system, resulting in an increased susceptibility to infection (Lovallo 2005). For example, studies of adolescents and medical students under exam and other stressful conditions have shown that they have an increased chance of falling victim to viral infections such as herpes, glandular fever (mononucleosis), or throat infections.

Unrelieved stress can in the long term induce or aggravate a number of other health problems. The increased demands on the heart and the constriction of blood vessels to the organs can contribute to high blood pressure (hypertension), the occurrence of migraines, and heart disease. Stress can have a number of effects on the gastrointestinal system. It can lead to excessive acid secretion in the stomach, which may contribute to the development of gastric ulcers, and aggravate irritable bowel syndrome and other related diseases. It can be associated with gastroesophageal reflux, in which the acid contents of the stomach rise into the esophagus. This causes heartburn and irritates the lining of the esophagus and may have particular consequences for singers (see chapter 5). It is not uncommon for asthma and skin conditions such as eczema to flare up. Finally, as discussed below, chronic stress can also trigger general or clinical depression.

HOW THE NERVOUS SYSTEM GENERATES
THE STRESS RESPONSE

The reaction of the nervous system to stress can be divided into two phases. The first is responsible for the recognition that a situation is threatening or stressful, while the second produces the appropriate physiological changes needed to cope with this. We will address these in turn.

The Limbic System

The recognition of a situation as being potentially stressful is the responsibility of the limbic system. This is a network composed of a number of areas in the forebrain (fig. 7-4C). We frequently worry about certain forthcoming events because of past experiences, so it should be no surprise to discover that two areas of the cortex that are involved in memory belong to the limbic system. One (the hippocampus) is responsible for laying down what is known as declarative memory—the memory of facts, events, and places, while another region (the amygdala) is responsible for the emotional aspects of memory. Activity in the amygdala is particularly associated with negative emotions such as fear. Both types of memory are inextricably linked to our interpretation of future situations. Clearly the emotional content of a memory will play a significant role in determining whether we regard situations as posing a threat or not. For example, hearing a particular piece of music may have little or no significance for one person, while for another, it may trigger strong positive (e.g., romantic) or negative (apprehensive) emotions depending on the circumstances in which it has been previously encountered. The hippocampus makes the association, while the amygdala indicates the emotional coloring. Associated with the limbic system are regions of the prefrontal cortex (the part of the brain lying just behind the forehead) where we plan our future actions. Through our imaginations we can construct a form of virtual reality through which we can play out various possible scenarios in order to consider what their consequences might be. This makes use of emotional memories and so, just by thinking about how a forthcoming performance may go, we can generate real physical responses. What we imagine will, of course, be shaped by past experience. If we have had a previous performance failure, we will worry more, whereas if our experiences were good, we will be more relaxed. These imagined scenarios may be quite irrational. For example, our apprehension may be greater at a venue where we once had a bad experience, even though everything has gone well since, but this doesn't make the feelings any less real. Clearly, the danger is that overanxiety about a negative outcome may contribute to the prophecy becoming self-fulfilling. This negative outlook is sometimes known as catastrophization—imagining only the worst possible outcome. On the other hand, with help it should also be possible to use our mental resources to reduce stress by reinterpreting potentially threatening situations that we know we will have to encounter.

The Hypothalamus and the Autonomic Nervous System

The physical manifestation of the emotional responses generated by the limbic system is controlled mainly by the hypothalamus (fig. 7-4A). This is the major center in the brain for maintaining what is known as homeostasis; that is, it regulates the metabolic processes of the body so that they are set at a level that is appropriate for the current situation. This control is exerted through the action of nerves and hormones. If the body becomes cold, mechanisms are set in motion by the hypothalamus to increase its temperature by mobilizing energy reserves and increasing muscular activity (including shivering) and through a reduction of heat loss by diverting blood away from the skin. It may also stimulate appetite to increase food intake. If the body becomes dehydrated, the hypothalamus increases fluid retention by the kidneys and generates a feeling of thirst to encourage drinking. In terms of the stress response, the crucial factor is that the hypothalamus also has the ability to switch body metabolism from a state that is compatible with passivity to one that will support the vigorous activity appropriate when facing a threat. It achieves its objectives through two executive arms. The first is the autonomic nervous system, which is described below. The second is through the release of hormones into the bloodstream, either from the pituitary gland, which hangs from the underside of the brain just below the hypothalamus, or from other hormone-secreting glands within the body. For the stress response, the most important hormonal response comes from what is known as the hypothalamic pituitary adrenal cortical system. Under the control of the hypothalamus, the pituitary gland releases a signal molecule into the bloodstream that activates the adrenal glands (fig. 10-2). These sit like a cap on top of the kidneys and are composed of two parts. The cores of the glands secrete adrenaline (which we will consider later), while the outer part (the cortex) secretes into the bloodstream hormones such as cortisol that play a major role in the stress response. Cortisol promotes the formation of glucose, which is the fuel that cells burn to produce energy from reserves stored in the body. However, it also suppresses the immune system, and though this is of little significance in the short term, we have seen that it may cause problems in chronic stress.

The autonomic nervous system regulates the distribution of blood to the muscles, organs, and skin and also controls the activity of glands such as those producing saliva, sweat, and digestive enzymes. It has two main divisions, known as the sympathetic and the parasympathetic systems (fig. 10-2). The parasympathetic system exerts its actions through many of the cranial nerves (see chapter 7) and through nerves that emerge from the lower (sacral) part of the spinal cord. When we are slumped on the sofa in front of the fire after a heavy meal, it is the parasympathetic nervous system that is ascendant. Under these circumstances, blood flow is directed to the gut, and we feel drowsy because less is going to the brain. Digestion is promoted through the secretion of saliva into the mouth and digestive enzymes in the gut, while the muscular walls of the stomach and intestines contract rhythmically to mix the food and enzymes together. The heart rate slows, the pupils become smaller, and the bronchioles in the lungs narrow as the oxygen demands of the body decline.

The sympathetic nervous system, by contrast, prepares the body for action or, as some would have it, "the three Fs"—fight, flight, or frolic! The nerves responsible emerge from the thoracic and upper lumbar segments of the spinal cord (fig. 10-2). These merge to form a strip of nervous tissue called the sympathetic trunk, which runs up into the neck and down into the abdomen and sends out branches to reach all regions of the body. The sympathetic nervous system generates many of the symptoms

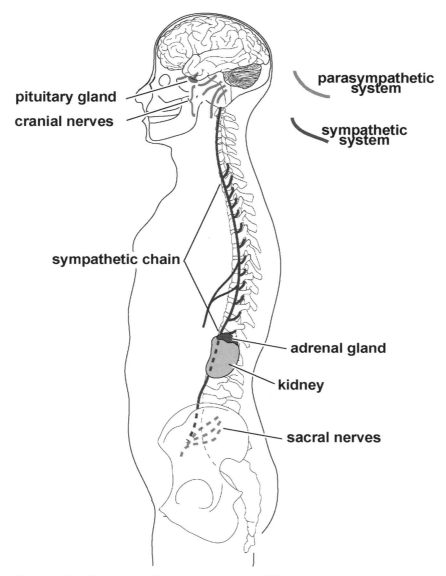

pituitary gland

cranial nerves

parasympathetic
system

sympathetic
system

sympathetic chain

adrenal gland

kidney

sacral nerves

Figure 10-2. The autonomic nervous system. This has two major divisions: the sympathetic and the parasympathetic systems. The sympathetic system prepares the body for action. Nerves from the thoracic and upper lumbar segments of the spinal cord combine to form the sympathetic trunk, which runs up the side of the vertebral column. This sends out branches to supply the organs, blood vessels, and glands. Its actions increase heart rate, open up the bronchioles of the lungs, enlarge the pupils, direct blood to the muscles and skin, and cause sweating and the rising of hairs in the skin. The parasympathetic system has the opposite action, preparing the body for a more passive role. It contributes to many cranial nerves and also to nerves that arise from the lower (sacral) regions of the spinal cord. It reduces heart rate and makes the pupils smaller and the bronchioles narrower. It also directs blood toward the internal organs and promotes digestive activity in the gut.

of the stress response. Nerves running to adrenal glands cause the release of adrenaline into the bloodstream. Heart rate increases and blood is directed away from organs such as the gut and toward the muscles of the limbs and trunk. One of the actions adrenaline can have is to produce muscle tremor, a problem many musicians are all too familiar with. The pupils enlarge and the bronchioles in the lungs widen to make it easier to take in air. The hair on the skin may rise, and we begin to sweat in preparation for cooling the body when the expected muscle activity starts. In addition, as the parasympathetic system shuts down, the mouth may become dry as the flow of saliva slows.

ANXIETY IN PERFORMANCE

A number of investigations have sought to reveal the physiological consequences of performance-related anxiety among musicians (Fredrikson and Gunnarsson 1992). In one study, the musicians were asked to take part in two playing sessions, one of which was a practice without an audience and the other a performance of the same music in front of an audience. The musicians were divided into two groups on the basis of how they themselves rated their typical level of performance anxiety. Interestingly, though the heart rate during performance was higher in the anxious group, the levels of adrenaline and cortisol did not appear to differ significantly between the more anxious and the less anxious musicians. Though many other studies have also reported a link between heart rate and self-assessed levels of confidence (Abel and Larkin 1990), one found that though heart rate increases during public performance, it is not related to subjective anxiety levels (Craske and Craig 1984). Assessment of performance quality by an adjudicating panel generally confirmed that the anxious students performed less well. This slightly confusing picture is probably a consequence of a number of differences between the design of the studies such as 1) the relatively small number of subjects in each study, 2) possible differences in the levels of experience and performance history between the groups of musicians studied, 3) a lack of standardization in how and when anxiety or confidence were measured, and 4) gender imbalances between some of the groups compared. This last point may have considerable significance as in one study, though the males were found to show greater increases in blood pressure immediately prior to performance, it was the females who reported greater levels of anxiety (Abel and Larkin 1990). However, the general trend that emerges from these studies is that performance anxiety is not related in a simple way to the physiological manifestations of stress. This emphasizes the importance of trait anxiety, whether intrinsic or reinforced by experience. We have already encountered the idea that a degree of stress is required to support high levels of performance, and this is well recognized by performers (Steptoe 1989). The crucial factor is therefore how one responds to it. Being inhibited by performance anxiety can be contrasted with the emotions reflected in phrases such as "being up for it," which are associated with a stressful situations where the negative aspects are overridden by positive strategies used to build self-belief. Consciously or unconsciously, self-congratulatory rituals are often used by sports teams for this purpose.

COPING WITH STRESS

There is no single magic bullet for dealing with stress. Surveys of coping strategies that are used by musicians to combat stage fright reveal a broad range of approaches. These include distraction techniques, the use of ritual, physical strategies including deep breathing and muscle relaxation, positive self-talk, and the use of drug treatments, preferably under medical supervision (Wolfe 1990; Steptoe 1989). Some techniques are directed primarily at stress management, while for the others this is just one of a broader range of objectives directed at the physical and emotional well-being of the performer. Because the origin as well as the nature of the stress response varies between individuals, so will the attraction and suitability of different coping strategies. There is no right or wrong approach; it is a matter of individual choice. Practical guidance in some of these techniques can be obtained from a variety of sources (e.g., Everly and Rosenfeld 1981; Connolly and Williamon 2004).

Exerting Control and Taking Responsibility

One factor that contributes significantly to how stressful a situation feels is the degree of control that the individual feels he or she can exert over the situation. Jobs that make high demands yet allow little control over decision making tend to lead to psychological stress. This is equally true of other life situations such as family relationships. An investigation into career stress in orchestral musicians suggested that many felt this to be a significant negative aspect of their working lives, though other factors such as irregular hours, the monotony of rehearsals, and separation from their families were also significant (Steptoe 1989). Being or feeling intimidated by the conductor is frequently cited as a major stressor (Wynn Parry 1998). On the other hand, unlike many stress-inducing occupations, a number of aspects of orchestral musicians' life provide sources of satisfaction and fulfillment (e.g., job variety, the pleasure of orchestral playing, and traveling). The long-term effects of control or the lack of it have been revealed in a series of fascinating studies of civil servants, which have found that senior grades, who exercise control to the greatest extent, live longer and have a lower risk of physical ailments such as heart disease than those in more junior positions (Marmot 1997). One way of reducing stress is therefore to find some way of exerting control. Some orchestras are now managed by the players, which should help matters considerably; however, this is not going to be a general solution. If one feels intimidated at work, taking a course in assertiveness that teaches individuals to make their feelings or wishes clear in ways that are firm but not based on anger may make a significant difference. With the increase in confidence this brings may come a realization that many perceived threats or criticisms are considerably exaggerated. If an orchestral player does several other things to make ends meet, such as teaching or session work, it may be that limiting or consolidating these activities will improve quality of life by reducing stress, even if income declines to some extent. The stress associated with the job should not be seen in isolation from life's other stressors such as balancing family commitments, and assertiveness training may help the performer manage these also. The other side of control is taking responsibility for one's actions (Everly and Rosenfeld 1981). Each person is to a large extent responsible for much of the stress in their daily lives in the sense that they themselves make the decision to take on certain work-related commitments, to adopt a given lifestyle, or to either put up with or resist particular patterns of behavior in others. A conscious acceptance of this is the first step in taking control.

Psychological Strategies

One popular approach to the treatment of performance-related anxiety is based on cognitive-behavioral therapy (Arcier 2000; Connolly 1997; Connolly and Williamon 2004). As the name suggests, this has two aspects, one of which is to change the subject's perceptions (cognition) of the stressful situation and hence the emotional response this engenders, while the second is to control the behavioral response to it. Stage fright is frequently associated with catastrophizing—being fixated on the worst possible outcome and its consequences. By contrast, effective coping strategies are best manifested by a realistic assessment that accepts that while small deficiencies may occur in a performance, these need not seriously affect audience perceptions and enjoyment or peer opinion (Steptoe and Fidler 1987). The therapy seeks to promote the realization that catastrophizing can become self-fulfilling and that in order to break the cycle it is necessary to replace the negative attitude with a more positive one. On the other hand, one will want to avoid the opposite extreme of being totally blasé, as this is unlikely to have a positive effect on performance quality! The behavioral arm of the therapy involves learning techniques to control the physiological response to stress. For example, the performer will be taught relaxation techniques and, once in a calm state of mind and body, will be taught to maintain this while being taken through a mental exploration of progressively more stressful situations leading up to a major performance scenario. This combines physical coping strategies (such as awareness of tension, muscle relaxation, and breath control) that can be used in the run-up to an actual performance, with an attempt to control the emotional response through familiarization (Connolly 1997). Of course these, and the purely physical strategies we will encounter next, also contribute to the feeling of being in control of the situation because the physical manifestations of stress are kept in check. The therapy may also involve actual performances, starting with small audiences that are known to be sympathetic (family, friends, or fellow students) and building up to more typical real-life audience situations. This may be particularly beneficial where stage fright has either been triggered initially or subsequently reinforced by bad experiences of public performance.

Meditation can be an effective means of stress reduction. Though it has been employed in many forms for centuries, it is only relatively recently that it has gained wide acceptance and respectability in the West. It may take place within the context of a religion or philosophy (e.g., Buddhism, certain forms of Christian prayer ritual) or be an entirely secular device (yoga and transcendental meditation). A central element of most systems is to focus the attention on a single subject. This can be a rhythmic physical activity, usually breathing (e.g., paranayama in hatha yoga) or the repetition of a phrase or syllable (e.g., a mantra such as the Buddhist "Om mani padme hum"). Alternatively, it may be a mental task such as the contemplation of an irresolvable problem (e.g., the Zen paradox of one hand clapping) or the visualization of an object or pattern such as a mandala (Everly and Rosenfeld 1981). Meditation serves to occupy the mind and reduce or eliminate the attention paid to other thoughts or sensations. There is growing evidence that the mental states brought about by the different forms of meditation are basically similar (Newberg and Iversen 2003). They are characterized by striking changes in the pattern of brain activity, which become more marked as the skill of the meditator increases (Lutz et al. 2004). In particular, there is a change in the frequencies of dominant rhythms of electrical activity in the cortex. The parasympathetic arm of the autonomic system gains the upper hand and metabolic rate falls. There is also an inhibition of areas of the sensory cortex that provide us with a three-dimensional awareness of the position of the body in space, and this may underlie the feeling of physical detachment or of a oneness with the external world that often results (Newberg and Iversen 2003). The areas of the brain whose roles in the stress response we have already discussed (the prefrontal cortex, limbic system, and hypothalamus) are all affected. Meditation tends to lower blood pressure, causing cells in the hypothalamus to release a hormone called vasopressin from the pituitary. Vasopressin narrows the arteries to return the blood pressure to normal levels, but it also appears to reduce feelings of fatigue and to have both a calming effect and a positive influence on mood (Newberg and Iversen 2003).

Physical Strategies

Some of the physical strategies utilized in stress management have already been encountered as elements of more psychological approaches. Two of the most common are breath control and muscle relaxation (Everly and Rosenfeld 1981). Used on their own, either of these techniques (but particularly breath control) can be useful during the period immediately before a performance. Breath control usually involves deep, slow breathing, which engages the muscles of the abdomen as well as those of the diaphragm and chest wall (see chapter 4). The duration of the various phases of breathing (inhalation, holding the lungs full, exhalation) is often regulated by counting. It is important to avoid overbreathing (breathing deeply and fast when the body is not active) because this can reduce the levels of carbon dioxide in the blood sufficiently to induce symptoms such as dizziness, tunnel vision, and even fainting. Though carbon dioxide is a waste product of respiration, it also plays an important role in controlling the acid-base balance of the blood. If levels of circulating carbon dioxide fall too far, the vessels supplying the brain start to shut down, reducing its blood supply. This is what produces the symptoms just described. Hyperventilation can also be seen as a symptom of the stress response, for which the simplest remedy is to breathe in and out from a paper or plastic bag. Rebreathing the exhaled air, which is rich in carbon dioxide, is the quickest way to return its concentration in the blood to the correct level.

The muscle tension that is associated with stress can be addressed through relaxation exercises. The feature that distinguishes this type of relaxation from simply slumping into your favorite chair is that attention is directed onto each of the major sets of muscles in turn and the tension in them is consciously observed before they are relaxed. Many systems advocate contracting the muscles strongly before relaxing them to make the release more obvious. It is necessary to do this because we are generally unaware of chronic muscle tension (indeed, if we were aware of it, the tension would probably never become chronic), so it is quite possible to be lying in bed thinking you are relaxed, with the muscles in your shoulders knotted and those of your face tightly contracted. An important element of all relaxation techniques is therefore to learn to recognize the muscle tension to which you have become oblivious. Once you are lying or sitting comfortably, muscle groups are worked through systematically in a simple, easily remembered order. For example, you might start first with the feet, then the ankles, lower legs, thighs, and so on. Initially one has to be constantly vigilant against the return of the habitual tension, not only in the large muscle groups, but also in the smaller ones, particularly those of the face, whose activity can be highly significant in stress. Apart from the unnecessary tension in postural muscles that is a feature of stress in everyday life, the musician also needs to seek out inappropriate tension in the muscles used in performance. Some of these may also be postural, but others will be those that control the arm or the hand. For example, in chapter 3, the negative consequences of excessive finger tension and of the co-contraction of antagonistic finger muscles were discussed. To eliminate this it is necessary to make a constant and conscious effort to reduce muscle activity to the minimum that is compatible with playing, something that is much more difficult than simple relaxation exercises performed outside the context of playing. One approach that could be more widely employed in treating chronic muscle tension in musicians would be to use a type of biofeedback in which information on muscle activity is collected from electrodes placed on the surface of the skin. This can then presented on a screen to give an objective and real-time indication of levels of muscle tension (Markison 1998; Levee, Cohen, and Rickles 1976).

Postural therapies such as the Alexander technique, tai chi, or yoga also have a role to play in stress reduction. These frequently incorporate breath control and muscle relaxation as part of their regimen but may offer other physical benefits. Followers of these therapies feel that they derive considerable benefit from them, and this belief alone may be sufficient to produce positive results. In conventional medicine nowadays, great emphasis is given to objective testing of new therapies, and it is felt that the same approach should be used for existing techniques that claim to provide specific health benefits. One of the difficulties in obtaining evidence of this type is that large numbers of participants are required by such studies if clear results are to emerge. Nonetheless, some recent preliminary investigations into the effectiveness of the Alexander technique on stress in musicians suggest that although it appears to have no effect on heart rate, it may produce a moderate reduction in levels of anxiety and an improvement in performance in low-stress situations (Valentine 1995, 2004; Valentine and Williamon 2003).

The general benefits of exercise and weight control are well known; however, in the context of stress relief their effect on heart rate and blood pressure is particularly relevant. Exercise, especially when accompanied by weight loss, reduces both resting heart rate and blood pressure and the degree to which these increase under conditions of stress, including those of musical performance (Georgiades et al. 2000; Taylor and Wasley 2004). Exercise also improves mental outlook or mood, an effect that becomes more pronounced and long lasting with increasing fitness (Petruzzello, Hall, and Ekkekakis 2001). In addition, the physical fatigue that results from exercise has a beneficial effect on sleep patterns. An important aspect of exercise and weight control through dieting is consistency. Following a strict diet or an intensive exercise program for a short period and then dropping it will have little or no long-term benefit. Exercise does not need to be an hour of intensive circuit training every day but should be tailored to your current level of fitness. Choose something that you can easily manage and hopefully enjoy and build up the intensity as you become able. For example, you might begin with one session of twenty to thirty minutes once a week for the first month, then two sessions of similar or slightly greater length for the next month, and so on (Taylor and Wasley 2004). As your physical condition improves, you will probably find that you are increasingly looking forward to these sessions and will not want to miss the feelings of well-being and satisfaction it gives. Exercise can be walking or cycling to work, swimming, team sports, or aerobics. It might be yoga, tai chi, or Pilates. It can be a solitary or a communal activity depending on inclination or convenience. You may also want to vary what you do, especially if some of your activities are likely to be affected by the weather or the season. The exercise sessions should be built into your daily activities so that they occur within a routine that allocates both to them and your other commitments adequate time for fulfillment. This will ensure that the benefits are not immediately dissipated by a stress-inducing rush at the beginning and end of each session. If you think you do not have time, you may need to reconsider your priorities! If you are often on tour, you will also want to devise a "portable" form of exercise such as regular walking or jogging. Some musicians exercise on the day of a performance as part of their preparation, but before such a scheme is implemented it is important to experiment carefully in order to work out the best time for this and how intensive it should be.

Detailed advice on diet is beyond the scope of this book, but the rules for successful weight loss are similar to those for gaining fitness. In the long term, losing weight means changing eating habits permanently, and this is most likely to be effective through combining a moderate reduction in food intake with a controlled increase in exercise. The result of this approach will be a relatively slow but sustained reduction in weight. It is better to eat a normal healthy diet, but less of it, than to follow one of the overhyped crash courses based on dubious nutritional premises that are constantly being publicized. The trouble with such diets is that even if they work, they are often so grueling that by the end you feel that you deserve the "reward" of returning to old habits! Instead, you should learn to become accustomed to food or drinks that are less sweet, to using reduced-fat milk, leaner meat, and unsaturated fats, and to eating more fruit and vegetables. Diet can also have a more direct influence on the stress response. Excessive amounts of caffeine can produce symptoms similar to stress and a high salt intake raises blood pressure, so it is important to control their consumption. A sustainable diet is not one without pleasure, but one in which overindulgence is resisted.

PHARMACOLOGICAL APPROACHES
TO STRESS MANAGEMENT

Drugs of one sort or another have been used in stress reduction for thousands of years. Some are so familiar to us that we don't even think of them in this way, but alcohol, caffeine, and nicotine are as much drugs as tranquilizers, antidepressants, and illegal drugs of abuse. They all have potent biological effects, and many can be used both for good and for ill. It is important to recognize the full range of effects that these drugs can produce and, even if they are prescribed for you by a doctor, to understand their action and possible side effects. It is up to you to take an active role in the decision about what is appropriate for you.

Alcohol and Nicotine

The most easily obtainable and traditionally used drugs for stress relief are alcohol and nicotine, and their use, past and present, has been widespread among musicians. While moderate drinking may be a perfectly acceptable means of reducing inhibitions and facilitating social interaction at the postperformance party, it is much less acceptable as a means of dealing with the anxiety of the performance itself. Even small amounts will impair the fine motor control needed for playing of a good standard as well as have an adverse effect on the ability to recall the music, though it may engender a frame of mind in which this doesn't appear to matter much at the time! One general effect of alcohol is to reduce the ability to perceive the loss of physical control, which makes it difficult for the drinker to find a balance between reducing anxiety and an unacceptable loss of technique. This will, however, be more obvious to fellow players and to the audience. Chronic excesses in alcohol consumption may ultimately lead to an increase in anxiety as well as other psychological problems such as addiction and physical damage to the liver and other organs. There are many better ways to deal with performance-related stress than this! It should also be appreciated that even socially acceptable levels of alcohol intake may be incompatible with other medications for stress such as tranquilizers and antidepressants. If these are prescribed for you, information on their compatibility with alcohol should be sought from your doctor.

Nicotine acts on the nervous system by mimicking one of the chemical neurotransmitters (acetylcholine) that nerve cells use to communicate. Contrary to common belief, nicotine acts as a stimulant and not a calming agent (Britton et al. 2000). It increases heart rate and blood pressure and the release of the stress hormone cortisol into the bloodstream. When the heart works harder, the blood vessels supplying its muscular walls become wider to increase the oxygen available to the tissue; however, nicotine can prevent this, especially in those whose arteries are already partly blocked with fatty deposits. Another effect is to increase hand tremor, which declines only as the nicotine gradually disappears from the circulation as it is broken down by the body. Nicotine also increases metabolic rate and suppresses appetite so that weight is reduced. On ceasing smoking, appetite and weight rise for six to twelve months; however, both should then return to presmoking levels. Smoking does not reduce anxiety, and the idea that it does is due to confusion about the origin of the physical symptoms seen in smokers who have not smoked for a short while or who try to quit. The feelings of irritability and restlessness that ensue are in fact withdrawal symptoms from nicotine dependence. Though nicotine is highly addictive, it does not in itself cause cancer. The high incidence of lung cancer among smokers is the result of exposure to a toxic cocktail of other compounds found in the smoke.

Prescription Drugs

Pharmacological treatment of serious chronic stress in the general population is based on tranquilizing drugs that reduce anxiety (anxiolytics) or promote sleep (hypnotics) and on antidepressants. We will deal with depression and antidepressants later in the chapter. The anxiolytics and hypnotics most widely prescribed today belong to a family of compounds known as benzodiazepines that include such well-known drugs as Valium (also known as diazepam) and Librium (West 2004). Though they vary to some extent in their properties, they all produce a degree of sedation, and this will clearly have a deleterious effect on the ability to carry out the type of complex behavior that underpins musical performance. In some of the newer benzodiazepines (e.g., buspirone) these symptoms are less severe; however, in one study of performance anxiety that compared buspirone treatment with cognitive-behavioral therapy in a group of musicians, the drug did not appear to have any marked effect (Clark and Agras 1991). Though the results must be treated with caution due to the small number of people involved in the study, there did appear to be a significant improvement in the group undergoing cognitive-behavioral therapy. Tranquilizers are potentially addictive and should never be prescribed for long periods. They should only be obtained on prescription and their use should be closely monitored by a doctor. Given the consequences of their side effects for the musician, their use in treating stress that is purely performance related is often questionable (James 1998).

Many musicians have encountered drugs known as beta blockers, which can be used to cope with the physical symptoms of performance-related anxiety. One much-quoted and extensive survey of the medical problems in orchestral musicians in the United States reported that up to 27 percent of the respondees had tried them at one time or another (Fishbein et al. 1998). Beta blockers act on the tissues that are the targets of the sympathetic nervous system. Most have relatively little effect on the brain, so while they reduce the physical symptoms of stress (e.g., increased heart rate and blood pressure, tremor), they have no direct effect on the psychological aspects of stress such as the inability to sleep or the presence of negative thoughts. The actions of the sympathetic nervous system during stress are brought about partly through the actions of a chemical neurotransmitter called noradrenaline (also known as norepinephrine), which is released from nerve endings, and partly through the release into the circulation of the hormone adrenaline (or epinephrine) from the adrenal glands. Noradrenaline and adrenaline bind to receptor proteins (called adrenoreceptors) in the heart and smooth muscle cells found in the walls of blood vessels or in the visceral organs to produce the physical manifestations of the stress response. There are several types of adrenoreceptors, but the stress response is mainly associated with a type known as beta-adrenoreceptors. Beta blockers work by interfering with the binding of adrenaline and noradrenaline to beta-adrenoreceptors. They were originally developed for the treatment of angina, where their role is to prevent the heart from becoming overtaxed during stress and to control high blood pressure, but their effectiveness in treating stress-related symptoms in normal individuals, particularly musicians, was quickly realized (Brandfonbrener 1990). There are now many beta blockers available. These each have slightly different properties; which one is prescribed will depend on the precise nature of an individual's stress symptoms (Nies 1990; West 2004). For example, not all are effective against tremor, which is likely to be an important concern for many players (James 1998). Beta blockers, like all prescription drugs, have powerful effects. You should therefore never use medication prescribed for someone else, but should always consult your doctor directly if you are considering these as an option. He or she will check that they are suitable for you and select the appropriate type, dosage, and pattern of use. Though quite safe when obtained and used in this way, they can be dangerous for those with certain medical conditions such as bronchial asthma, low blood pressure, and some other problems. In the case of asthma, for example, they will counteract the effect of the drugs in inhalers, leaving the patient in a dangerous situation during an attack. They are also not appropriate for performers who must be physically active, such as dancers, because their effect on cardiac output will curtail the ability to sustain high levels of muscular activity.

A consideration of the effects of drugs of abuse is beyond the scope of this book, but an informed and thoughtful consideration of the risks these present, together with further information on the drugs already mentioned, can be found in West (2004).

DEPRESSION

We all get fed up from time to time and may complain about being depressed. This mood generally only lasts for a few hours or days at most and we remain perfectly capable of continuing our normal daily lives. We may respond to feeling down by indulging in some energetic exercise or by seeking out pleasurable experiences of one sort or another, for example, taking a holiday or perhaps indulging in "retail therapy." Stress can cause this type of depression. For example, it can be triggered by an unpleasant incident at work that knocks our self-esteem, or the feeling of being undervalued. Musicians, whose performance is under constant scrutiny not only by others, but also by themselves, may feel particularly vulnerable. However, prolonged stress can also lead to a group of altogether more serious conditions that are classified under the heading of clinical or major depression. There are several types of clinical depression, but they are usually divided into two broad categories. The first is unipolar depression, in which the changes in mood are entirely negative. By contrast, bipolar depression (also known as manic depression) is characterized by violent mood swings between the extremes of depression and overexcitement.

Unipolar Depression

The main classification scheme used for depression in the United States, the *Diagnostic and Statistical Manual of Mental Disorders* (*DSM-IV*; see American Psychiatric

Association 1995) requires the presence of five of the following symptoms over a period of two weeks for a diagnosis of clinical depression:

- Depressed mood most of the day
- Diminished interest or pleasure
- Significant gain or loss of weight
- Inability to sleep or sleeping too much
- Reduced control over bodily movements
- Fatigue
- Feelings of worthlessness or guilt
- Inability to think or concentrate
- Thoughts of suicide or death

However, such phrases give little idea of what clinical depression actually feels like; indeed, depressed individuals find it almost impossible to describe their feelings in words. In severe cases it is an overwhelming sadness and apathy generally coupled with a total lack of energy so that even simple tasks such as getting out of bed and taking a shower present insuperable obstacles. This is difficult for the family or friends of the depressed person to cope with because it represents a mental state so far outside the bounds of normal experience that it makes it very hard for them to empathize with it. The natural reaction is to tell the depressed person to "snap out of it," which is how we try to respond to a normal bout of the blues, but a request like this to take control of the situation encapsulates precisely what is impossible for someone suffering from clinical depression. Clinical depression is a common condition. Approximately 5 percent of the population is likely to be affected at any one time, with women being twice as likely to experience it as men. The prevalence of depression may come as a surprise, but even today there is a considerable and completely unjustified stigma against it, which stops many sufferers from wanting to talk about it. Recently, however, some very eloquent books have been written about depression by individuals who have suffered from it. Two of these are *Malignant Sadness* by Lewis Wolpert (1999) and *An Unquiet Mind* by Kay Jamison (1996), and anyone who wishes to understand more about its various forms and how it can be treated will find these to be invaluable sources of information.

Bipolar Depression

As the name suggests, a person with bipolar or manic depression experiences abrupt swings between two extreme emotional states. The depressed state is similar to the one we have just encountered in unipolar depression. The symptoms of the manic phase as listed in *DSM-IV* are given below. The presence of any three is regarded as being indicative of the condition:

- Overactivity
- Increased talkativeness or pressure of speech
- Flight of ideas or racing thoughts

- Inflated self-esteem
- Decreased need for sleep
- Distractibility
- Indiscreet behavior with poor judgment
- Marked impairment in occupational or social function

This is probably best illustrated by an example. The writer Virginia Woolf suffered from bipolar depression, and Wolpert (1999) presents a description that her husband, Leonard, gave of the manic phase. "She talked almost without stopping for two or three days, paying no attention to anyone in the room or anything said to her. For about a day what she said was coherent; the sentences meant something though it was nearly all wildly insane. Then gradually it became completely incoherent, a mere jumble of dissociated words." Though the mania may be characterized by great energy and resistance to fatigue, the ideas that flood the mind are constantly changing, so while great enthusiasm may be put into various schemes the individual devises, most are never carried to fruition. The level of mania is variable, however, and in some cases a sufficient level of control may remain to allow life to be lived almost normally. Indeed, it has even been suggested that certain historical figures such as Winston Churchill, Abraham Lincoln, and Theodore Roosevelt may owe some of their political success to the prodigious workload that a mild manic state allowed them to maintain for at least some part of their lives (Snyder 1986).

Many factors may contribute to the onset of depression, and there is still considerable controversy about their relative importance. There is undoubtedly a genetic component to the susceptibility to depression. In addition, there is evidence that a variety of social stresses, whether within or outside the family, can be significant contributing factors. For example, bereavement in childhood or the loss of a supportive partner are possible triggers, as are the perceptions of constant criticism or stress within the family setting, either in childhood or adulthood. As in our discussion of general stress earlier in this chapter, a feature of many of these situations as perceived by the individual concerned is a lack of control over events and an inability to escape them. In women, depression may also be associated with pregnancy or childbirth. Many people suffer from recurrent bouts of depression at more or less regular intervals. This is sometimes, but by no means always, related to light intensity and day length. Depression of this type is called seasonal affective disorder and in northern latitudes is thought to underlie annual mood swings, which are seen to some degree in much of the population. Treatment is often based on daily exposure to short periods of intense artificial light, and though this is not effective for all patients, many show significant mood improvement as a result.

In order to develop treatments for any medical condition, it is necessary to understand not only the external causes but also the organic changes within the body that underlie it. In the case of depression, current theories and treatments are based on the belief that the changes in mood are the result of problems in brain chemistry, and in particular with the activity of one small group of the neurotransmitters that neurons use to communicate with each other. The main neurotransmitters involved (noradrenaline and serotonin) appear to modulate the activity of neural circuits; that is, they make them more or less responsive to stimulation. Intuitively, fluctuations in the effectiveness of these transmitters appear to offer a logical explanation for changes in mood. Mania and depression can be seen as extremes of the normal range of moods that we all experience; however, the level at which the "thermostat" is set differs for each of us. Those of us who exist closer to the manic end are regarded as extroverts, while those whose moods lie nearer the depressive end are described as introverts. Individuals with manic depression may therefore perceive their transitions between high and low moods as a movement between two distinct personalities. Normally the activity of the neurotransmitters responsible for mood is self-regulating so that though our feelings normally fluctuate, they do so around an average value that is typical of our personality type. During manic or depressive episodes, the self-regulating mechanism appears to become locked at one extreme or the other.

As depression appears to be caused by abnormally low levels of noradrenaline or serotonin in the brain, antidepressant drugs are designed to increase their availability within the brain. When two nerve cells communicate with each other, a neurotransmitter released from the axon on one side of the synapse binds to receptor molecules on the surface of the dendrite that forms the other side to induce some change in its activity. After a while the transmitter falls off the receptor, but if it is allowed to remain in the vicinity of the synapse it will soon bind to another receptor, making the size and duration of the signal between the two neurons difficult to control. In order to prevent this from happening, the transmitter is removed, usually by pumping it back into the axon it came from and/or by destroying it with an enzyme. If not enough transmitter is being released in the first place, blocking either of these two processes will make the small amount that is available more effective. Antidepressant drugs target both of these processes. Those that prevent the transmitters from being pumped back into the axon may act on both serotonin and noradrenaline (e.g., tricyclic antidepressants) or on serotonin alone (selective serotonin reuptake inhibitors). Others (the monoamine oxidase inhibitors) block the enzyme that breaks down both transmitters. These are the main classes of drugs used to treat unipolar depression. There is, however, a paradox in the action of antidepressants that, despite intensive research, remains unresolved. It is that although the effects of these drugs on neurotransmitter levels can be seen soon after they are first given, changes in mood do not appear for an additional four to six weeks. This is just one indication that our understanding of the mechanism of depression is far from complete (Castren 2005). Manic (bipolar) depression is usually controlled by the administration of antidepressants and of Lithium, a mood stabilizer whose precise mechanism of action is unknown and whose therapeutic properties were discovered by chance (Snyder 1986). Because of the wide role played by noradrenaline and serotonin, within both the brain and the autonomic nervous system, antidepressants can have many side effects. How severe these are is often unpredictable, so finding the most suitable drug is to some extent a matter of trial and error. In this search, the long time lag between first taking the drug and any resultant change in mood is a major problem. Furthermore, a treatment used successfully to treat one bout of depression may not be effective for a subsequent bout and so the search for a suitable drug must begin all over again.

A number of non-drug-based therapies are also used in the treatment of depression today. The most notorious of these is electroconvulsive shock therapy (ECT), in which a seizure-inducing electric shock is applied to the head. Prior to the procedure the patient is anesthetized, given a muscle relaxant to prevent overt convulsions, and ventilated with oxygen. The mechanism of its action is unknown, but its therapeutic effects appear to result from the induced seizure rather than the shock itself. ECT has a rather lurid history, but despite this it can prove a highly effective treatment when used with today's knowledge and under controlled conditions. It is generally indicated when drug treatments have proved ineffective, especially if there are suicidal tendencies. The main side effect is some temporary loss of memory.

Another approach to depression is psychotherapy, either used alone or in combination with drug treatment. The term *psychotherapy* covers a variety of approaches, including cognitive and behavioral therapies like those already described, and interpersonal therapies that concentrate on analyzing relationships and conflicts with other individuals, which may contribute to the triggering of depression. The evidence that is currently available suggests that psychotherapy can be as effective as drug treatment in bringing about a remission from depression (Casacalenda, Perry, and Looper 2002), though there may be factors in some cases (e.g., suicidal tendencies) that make the use of antidepressants either strongly advisable or necessary. There is some evidence that a combination of drug treatment and psychotherapy may be more effective than either treatment alone and that psychotherapy may help to reduce the chance of recurrent episodes of depression, but more extensive and objective studies are needed to support these claims.

REFERENCES

Abel, J. L., and K. T. Larkin. 1990. Anticipation of performance among musicians: Physiological arousal, confidence, and state anxiety. *Psychol Music* 18:171–82.

American Psychiatric Association. Task Force on DSM-IV. 1995. *Diagnostic and statistical manual of mental disorders (DSM-IV): Iinternational version with ICD-10 codes.* 4th ed. Washington, DC: Author.

Arcier, A. F. 2000. Stage fright. In *Medical problems of the instrumental musician*, ed. P. C. Amadio. London: Martin Dunitz.

Brandfonbrener, A. G. 1990. Beta blockers in the treatment of performance anxiety. *Med Prob Perform Artists* 5:23–26.

Britton, J., C. Bates, K. Channer, L. Cuthbertson, C. Godfrey, M. Jarvis, and A. McNeill. 2000. *Nicotine addiction in Britain: A report of the tobacco advisory group of the Royal College of Physicians*, ed. Royal College of Physicians of London, Tobacco Advisory Group. London: Royal College of Physicians of London.

Casacalenda, N., J. C. Perry, and K. Looper. 2002. Remission in major depressive disorder: A comparison of pharmacotherapy, psychotherapy, and control conditions. *Am J Psychiatry* 159 (8):1354–60.

Castren, E. 2005. Is mood chemistry? *Nat Rev Neurosci* 6 (3):241–46.

Clark, D. B., and W. S. Agras. 1991. The assessment and treatment of performance anxiety in musicians. *Am J Psychiatry* 148 (5):598–605.

Connolly, C. 1997. Mental skills to optimise musical performance. In *Proceedings of the 7th International Conference on Music Perception and Cognition*, ed. J. Renwick. Adelaide, Australia: Causal Productions.

Connolly, C., and A. Williamon. 2004. Mental skills training. In *Musical excellence: Strategies and techniques to enhance performance*, ed. A. Williamon. Oxford: Oxford University Press.

Craske, M. G., and K. D. Craig. 1984. Musical performance anxiety: The three-systems model and self-efficacy theory. *Behav Res Ther* 22 (3):267–80.

Everly, G. S., and R. Rosenfeld. 1981. *The nature and treatment of the stress response: A practical guide for clinicians*. New York: Plenum Press.

Fishbein, M., S. E. Middlestadt, V. Ottati, S. Straus, and A. Ellis. 1998. Medical problems among ICSOM musicians: Overview of a national survey. *Med Prob Perform Artists* 3 (1):1–8.

Fredrikson, M., and R. Gunnarsson. 1992. Psychobiology of stage fright: The effect of public performance on neuroendocrine, cardiovascular and subjective reactions. *Biol Psychol* 33 (1):51–61.

Georgiades, A., A. Sherwood, E. C. Gullette, M. A. Babyak, A. Hinderliter, R. Waugh, D. Tweedy, L. Craighead, R. Bloomer, and J. A. Blumenthal. 2000. Effects of exercise and weight loss on mental stress-induced cardiovascular responses in individuals with high blood pressure. *Hypertension* 36 (2):171–76.

James, I. 1998. Medicines and stage fright. In *The musician's hand: A clinical guide*, ed. C. B. Wynn Parry. London: Martin Dunitz.

Jamison, Kay R. 1996. *An unquiet mind: A memoir of moods and madness*. London: Picador.

Kendrick, M. J., K. D. Craig, D. M. Lawson, and P. O. Davidson. 1982. Cognitive and behavioral therapy for musical-performance anxiety. *J Consult Clin Psychol* 50 (3):353–62.

Levee, J. R., M. J. Cohen, and W. H. Rickles. 1976. Electromyographic biofeedback for relief of tension in the facial and throat muscles of a woodwind musician. *Biofeedback Self Regul* 1 (1):113–20.

Lovallo, W. R. 2005. *Stress and health: Biological and psychological interactions*. 2nd ed. Thousand Oaks, Calif.: Sage Publications.

Lutz, A., L. L. Greischar, N. B. Rawlings, M. Ricard, and R. J. Davidson. 2004. Long-term meditators self-induce high-amplitude gamma synchrony during mental practice. *Proc Natl Acad Sci USA* 101 (46):16369–73.

Markison, R. E. 1998. Adjustment of the musical interface. In *The musician's hand: A clinical guide*, ed. C. B. Wynn Parry. London: Martin Dunitz.

Marmot, M. 1997. Contribution of job control and other risk factors to social variations in coronary heart disease incidence. *Lancet* 350:235–39.

Newberg, A. B., and J. Iversen. 2003. The neural basis of the complex mental task of meditation: Neurotransmitter and neurochemical considerations. *Med Hypotheses* 61 (2):282–91.

Nies, A. S. 1990. Clinical pharmacology of beta-adrenergic blockers. *Med Prob Perform Artists* 5:27–32.

Petruzzello, S. J., E. E. Hall, and P. Ekkekakis. 2001. Regional brain activation as a biological marker of affective responsivity to acute exercise: Influence of fitness. *Psychophysiology* 38 (1):99–106.

Smith, A. M., A. Maragos, and A. van Dyke. 2000. Psychology of the musician. In *Medical problems of the instrumental musician*, ed. P. C. Amadio. London: Martin Dunitz.

Snyder, S. H. 1986. *Drugs and the brain, Scientific American Library series no. 18*. New York: Scientific American Books.

Steptoe, A. 1989. Stress, coping and stage fright in professional musicians. *Psychol Music* 17:3–11.

Steptoe, A., and H. Fidler. 1987. Stage fright in orchestral musicians: A study of cognitive and behavioural strategies in performance anxiety. *Br J Psychol* 78 (Pt 2):241–49.

Taylor, A., and D. Wasley. 2004. Physical fitness. In *Musical excellence: Strategies and techniques to enhance performance*, ed. A. Williamon. Oxford: Oxford University Press.

Valentine, E. R. 1995. The effect of lessons in the Alexander technique on music performance in high and low stress situations. *Psychol Music* 23:129–41.

———. 2004. Alexander technique. In *Musical excellence: Strategies and techniques to enhance performance*, ed. A. Williamon. Oxford: Oxford University Press.

Valentine, E. R., and A. Williamon. 2003. Alexander technique and music performance: Evidence for improved "use." In *Proceedings of the Fifth Triennial ESCOM Conference*, ed. C. Wolf. Hannover, Germany.

West, R. 2004. Drugs and musical performance. In *Musical excellence strategies and techniques to enhance performance*, ed. A. Williamon. Oxford: Oxford University Press.

Wolfe, M. L. 1990. Coping with musical performance anxiety: Problem-focused and emotion-focused strategies. *Med Prob Perform Artists* 5:33–36.

Wolpert, L. 1999. *Malignant sadness: The anatomy of depression*. London: Faber and Faber.

Wynn Parry, C. B. 1998. The musician's hand and arm pain. In *The musician's hand: A clinical guide*, ed. C. B. Wynn Parry. London: Martin Dunitz.

Index

References to figures and tables are indicated by italics, and entries in square brackets refer to material on the accompanying CD-ROM.

abdomen, 18, 27, 32, 104–5, 108, 113–20, 123–24, 166, 183, 308, 324, 336, 341
abdominal wall, 4, 25–26, 104, 106, 108, 113–15, *116*, *119*, 120–29, 133 abduction, *43*, 46, 48, 51, 77, 90
absolute pitch, sense of, *236*, 248, 314–16
acoustic bass stop, of organ, 288, 305–6
acromium, 44, *45*, 46, 48, 77
Adam's apple, 145, 179
adduction, *43*, 51, 90
adhesive capsulitis, 81
adrenal glands, 184, 336, 338, 345
alcohol, 83, 172, 243, 295, 344
Alexander technique, 40, 69, 73, 84, 342
allergic reactions, 7
allodynia, 15
alto voice (castrato), 186
alveoli, *102*, 103, 132
amusia, 316–17
amygdala, *222*, *322*, 333, 335
anaesthesia, local/topical, 73–74, 78, 161,163, 173–74, 210
anatomical snuff box, 59, 78
androgens, 179,181–85, 223
annulus fibrosus, 18, *19*, 20, 23, 28
anterior cingulate gyrus, 323
antidepressant drugs, 344–45, 349–50
antihistamines, 173
anxiety, 14–15, 29, 40, 69, 91, 104, 229, 264, 266, 332, 335, 338, 340, 344–45

anxiolytic drugs, 345
aponeurosis, palmer, 79
appoggio, 113
arachnoid, 217
armpit. See axilla
artane, 268
arthritis, 92; rheumatoid arthritis, 78, 80; osteoarthritis, 46, 80
articulator (voice), *144*, 145, 171–72
arytenoid cartilage. See cartilages, of the larynx
aspirin, 15, 173, *182*, 299
Association of British Orchestras (ABO), 66, 299
asthma, 7, 334, 346; and wind playing, 132, 135–36
astrocytes, 216
atemstütze, 113
athetosis, 243
autonomic nervous system, 13, 224, 229, 321, 323, 335–36, *337*, 341, 349, auditory system, 163, 218, 220–21, 227–28, 230, 248–49, 254–55, 257, 276–331
auxiliary muscles of respiration, 108–111
axilla (armpit), 46, 82, 110, 181
axon, *6*, 9–13, 81–82, *214*, 215–16, 219–20, 224, 238, 241, 288, 302, 332, 249

back pain, 17, 27–29, 38–40, 75
baclofen, 268

bagpipes, 73, 79, 321, 326
Baillot, Pierre, 35
baritone voice, 120, 154, 167
basal ganglia, *222*, 224, 233, *237*, 243, 246, 252, 265, *310*, 311–12, 323
basilar membrane, *283*, *284*, *287*
bass voice, 125, 161, 165, 167
bassoon, 78–79, 92, *126*, 132, *195*, 209, 280
bed rest, 28
Bell's palsy. *See* facial nerve palsy
benzodiazepines, 268, 345
beta blockers, 345–46
blood: clotting of, 173, 182; plasma, *102*, 104; supply, 2, 5–6, 33, 38, 82, *102*, 103, 174, 180, *181*, 184, 203, 207, 216–17, *221*, 223–24, 230, 233, 265, 293, 295, 317, 336, 338, 341; pH, 103, 341; pressure, 7, 131, 207, 334, 338, 341–46; red blood cells, 2, *102*; vessels, 5, 64, 71, 82–83, 102, 104, 172–73, *175*, 180, 182, 207, 210, 217, 293, 317, 321, 334–35, *337*; white blood cells, 2, 175
BOLD (blood oxygen level dependent signal), 233
bone, 1–4, 8, 13; alveolar, 102, 193, 196
bones, named: carpal, 50–51, *52*, 57, 78, 85; clavicle (collarbone), 8, *23*, 24, 44, *45*, 46, *63*, 64, 83, 106, 111–12, 122, 194; femur (thigh bone), 25–26; humerus, 33, 44, *45*, 46, 48–49, 53, 55, 65, 77, 84, 110–11; hyoid bone, 141, *142*, 143, 165–66; jaw (mandible), 27, 36, *142*, 143, 166, 193–94, 196–99, 203, 206, 209, *221*, 282; metacarpal, 50–51, *52*, 57; phalangeal (finger bones), 51, *52*, 53, 55, 57, 85; radius, 44, *50*, *51*, *52*, 53; rib, 26, 64, 83, *102*, 111; scapula (shoulder blade), 24–25, 33, 44, *45*, 46, 49, 75, 77, 109, 111, 143, 195; sternum (breastbone), 22, 24, 44, *45*, 105–6, 111–12, 143, *156*, 194; ulna, 49, *50*, *51*, *52*, 51, 53; zygomatic (cheek bone), 193
botox, focal dystonia and, 209, 268–70
bow, 35–36, 253; design of, 87, 95, *96*
boxwood, 7
Bernouilli effect, 153
Beethoven, Ludwig van, 36, 254, 293, 300, 326

brass instruments, 7, 31, 49, 66, 91, 93, 114, *123*, 126, *127*, 129, *131*, 132–33, 135, 144, *195*, 196, 198–99, 200–209, 256, 265, 280, 298–99. See *also* individual instruments; ergonomic supports for, 93
brace, for teeth, 196
brachial plexus, 8, *63*, 83–84, 93
Braille reading, 265, 269
Brain: cortex of. See cortex; gender differences in, 230–31, 235, *236*, 248–49, 314–16; imaging of, 233–34, 248; nerve cells of, 213, *214*, 215; organisation of, *218*, 219, *220*, 221, *222*, 223–24, *225*, 226–31; tumors of, 78, 217, 293
brainstem, 219, *220*, 221–23, 238, 241–42
breast bone. *See* bones, named
breathing: [Animation 4-1 breathing]; [Animation 4-2 breathing, continuous]; body type and, 114–17, *118*, 119–20; posture and, 31, 37, 39, 106, 109–20, 123–24, 166; in singing, *109*, 110–20, *123*, 124–25, *126* (*see also* plethysmography and Konno-Mead diagrams); in speech, 115, 117–18, 120, *121*; in stress, 341; in wind playing, *123*, 125, *126*, 12–29, *130*, 131–33, *134*, 135–36 (*see also* plethysmography and Konno-Mead diagrams); quiet, *103*, 104, 112, *116*, 118, 120, *121*
breathy phonation. *See* phonation, breathy
British Association of Performing Arts Medicine (BAPAM), xiii, 66, 69
Broca's area. *See* cortex, areas of
Broca, Pierre Paul, 312
bronchi, *102*
bronchioles, *102*, 132, 221, 336, 338
Broschi, Carlo. *See* Farinelli
burning mouth syndrome, 210
"butterflies" in the stomach, sensation of, 334
bursa, *45*, 48–49, 80, [Animation 3-2 shoulder problems]
bursitis, 49, 80, [Animation 3-2 shoulder problems]
buspirone, 345

Cafferelli, 185
calcium, 2, 184

carpal tunnel, 59, 61, *64*, 65, 82, 85, [Animation 3-5 wrist position]

carpal tunnel syndrome, 85

carrying, 28–29

carbon dioxide, 102, 132, 341

cartilage, 1–4, 18, 22, 80, 102, 105, 111, 139, 141, 145; articular, 3; hyaline, *3*, 4, 6, [Animation 3-1 shoulder]

cartilages of the larynx arytenoid, 148, *149*, 150, 155, 157, 160, 162–63, 176, *178*, 179, [Animation 5-2 larynx breathing], [Animation 5-3 larynx, voice quality], [Animation 5-4 larynx, pitch], [Video 5-1 normal larynx]; cricoid, *140*, 145, 148, *149*, 150, 160, 163, 179, [Animation 5-2 larynx breathing], [Animation 5-3 larynx, voice quality], [Animation 5-4 larynx, pitch]; thyroid, *140*, 145, 148, *149*, 150, 159, *178*, 179, 206, [Animation 5-2 larynx breathing], [Animation 5-3 larynx, voice quality], [Animation 5-4 larynx, pitch]

castrati, 185–87

catastrophization, 15, 232, 335, 340

cauda equina, 9

cell body, *9*, 12, *214*

cello, 13, 37–38, 40, 52, 77, 92–93, 252–53; spike, 40

central sulcus. *See* sulcus, central

cerebellum, *218*, 219, *220*, 231, *236*, *237*, 238–39, 243, 246, 249, 252, *310*, 311

cerebral hemispheres, 219, 228, 247, 249

chairs, 22, 27, 37–39

cheilitis, 7

chest. *See* thorax

"chills," sensation of, 323

chin rest (violin/viola), 7, 34–36, [Animation 2-2 violin posture]

chorea, 243

chunking. *See* memory

Churchill, Winston, 348

cingulate gyrus, *222*, 229, *322*, 333

circular breathing, 131, *134*, 135, 141

clarinet, 7, 92, *126*, 131, *195*, 203–4, 208, 299; harmonics of, 280; thumb support, 71, 78, 80

clavicle. *See* bones, named

cleft palate, loss of seal and, 205

coccyx, *18*

cochlea, *283*, 286, *287*, 288–91, 297, 299–300, 302, 304–6

cochlear amplifier, 288, *289*, 291, 296

cochlear duct. *See* scala media

cocobola, 7

cognitive behavioral therapy, 230, 340, 345, 350

cold packs, 71

cold sweat, 229, 334

collar bone. *See* bones, named

colliculi, 220, 302, 320

colophony, 7

conductors, 39, 77, 243, 300, 332, 339; sound localization in, 320

coloratura singing, 123, 186

compression. *See* nerves

compression, as treatment, 71

conchae, 172

consonance, 313, 321

contraceptives, voice and, 173, 183

coracoid process (of shoulder blade), *45*, 46, 111

corpus callosum, *218*, 222, 224, 229, 231, *236*, 247–49, 323

corpus striatum, 323

cortex (of brain), 215, 219–20, *222*, 223–30, 291

cortex, areas of: auditory, *225*, 228, 255, 291, 300, 302, *303*, 306, *307*, 308, 309, *310*, 311–17, 323, 327; Broca's area, *237*, *310*; primary motor, *225*, 227, *237*, *240*, 241–46, *247*, 248, 252, 254, 265–66; orbitofrontal, *322*, 323; prefrontal, 312, 335, 341; premotor, *237*, *240*, 242, 246, 248, 250, 252, 255, 265, *310*, 312; presupplementary motor, *237*, *240*, 242; primary sensory (somatosensory), *225*, 227, *237*, 238–39, *240*, 242, 246, 249, 264, 269, 341; sensory association, 230, *237*, *240*, 249; supplementary motor, *237*, *240*, 242, 246, 248, 250, 252, 255, *310*, 311; visual, *225*, 228–29, 230, 242; Wernicke's area, 228, *307*, 309, *310*

Corte, Marchese, 286. *See also* organ of Corti

cortical maps: sensory, *226*, 227, 239–40, 264–65, 269; motor, *226*, 227, 246, *247*, 264, 269; auditory, *307*, 308

cortisol, 336, 338, 344

collar bone. *See* clavicle

colophany, 7

propolis, 7

cover (of vocal folds), 147, *148*, 150, 153, *156*, 161, [Animation 5-5 vocal fold cycle], [Animation 5-6 vocal fold cycle, continuous], [Video 5-1 normal larynx]

cerebrospinal fluid, 217, 219

cranial nerves, 220, *221*, 223–24, *226*, 241, 336, *337*. *See also* nerves, named

cricoid cartilage. *See* cartilages, of the larynx

cubital tunnel, 65, 84, [Animation 3-6 ulnar nerve]

curse of the MacCrimmons, 79

cushions: support (for guitar), 37; wedge, 38

de Quervain's syndrome, 78

deafness, 292–93; age-related (presbycusis), 295; conductive, 291; drug induced, 292; in musicians, 297–300; nerve, 291; noise-induced, *296*, 297

decibel (dB), 278

dendrites, 9, 10, *214*, 216

dental problems, and wind playing, 196–97, 203–4

depression, 268, 334, 346–50; bipolar, 347–49; unipolar, 346–47

dermatitis, contact, 7

dermatome

dermis, 5, *6*

Deutsche Gesellschaft für Musikphysiologie und Musikermedezin, xiii

deviation of wrist, [Animation 3-5 wrist position]; radial, 50; ulnar, 50, 88, *90*

diabetes, 78, 81, 85

diaphragm, 104, *105*, 106; role in breathing, 106, *107*, 108; role in singing, 113–22, *123*, 124, 166; role in wind playing, 128–29

diet, 172–73, 179

didgeridoo: circular breathing and, 135; vocal tract resonances and, 203

difference tones. *See* Tartini tones

disks: intervertebral, *18*, *19*, 20–21, 23, 26–27, 29, 39; prolapsed ("slipped"), *19*, 28, 36

dissonance, 313, 316, 321, 323

dorsal horn (of spinal cord), 9, 12

dorsal root ganglion, 9, 12,

double jointedness. *See* joint hypermobility

double bass, 36–37, 93

DPOAE (distortion product oto-acoustic emissions), 240

DSM-iv, 346–47

Dupuytren's contracture, 79, 81

dura, 217

ear, 278, 282, *283*, 284–300; external, 282; middle, 282, 285; inner, 219, 221, 243, 282, 286–91

eardrum (tympanic membrane), 282, *283*

earplugs, 299

ear wax, 292–93

ebony, 7

eczema, 7, 334

electroconvulsive shock therapy (ECT), 349

ectomorph, *118*, 120

edema. *See* Reinke's edema

embouchure, 4, 114, 127–28, 131, 134–35, 193, *194*, *195*, 196–204; muscles of, 198–99. *See also* muscles, named; muscles, recording activity in

emotional responses to music, 6, 320–21, *322*, 323–24

endometrium, 180, *181*

endometriosis, 185

endomorph, 117, *118*, 119–20

endorphins. *See* neurotransmitters

enkephalins. *See* neurotransmitters

epicondyl, 77, 84

epidermis, 5, *6*

epiglottis, 139, *140*, 143, 145, *146*, *149*, 202

epilepsy, music and, 326–27

epithelium, 5, *6*, 172; of pharynx, 141; of larynx, 141, 145, *146*, 147, *148*, 161, 173–74, 176; mucosal, 141

Erdesz, Otto, 95, *96*

ergonomics, of instruments, 91–93, *94*, 95, *96*, 97

esophagus, 125, 139, *140*, 141–42, 174, 221–22

estrogen, 180, *181*, 182–84, 223

Eustachian tube, 139, *283*, 285, 292

exhalation. *See* expiration

extension, *20*, *43*

exercise, benefits of, 28, 34, 73–76, 78, 106, 172, 187, 342–43, 346

exercises, for rehabilitation and mobility, 39–40, 52, 62, 73, 80–81, 84, 86–87, 113, 205, 270
exteroception, 12
expiration, 101, 104, 106, *109*, 108, 111, 115, 116, 122, 127–28
expiratory reserve volume, *103*, 104, 132
eyesight: and posture, 29; in wind players, 207–8

facial nerve palsy, 210, 285
falsetto register, 153, 155, *156*, 157, *158*, 159–60
Farinelli, 185–86
false teeth, and wind playing, 204
fascia, deep, 49
Feldenkrais, 40, 69, 73
fiddler's neck, 6–8
fingers, 4, 12–13, 39, 51, *52*, *54*, *56*, *58*; 59–63, 72–95; bones of (*see* bones, named; limitations to movement of); pads of, 6, 12, 73, 239, 251, 263; relaxation of, 11, 29, 36, 342
flexion, *43*, 20
flow glottogram, *152*, 153, *154*, [Animation 5-5 vocal fold cycle], [Animation 5-6 vocal fold cycle, continuous]
flow phonation. *See* phonation, flow
flute, 7, 31, *32*, 33, 49, 85, 87, 93, *94*, *126*, 128–29, 133–35, *195*, 196, 198–99, 202, 269
fMRI (functional magnetic resonance imaging), 233, 235
focal dystonia, 261–70; brain mapping and, 264–66; of embouchure, 204; history of, 261–62; incidence of, 209, 262; injury and, 263–64; predisposing factors, 266–67; symptoms of, 262–63; theories of, 263–66; treatment of, 267–70; of upper limb, 253, 263–64
forebrain, *218*, 219, *222*, 223–25, *237*, 243, 306, 335
formants, 124, *144*, 165–66, 170, 172, 203; singers', 124, 154, *164*, [Video 5-2 singers formant]; tuning, in sopranos, *164*, 166, *170*; vowels and, 167, *168*, 169, *171*
French horn, 33, 87, *126*, *130*, 131, 135, 199, 209

frontal lobe (of brain), *218*, 224, *225*, 306, 309, 311–13, 323
frozen shoulder. *See* adhesive capsulitis
functional residual capacity, *103*, 104, 120, *121*

ganglion, dorsal root (of spinal cord), *9*, 12
ganglion cysts, 78–79
gastric ulcers, 334
gastroesophageal reflux, 173–76, 180, 334
guitar, 6, *32*, 37, 52, 78, 80, 85, 88, *89*, 248, 262–63, 269–70; electric, strings of, 8
glands, 174, 180, 292, 321, 336; adrenal, 181, 184, 336, *337*, 338, 345; of larynx, *146*; pituitary, 180, *218*, 222, 224, 321, 336; salivary, 7, 13, 199, *206*, 207, 209, *221*; sebaceous, 6; sweat, 5, *9*,13; thyroid, 151
glandular fever, 334
glenoid, 44, 46
glial cells, 81, *214*, 216–17
glottis, 114–15, 124, 129, 133, 139, 145, 148, *149*, 151, 153–54, 157, 159–63, 176, 201–2
glottogram. *See* flow glottogram
glue ear, 292–93
Golgi tendon organs, larynx, 162
Grant, Ulysses S., 316
gray matter, *9*, 10, 216, 219, *222*, 224–25, 229, *236*, 238, 243, 245–46, 249–50, 308, 317
growth hormone, 224
Guercino, 92
Guyon's canal, *64*, 65, 85
gyri (of brain), 227

habituation, 252, 293
halitosis, 174
hair cells, of the inner ear, 286, *287*, 288, *289*, 290–97, 302; damage to, 291–95, *296*
hair follicles, 5, *6*, 12
handedness, 52, 229, 231, 246, 249
hand, 4, 31, 42, 49, 51–65, 71, 73–74, 76–80, 84–86, 88–93, 95, 334, 344; cortical representation of, 227, 229–30, 239, 241–42, 245–49, 252, 264–65; anatomy of, *43*, 50, *51–56*, 57, *58*, 59–62, *63–64*, 65–67, *72*, *89*

Handel, George Frederic, 185
Haydn, Joseph, 326
hemoglobin, 102, 104, 233
hemorrhage, in vocal folds, 173, 175, 179
hard palate, *140*, 141, 205
harmonics, 124, 202–3, 235, 280, *281*, 286,
    290–91, 297, 302, 304–6, 309, 311–15;
    of the voice, 144, 154–55, 157, *164*,
    165, 167, 170, *182*, [Video 5-2 singers
    formant]
harp, 34
harmony, perception of, 235, 249, 255, 306,
    314
harpsichord, 39
Healthy Orchestra Charter, xii, 66
hearing. *See also* sound, 276–91; loss of,
    291–300 (*see also* deafness); normal
    frequency range of, *279*, 280
heart rate, 104, 135, 217, 221, 224, 336,
    343–44; stress and, 334, 338, 342
heartburn. *See* gastroesophageal reflux
herpes, 334
Heschl's gyrus. *See also* cortex, auditory,
    307
blood pressure, 71, 131, 207, 334, 338,
    341–46
hindbrain, *218*, 219
hippocampus, *222*, 229, 250, 311, *322*, 323,
    335
histamine, 14
homeostasis, 336
homunculus: motor, *226*, 227, 241–42;
    sensory, *220*, *226*, 227, 238
hormone replacement therapy, 183–85
hormones. *See also* menopause, menstrual
    cycle, puberty, 26, 179–86, 223–24;
    effect on voice/larynx, 179–86
Horowitz, Vladimir, 253
humerus. *See* bones, named
Huntingdon's chorea, 243
hypertension, 334
hyperventilation, 120, 341
hypnotic drugs, 345
hypothalamic pituitary adrenal cortex system
    (HPAC), 336
hypothalamus, *218*, *222*, 223–24, 229, 231,
    322, 323, 335–36, 341
hypothenar eminence, 57
hysterectomy, 184–85

ibuprofen, 15, 71, 182
incus. *See* ossicles
inertive reactance, 153
inflammation, 15, 59, 62, 70–71, 76–78,
    80–81, 85, 173, 182, 292
inhalation. *See* inspiration
injury, performance-related, xii, xiii, 1, 14,
    65–67
inspiration, in breathing, *105*, *107*, 110, 112,
    115, 118–21, 132, *134*, 135, 341,
inspiratory capacity, *103*
inspiratory reserve volume, *103*, *109*
insula, 323
interaural intensity difference, 318, *319*
interaural time delay, 318, *319*
interneuron, 9, 10, 13, *214*, 215–16, 223, 238
irritable bowel syndrome, 334
ischial tuberosities, 27, *30*, *32*
isovolume line, 115, *116*, [Video 4-3 Konno
    Mead sing], [Video 4-4 Konno Mead wind]

jaw. *See* bones, named
joints, 2–4; capsule of, *3*, 29, 46, 49,
    78–81, 194, [Animation 3-1 shoulder];
    hypermobility of, 79–80; synovial, *3*, 23,
    46, 49, 59, 76, 78, 80, 85, 193
joints, named: elbow, 4, *32*, 39, 49, *50*, 53,
    55, *63*, 64–65, 77–78, 80, 82–84, *90*;
    intervertebral, 29; interphalangeal, distal
    (DIP), 51, *52*, 53, 90; interphalangeal,
    proximal (PIP), 51, *52*, 53, 81;
    metacarpophalangeal (knuckle), 51, *52*,
    53, *58*, 90, 92; shoulder, 3–4, 22, 44, *45*,
    46, 49, 80–81, [Animation 3-1 shoulder];
    temporomandibular (jaw), 3, 36, 193;
    wrist, 39, 59; zygapophysial, 21

keratin, 5, 196
keyboard, *32*, 39, 49–50, 61–62, 66, 77–78,
    80, 87–89, *90*, 95, 97, 241, 246–48, 251,
    254–56, 259, 262–63, 269
Konno-Mead diagram, 115, *116*, 117, 119,
    127, [Video 4-3 Konno Mead sing],
    [Video 4-4 Konno Mead wind]
Kung, Tzu Chen, 326
kyphosis, *18*, 22, 26–27, 39

lamina propria (of vocal folds), *146*, 147,
    148, 150, 173, 177

language, brain areas associated with, 228, 230, *237*, 309, 314, 316

laryngocoele, 205, *206*

larynx, 2, 5, 102–3, 108, 124, 139, *140*, 141–43, *144*, 145–63; breathing and, [Animation 5-2 larynx, breathing]; control of, *149*, 161–63; growth of, 177, *178*, 179–80; height of, 112, 124, *142*, 143, [Animation 5-1 larynx height]; innervation of, *142*, 151, 161; joints of, 160–63, 179; muscles of (*see* muscles, named); sensation in 151, 161–63, 174; structure of, 139, 145, *146*, 147–50; wind playing and, 129, 131, 133–34

laryngitis, 173–74, 176

laryngopharynx, *140*

laryngoscope, 131, 145

lentiform nucleus, *237*. *See also* basal ganglia

learning, of motor skills. *See* motor learning

librium, 345

lifting, 28–29, *30*, 133

limbic system, *222*, 229, 266, *322*, 335, 341

Lincoln, Abraham, 348

Linburg-Comstock syndrome, 62, [Video 3-1 tendon linkages]

lip, 8, 131, 196, 198–200, 203, 209, 265

lip shield, 197

lips, pressure of mouthpiece on, 201

ligaments, 3; annular, 49; ligamentum flavum, 22; nuchal, 23, 25, 44; vocal, *146*, 147, *148*, *149*, 150, 153, 157, *158*, 159, 177, *178*

lithium, 349

long bones, 2, 186

longbowmen, 2

lordosis, *18*, 22, 26–27, *30*, *32*, 37–39, [Animation 2-1 stand sit]

loss of seal, 135, 204–5, 208

lumbar support, 27, 37–38

lung pressure: in singing, 115, 120; in wind playing, 132–33, 207

lungs, 5, 102–5, 115, 120, 124–25, 127–29, 132–33, 135, 184, 207, 345

magnetoencephalography (MEG), 233

Majorano, Gaetano. *See* Cafferelli

malleus. *See* ossicles

mandible. *See* bones, named

manic depression. *See* depression, bipolar

Manzuoli, Giovanni, 185

Mary Rose, Tudor warship, 2

marrow, 2

Mavron quartet, ix, xv, xvii, 293

Médecine des Arts, xiii

meditation, stress and, 340–41

medulla (oblongata), *218*, 219, *220*

Meissner's corpuscle, *6*, 12,

melody, perception of, 235, 249–50, 255, 309, *310*, 311–12, 314, 316–17, 320

memory, 87, 163, 228, 234, 252, 254, 256, *258*, 259–60, 268, *310*, 311, 314, 317–18, 355; associative, 229, 250, 335; auditory, 257; chunking in, 257; emotional coloring of, 322, 355; lapses of, 257, 334, 350; motor, 13, 242, 252, 257, 266; of the score, 251, 253, 257, 260; working, 311–12, 315, 334

meninges, 217, 219

Menière's disease, 293, 295

menopause, 2, 26, 183–85, 187, 292

menstrual cycle, *181*, 213, 316; voice and, 180–81, *182*, 183–84

mental rehearsal, 71, 87, *244*, 253–55

Merkel ending, *6*, 12

mesolimbic pathway, 322–23

mesomorph, 117, *118*, 120

Messaien, Olivier, 318

Meyerbeer, Giacomo, 185

mezzo-soprano voice, 125, *164*, 167, 186

microglia, 217

midbrain, *218*, 219, *220*, 224, 243, 302, *322*, 323

migraine, 334

mirror neurons, 228, 312

missing fundamental illusion, 304–6, 308, 313, [Sound Presentation SP9-3 missing fundamentals]

modal register, 155, *156*, 157, *158*, 159

Modigliani figure, voice and, 184

modiolis, of embouchure, 199

mononucleosis. *See* glandular fever

Moreschi, Alessandro, 185–87

motor neuron, *9*, *10*, *11*, 13, 210, 215, 241, 245, 268,

motor neurons, synchrony of, 61

motor pool, 10, 241–42, 245

motor skill, acquisition of, *237*, *240*, 243, *244*, 246, 251–52, *258*
motor unit, 10, *11*, 241
mouthpiece, 7–8, 127, 131, 144–45, *195*, 196–97, 199–201, 203, 308, 280, 299
"Mozart effect," 324–26
Mozart, Leopold, 185
Mozart, Wolfgang Amadeus, 185, 245, 324–26
MRI (magnetic resonance imaging), 233, 235, 245, 248
mucosa. *See* epithelium, mucosal
mucosal wave (of vocal fold), *152*, 153, [Animation 5-5 vocal fold cycle], [Video 5-1 normal larynx]
muscle, 4–6, 10, 12, 14; cardiac, 5; composition of, 4; fast fibers, 4; fibers of, 4, 10, *11*; slow fibers, 4; smooth, 5,13; striated, 4, *11*
muscle wasting, 65, 85
muscles, co-contraction of, 91, 114, 261, 263, 342
muscles, named, of back and neck: erector spinae, *20*, *23*, 24–26, 28–29, *30*, 39; longus capitus, *23*, 24; longus coli, *23*, 24–25; quadratus lumborum, *23*, 26; rectus abdominus, *23*, 25–26, 29, *32*, *105*, 106, 108, *109*; psoas, *23*, 25; scalenes, 33, 83, 93, *110*, 111–12, 195; splenius capitus, *23*, 24; sternocleidomastoid, *23*, 24, 33, 35, *110*, 111–12, 194, 206; transversospinalis, *23*, 24
muscles, named, of ear: stapedius, *283*, *284*, 285, 295; tensor tympanum, 282, *283*
muscles, named, of embouchure, jaw, and palate, *194*; buccinator, 135, 198–99, *194*; depressor anguli oris, 199, 200, [fig 6-1 latin]; depressor labii inferioris, 199, [fig 6-1 latin]; levator anguli oris, 199, 200, [fig 6-1 latin]; levator labii superioris, 198, [fig 6-1 latin]; orbicularis oris, 198–200, [fig 6-1 latin]; orbicularis oris, rupture of (*see* Satchmo's syndrome); masseter, 36, 193, *194*, 197–99 [fig 6-1 latin]; platysma, 199, 200, [fig 6-1 latin]; pterygoids, 194, 198; risorius, 199, [fig 6-1 latin]; levator palati, 141, 204; tensor palati, 141, 204; temporalis, 36, 193, *194*, 197–99, [fig 6-1 latin]

muscles, named, of larynx (or acting upon it): cricoarytenoid, lateral, 124, 148, *149*, 157, 160, [Animation 5-2 larynx breathing], [Animation 5-3 larynx, voice quality]; cricoarytenoid, posterior, 148, *149*, 151, 155, *158*, [Animation 5-2 larynx breathing], [Animation 5-3 larynx, voice quality]; cricothyroid, 124, *149*, 150–51, *156*, 157, *158*, 159–60, [Animation 5-4 larynx, pitch]; interarytenoid, 148, *149*, 155, 157, 162, 179, [Animation 5-3 larynx, voice quality]; omohyoid, *142*, 143, 166; sternohyoid, *142*, 143, 165; sternothyroid, *142*, 143, 165; thyroarytenoid, *142*, *146*, 148, *149*, 150, *156*, 157, 159–60, 162, [Animation 5-4 larynx, pitch]; thyrohyoid, *142*, 143, 165; transverse arytenoid, 124, *146*, *149*, 150, 153, 159–60, [Animation 5-7 vocal timbre] (*see also* interarytenoid; vocalis)
muscles, named, of lower limb: gluteus maximus, *20*, 26, *30*, 112; hamstrings, *3*, *24*, 26; psoas, *23*, 25; quadratus femorus, *30*
muscles, named, of respiration: auxiliary, 108–13; diaphragm, *102*, *103*, 104–8, *109*, 113–15, 117, 119–24, 128–29, 133, 166, 341, [Animation 4-1 breathing], [Animation 4-2 breathing, continuous] (*see also* diaphragm); intercostals, *102*, *105*, 106–8, 113–15, 120, 122, 166, 341; intercostal, external, *105*, 106, *109*, 115; intercostal, internal, 105, 108, *109*; lateral abdominal, *105*, 106, 108, *109*, 125, [Animation 4-1 breathing], [Animation 4-2 breathing, continuous] (*see also* internal and external oblique and transverse abdominal); latissimus dorsi, *47*, *110*; oblique, external, 106, 125; oblique, internal, 106, 125; pectoralis major, 33, *50*, *110*, 101; pectoralis minor, 46, *48*, *110*, 101; rectus abdominus, *20*, 25–26, 29, *30*, *105*, 106, 108, *110*; scalenes, 33, 83, 93, *110*, 111–12, 195; serratus posterior inferior, *110*; serratus posterior superior, *110*; sternocleidomastoid, *23*, 24, 33, 35, *110*, 111–12, 194, 206; subclavius, 109, *110*, 111; transverse

abdominal, 106; trapezius, 23–25, 44, *47,
48, 110,* 111–12, 206
muscles, named, of upper limb and shoulder:
abductor of thumb (long), *55, 56,* 57, 59,
78; abductor of thumb (short), *54,* 57,
59, 78; adductor of thumb, 59, *63,* 65;
biceps, 4, 44, 49, *50,* 65; brachilis, 49, *50;*
brachioradialis, 49, *50;* coracobrachialis,
49, *50;* deltoid, 33, 35, *45,* 46, *47, 48,*
49, 80; extensors of the wrist, 50, *55;*
extensors of the fingers, *55, 56, 57,* 61,
77, 91, 263, 267; extensors of the thumb,
55, 56, 57, 59, 78; flexors of the wrist,
50, *53,* 64, 84; flexors of the fingers, *53,
54,* 55, 57, *58,* 61–62, 65, 90–91, 263,
167; flexors of the thumb, *53, 54,* 57,
62; infraspinatus, *45,* 46, *47* (*see also*
rotator cuff); interosseus muscles, *54, 56,*
57, *58,* 62, *64,* 65, 77; latissimus dorsi,
47, 110; levator scapulae, 24, 33, 44, *47;*
lumbricals, 10, *54,* 57, *58,* 62, *64,* 65, 77,
[Animation 3-3 lumbricals]; opponens, of
little finger and thumb, 57, 59; pectoralis
major, 33, *50, 110,* 111; pectoralis
minor, 46, *48, 110,* 111; pronator teres
and quadratus, 49, *51,* 65; rhomboids,
24, 44, *47;* serratus anterior, 46, *47, 48;*
subscapularis, 46, *48* (*see also* rotator
cuff); supinator, *51;* supraspinatus, 33–34,
45, 46, *48,* 49, 77, 80, [Animation 3-2
shoulder problems] (*see also* rotator cuff);
teres major, *48;* teres minor, 46, *48* (*see
also* rotator cuff); trapezius, 23–25, 44,
47, 48, 110, 111–12, 206; triceps, 49, *50,*
64–65, 245
muscles, named, of vocal tract and mouth:
constrictors of the pharynx, 141, 143,
198; digastric, *142;* genioglossus, 143,
142; geniohyoid, *142;* hyoglossus, *142,*
143; myelohyoid, *142;* palatoglossus,
143; levator palati, 141, 204; styloglossus,
143; stylohyoid, *142;* stylopharyngeus,
141, *142,* 143, 166; tensor palati, 141,
204
muscle spindles, of larynx, 162
muscle tension, 25, 27, 29, 36, 39, 40, 44,
69, 86–88, 94, 111, 120, 131, 196, 198,
267, 340–42
musici. *See* castrati

Musician's Benevolent Fund (MBF), xiii, 66
Mustafa, 185
myelin, 81–82, *214,* 216, *236,* 248

naked sensory ending, *6,* 12
Napoleon Bonaparte, 186, 206
nasopharynx, 141, 171, 204
neck, 24–25; breathing and, 106, 111–12;
muscles of. (*see* muscles, named); nerves
of, 64, 83–84, 222, 241, 336; vertebrae
of, *20,* 21, 23, 44, 109; posture and, 31,
32, 34–35, 37, 66, 86; structure related
to voice, *140,* 151, 165–66, 179, 194;
tension in, 27, 29, 36–37, 39, 111; wind
playing and, 195, 205–6; dystonia and,
261
nerve root, *18, 19,* 128, 35, 64, 83
nerves: compression of, 8, 13, *19,* 33, *63,
64,* 65, 69, 78, 81–85, 207, 210, 263–64,
267, [Animation 3-6 ulnar nerve]; axons,
regrowth in, 13, 82, 210; cranial, 202,
220, 221, 223–24, *226,* 241, 302, 336,
337; double crush of, 82; segmental, 8, *9,*
10, *18;* structure of, 81–82
nerves, named: abducent, *220;* auditory,
221, *287,* 241, *303,* 313 (*see also*
vestibulocochlear); digital, 85; facial,
198–99, 209–10, *220, 221, 226,* 285;
glossopharyngeal, *220, 221, 226;*
hypoglossal, *221, 220, 226;* laryngeal
(superior and recurrent), *142,* 151;
median, *63, 64,* 65, 83, 85, *89,* 264;
oculomotor, *220, 221;* olfactory, *221;*
optic, 207, *221;* radial, 64–65, *72;*
trigeminal, 198, 210, *220, 221, 226,* 282;
trochlear, *220, 221;* ulnar, *63, 64,* 65, 82–
85, 263–64, [Animation 3-6 ulnar nerve];
vestibulocochlear, *220, 221,* 302 (*see also*
auditory); vagus, *220, 221,* 222, *226*
nerve entrapment. *See* nerve compression
neurotransmitter: acetylcholine, 344, 268,
270; adrenalin (epinephrine), 333, 336,
338, 345; dopamine, 268, 322–23;
endorphin, 15, 323; enkephalin, 15,
323; CGRP, 14; glutamate, 14, 287;
noradrenalin (norepinephrin), 345,
348–49; serotonin, 348–49; substance P,
14, 15
nickel, 7–8

nicotine, 344–45
19-norsteroids, 183
noble posture, in singing, 120
nucleus accumbens, *322*, 323
nucleus pulposus, *19*, 20–21, 27–28, 39

oboe, 7, 92, 103, *126*, *130*, 131, *195*, 202, 204, 207–8, 269, 280, 297
occipital lobe (of brain), *218*, 224, *225*, 227
oligodendrocytes, 216
omega sign (in primary motor cortex), *247*
opposition, *43*, 51, *164*
organ of Corti, 286, *287*, 288, 290–91, 295, *296*
organ pipes, 280, 288, 290–91, 295
oropharynx, *140*, 141, 172
Ositrakh, David, 36
ossicles of ear, 282, *283*, 285, 291–93, 300; malleus, 282, *283*; incus, 282, *283*; stapes, 282, *283*, *284*, 285, 292
osteoporosis, 2, 26, 184
otitis media, 292
otoacoustic emissions, 288, 290
otosclerosis, 292–93, 295, 300
oval window, 282, *283*, 286, 292
overbreathing. *See* hyperventilation
overbite, of teeth, 196, *197*, 203
overjet, of teeth, 196, *197*
overuse syndrome, 74–76
oxygen, 2, 5, 82, 102–4, 120, 180, 216–17, 233, 285, 295

Pacinian corpuscle, *6*, 12
Paganini, Niccolò, 79
palate, 139, 143, *144*, 145; soft, *134*, 135, *140*, 141, 144, *171*, 204–5, *221*
pain, 12, 13–16, 22, 36, 2, 46, 49, 62, 65, 67, 70–71, 80, 83, 105, 111, 161, 174, 182, 185, 196, 208–10, 215, 263, 278, 334; allodynia, 15; burning mouth, 210; back, 17, 27–29, 38–40, 75; chronic, 15–16, 28–29, 33, 76; gate theory of, 15; hyperalgesia, 15; windup, 15
painkillers, 15, 182; aspirin, 15, 173, *182*, 292; ibuprofen, 15, 71, 182; nonsteroidal anti-inflammatories (NSAIDs), 15; opiates, 15
parietal lobe (of brain), *218*, 224, *225*, 227–28, 242, 249, 309

paraphenylenediamine, 7
parasympathetic nervous system, 336, *337*, 338, 341
Parkinson's disease, 224, 243, 268, 312
pear-shaped down posture, *119*, 120, 166
pear-shaped up posture, 118, *119*, 120, 123, 166
perfect pitch. *See* absolute pitch, 314–16
Performing Arts Medicine Association (PAMA), xiii, 70
peripheral nervous system, 8, 12, 13–15
phalangeal cells, *289*
phalangeal bones (phalanges), 51, *52*, 53, 55, 57
pharyngocoele, 205, *206*
pharynx, 114, 125, 131, 133–34, 139, 141, 143, *144*, 145, 151, 165–67, 169, 171–72, 174, 179, 193–94, 198, 201, 204–6, 221, 227
phonation: breathy, 153, [Animation 5-3 larynx, voice quality]; flow, 124, 155, [Animation 5-3 larynx, voice quality]; pressed, 124, 155, 176–77, [Animation 5-3 larynx, voice quality]
phrenology, 234
physiotherapy, 69–70, 72–73, 78–79, 84
pia, 217
piano, 29, 31, *32*, 33, 39, 50, 57, 62, 79, 85, 88–89, *90*, 91–92, 95, 161, 241, 246, *247*, 248, 252–54, 256–57, 260, 262–63, 266, 269–70, *279*, 280, 302, 315–16, 320, 324, [Animation 2-3 piano posture]. *See also* keyboard
piano playing, analysis of, 89–90, 256, *258*, 259–60
piccolo, *130*, *195*
Pilates, 40, 106, 343
piriform recess, 165–66
pitch: absolute, 253, 255, 280, 300, *301*, 302, 304–6; 308, 314. *See* absolute pitch, sense of; amusia; relative pitch, sense of
pitch contour, 306, *310*
pituitary gland, 180, *218*, *222*, 224, 336, *337*, 341
planum polare, 309, *310*, 311
planum temporale, *236*, 306, *307*, *310*, 311, 313, 315, 318, 320
pleasure, pathways mediating, *322*, 323–24

plethysmography, 114–15, *121*, [Video 4-1 plethysmography sing], [Video 4-2 plethysmography wind]

pleura, *102*, 105–6

pleurisy, 105

pneumoparotitis, *206*, 207

pons, *218*, 219, *220*

posture: in instrumental playing, 17, 22, 24, 28, 29–31, *32*, 22–39, 59, 61, 67–68, 76–78, 83–84, 87–88, *89*, *90*, 91–93, [Animation 2-2 violin posture], [Animation 2-3 piano posture]; in singing, 106, 109–10, 112, 117–18, 120, 123–24, 166. Refer also to individual instruments

postural training and exercises, 36, 39–40, 342

practice, 13, 186, 196–97, *236*, 248–51, 264; deliberate, 240, *236*, 259–60; learning and, 242, 251–52, 255–57, 259–60; mental, 29, 37, 40, 75–77, 86–87, 260–61 (*see* mental rehearsal)

presbycusis. *See* deafness, age-related

pressed phonation. *See* phonation, pressed

pressure: in airway (singers), 143, 151, 153–54, 161–63; in airway (wind players), *126*, *130*, 199, 200, 202, 204–8; of mouthpiece, 196, 200–201; on teeth, 196, 203–4

progesterone, 180, *181*, 182–84

Prinner, Johann Jacob, 92

pronation, 35, *43*, 49, *51*, 65, 95, *96*

propolis, 7

proprioceptor, 12–13

prehensile grip (hand), 57

prephonatory posturing, 115, *116*, 120, *121*

pressed phonation. *See* phonation, pressed

puberty, the voice and, 177, 179–82, 186

pulse register, 115, *156*, 157

pyramidal tract, 241

Quantz, Joachim, 186

Rachmaninov, Serge, 79, 254

radius, 49, *50*, *51*, 53

Ramazzini, Bernardini, 66, 261

Ravel, Maurice, 317

recorder, 114

reed, 103, 108, 114–15, 127, 129, 132–35, 141, 144–45, 196–97, 199, 203

reed instruments, 132–35, 196, 199, 202, 204

reflexes, 13, 134, 220, 245, 285, 302; of larynx, 162–63; stapedius, 285, 295

register. *See* vocal register

Reinke's edema, 173–75, *182*, [Video 5-3 edema nodules]

relative pitch, sense of, 314–15

relaxation line, 108, *109*, 115, *116*, [Video 4-3 Konno Mead sing], [Video 4-4 Konno Mead wind]

relaxation, stress and, 339–42

repetitive strain injury, 74, 76, 263

residual volume, *103*, 104

resonator (voice), *144*, 145, 165–70, *171*

respiratory braking, 108, *109*, 122, 127–29

respiratory movements, 105, *107*

rest (as treatment), 28, 70–71

retinaculum, [Animation 3-4 retinacula of wrist]; extensor, *56*; flexor, *54*, 59, *64*, 65, 79, 85

rhythm, perception of, 235, 249–50, 306, 308–9, *310*, 311–12, 316, 326

rib cage, 8, *20*, 46, 104, 111, 117, 120, 123, 127–28, 204

rib movements, in breathing, 105–6

rima glottis. *See also* glottis, 145

Rimsky-Korsakoff, Nikolai, 318

ring splints, *72*, 78, 80

ring, vocal, 124, 167

Rivinus, David, 95, *96*

Roosevelt, Theodore, 348

rosewood, 7

rosin, 7

Rossini, Gioachino, 185

rotator cuff, 46, *47*, 48, [Animation 3-1 shoulder]; syndrome, 34, 36, 68, 77, 81, [Animation 3-2 shoulder problems]

round window, 282, *283*

Rubinesque figure, voice and, 184

Rubenstein, Arthur, 253

Ruffini ending, *6*, 12

Sacks, Oliver, 229

salivary gland, 7, 13, 141, 199, *206*, 209, *221*

"Saturday night" palsy, 82

Satchmo's syndrome, *206*, 208–9

saxophone, 92, 132, 202–3, 208, 280

scala media, 286, *287*

scala tympani, 286, *287*

scala vestibuli, 286, *287*

scapula (shoulder blade), 24–25, 33, 44, *45*, 49, 75, 77, 109, 111, 143, 195

Schumann, Clara, 256

Schumann, Robert, 293

Scriabin, Alexander, 318

Score: learning, 71, 87, 253, 255–57 (*see also* memory); reading, *221*, 250, 253–54

scoliosis, 22, 34

scrivener's palsy, 261 (*see also* focal dystonia)

Schwann cells, 216

seasonal affective disorder, 348

seating, posture and, 37–39, [Animation 2-1 stand sit]

semicircular canals, *283*

sensory neuron, *9*, 10–14, 215, 243, 245

setup, instrumental, 7, 36, 40

Shakespeare, William, 326

Shebalin, Vissarion, 317

Shostakovitch, Dimitri, 317

shoulder blade. *See* bones, named, scapula

shoulder rest, 8, 35, 95, [Animation 2-2 violin posture]

shoulder joint. *See* joints, named

skill learning. *See* motor skill, acquisition of

skin, 4–5, *6*, 7–8, *64*, 65, 73, 78, 81, 215, 238–39, 243, 245, 263, 306, *337*; sensation in, *6*, 11–14, 73, 183, 186, 198, 224, 268; callus on, 6; reaction to metals, 7. *See also* dermatitis, contact

slipped disk. *See* disk, prolapsed

Smetana, Bedřich, ix, xv, 293, *294*, [Smetana quartet, Mavron.wma]

smoking, 127, 173, 344. *See also* nicotine

soft palate. *See* palate, soft

somatization, *68*, 334

somatotype, 83, 91; breathing and, 117, 128

soprano voice, 124–25, 161, *164*, 166–67, 169, *170*, 179, 186

sound: frequency, coding in the nervous system, 286, 300, *301*, 302, 304–6, *307*; harmonic structure of, 280, *281*, 282, [Sound Presentation SP-1 sound identification]; intensity, 278; localization of, 318, *319*, 320; nature of, 276, *277*, 278–82; occupational exposure limits, 299; pressure, 278

Sound Ear Initiative, xii, 298

speech, breathing in, 117, *118*, 120, *121*

Spohr, Louis, 34

spine (vertebral column), 8–9, 17, *18*, *19*, *20*, 21–22, *23*, 24–31, 34–35, 37, 39, 44, 83, 105–6, 111, 139, 150, 184, 195, 217, 337

spinal cord, 1, 8, *9*, 10–11, *12*, 13–15, *18*, 22, 28, 64, 76, 81, 217, 219–20, 223–24, *237*, 238, *240*, 241–45, 336

splinting, 71, *72*, 81

selective serotonin re-uptake inhibitors, 349

stage fright, 332, 339–40

standing, 22, *20*, 26–27, 29, 31, 36, 106, 112, 122, [Animation 2-1 stand sit]

stapes. *See* ossicles of ear

stapedius reflex, *283*, *284*, 285, 295

state anxiety, 332

stereocilia, 286–88, *289*, 290, 295, *296*

steroid hormones, 26. *See also* androgens and testosterone

sternum. *See* bones, named

stress, 13, 25, 27, 36, 36, 44, *68*, 69, 76, 91, 111, 135–36, 172, 205, 210, 229, 257, 266, 295, 332, *333*, 334–38, 348; acute, 332; chronic, 332; management of, 36, 40, 67, 339–46

stretching, 37, 39–40, 52, 76, 80–81, 86–87

stringed instrument, 6, 13, 31, 34, 36–37, 39, 44, 46, 52, 57, 61, 66, 73, 77, 79–80, 85, 87–88, 91, 93, 95, 132, *236*, 239, 248, 250, 253, 262–63, 269, 279–80, 282. Refer also to individual instruments

string playing, analysis of, 88, 25–26, 252–53

"strohbass" register. *See* pulse register

strokes, 230, 233, 261, 265, 270, 317

stool, 36–37; kneeling, *32*, 38; piano, *32*, 39, 88, [Animation 2-3 piano posture]

styloid process, *142*

subglottal pressure, 122–24, 153–54, 163

substantia nigra, 224

sulcus, 224–25, 234, 239; central, *218*, 225, 227, 238, 241, 246, *247*

superior olivary nucleus, 291, 302, *303*

superior temporal gyrus, 311–13, 317

supination, *43*, 49, *51*, 77, 93, *94*

support, in singing, 110, 112–15, 124–25, 177, 183

supraglenoid tubercle, 49

surgery, 62, 67, 70, 73–74, 78–79, 81, 83–85, 151, 175–76, 205, 241, 267, 292–93, 317

swallowing, 139, 141–43, 145, 174, 205, 221–22, 285, [Animation 5-1 larynx height]

sweat, 5, 17, 86, 224, 295, 338; cold, 229, 334; gland, 5, *6*, 13, 321, 336

sympathetic nervous system, 336, *337*, 345

synesthesia, 318

synapse, *214*, 215–16, 349

syncope, in wind players, 207

synovial fluid, 3, 23, 46, 59, 80

tai chi, 40, 69, 73, 342–43

Tartini, Giuseppe, 288

Tartini tones, 288, 290, 304, [Sound presentation SP9-2 Tartini tones]

taxi drivers, memory of, 250

tectorial membrane, 286, *287*, 295–96

teeth: grinding of, 36, 91; wind playing and, 193, *195*, 196–98, 203–4, 210, 299

tempo, 256, 311–12, 314, 324–25

temporal lobe (of brain), *218*, 224, *225*, 227–29, 250, 282, 306, *307*, 308–9, *310*, 311–12, 323

tendon, 2, *3*, 4–5, 12, 26, 49, *60*, 62, 70–80, 85, 88, 219, 238–39, 243, 245; inflammation of, 55, *56*, 57, 61–62 (*see also* tendonitis); sheath (*see* tenosynovium; trigger finger)

tendons, named: biceps, 49; extensor (of fingers), 55, *56*, 57, [Animation 3-3 lumbricals], [Animation 3-4 retinacula of wrist]; extensor expansion (of fingers), 55, *58*, [Animation 3-3 lumbricals]; flexor, deep (of fingers), 53, *54*, 55, 57, 90, [Animation 3-3 lumbricals], [Animation 3-4 retinacula of wrist]; flexor, superficial (of fingers), 53, *54*, [Animation 3-3 lumbricals]; interosseus, 57; lumbrical, *45*, 57; of long muscles of the thumb, 57, 59, 78; supraspinatus, 34, 46, 48, 77, [Animation 3-2 shoulder problems]

tendonitis, 76–79

tenor voice, 125, 161, 165

tenosynovia, *54*, *56*, *60*, 61, 76, 78

tenosynovitis, 76–78

tension. *See* muscle tension

testosterone, 179, 183, 186, 229, 235

total lung capacity, *103*, 104, 129, 132

temporomandibular joint syndrome, 36

thalamus, *218*, *222*, 223, 229, *237*, 238, 243, *322*

thenar eminence, 59, 65, 85

thoracic outlet, *63*, 64, 83; syndrome, 64, 83–84

thoracic recoil, 108, 114, 120, 122, 128–29, [Animation 4-1 breathing], [Animation 4-2 breathing, continuous]

thorax (chest), 8, 22, 25, 31, 39, 44, 46, *47*, 75, 92, *102*, 104, *105*, 106–15, *116*, 117–18, *119*, 120, 122–23, 125, 136, 179, 204–5, 207, 306, 334, 341

throat infection. *See* laryngitis

throat singing, 169

threshold shift, temporary (of hearing), 296, 298

thyroid cartilage. *See* cartilages, of the larynx

thyroid notch, 145, 150

tics, 243

tidal breathing, *103*, 104, 117

tidal volume, *103*, 104

timbre, 235, 280, 302, 305–6; perception of, 255, *310*, 311–12; vocal, 144, 154–55, 157, 159–60; wind playing, in, 128, 202–3

tinnitus, xv, 292–93, *294*, 295–96, 300, [Smetana quartet, Mavron.wma]

tip links, of hair cells, 287, 290, 295

tone deafness. *See* amusia

tongue, 124, 131, *134*, 133–35, 139, *140*, 141, *142*, 143, *144*, 145, 166, 169, 199–203, *214*, 221, 227, 238; vowels and, *168*, 169–70, *171*

tonsils, *140*, 179, 205

tonotopy, *284*, 286, 300, *301*, 302, *303*, 305–6, 308

trachea, *102*, 104, 106, 139, *140*, 141–42, 145, *146*, *149*, 150, 161, 166, 170, *175*, 205, 223

trait anxiety, 332, 338

treatment, forms of, xii–xiii, 13–16, 28, 36, 66–67, *68*, 69–74, 76, 78–81, 84–85, 175–76, 182, 185, 196, 210, 264, 267–70, 292–93, 295, 334, 340, 345–46, 348–50

tricyclic antidepressants, 349

trigger finger, *60*, 78
trigeminal neuralgia, 210
trillo, in Renaissance music, 123, 129
trombone, 33, *126*, *131*, 166
trumpet, 33, 49, *126*, *131*, 135, 145, 166, 198, 200–202, 204, 207–9, 297–98
tympanic membrane. *See* eardrum
tuba, *126*, 129, *131*, 132, 202
turbinate bones, 172
Tuva, 170

ulna. *See* bones, named
underbite (of teeth), 196, *197*
underjet (of teeth), 196, *197*
uterus, 80, *181*, 182
uvula, *140*, 141

valium, 345
valsalva manoeuvre, 133–34, 202
vasopressin, 341
varnish, 7
velopharyngeal insufficiency. *See* loss of seal
ventral horn (of spinal cord), *9*, 10, 245
ventral roots, 8, *9*
ventral striatum, *322*, 323,
ventral tegmental area, *322*, 323
ventricles: of the larynx, *140*, 145, *146*, 206; of the brain, *218*, 219, *222*, 223, 229
vertebrae, 8, 17, *18*, *19*, *20*, 21–26, 69, 109–10, 112, 220
vertebral column. *See* spine
vestibular fold, *140*, 145, *146*, 206, 222
vestibular system, 219, 243, 292
vibrato in: singing, 124–25; flute playing, 124, 128–29; reed instruments, 133, 202; brass instruments, 202; stringed instruments, 12, 93
vibrator (voice), 143, *144*, 145–55
viola, 6, 8, 13, 24, 34, 36, 49–50, 77, 84, 92, 95; Erdesz design, 95, *96*; "Pelligrini" design, 95, *96*
violin, 6, 8, 13, 24, *32*, 34–36, 49–50, 84, 92, *247*, 279, 293; design of, 95, *96*, [Animation 2-2 violin posture]
vital capacity, *103*, 104, 106, 112, 120, *121*, 122, 125, *126*, 127, 129, 132–33
vocal cords. *See* vocal folds
vocal folds; breathing and, [Animation 5-2 larynx, breathing]; changes through life,

177–84, 187; chink between, 155, *182*, [Animation 5-3 larynx, voice quality]; in singing, 108, 114, 120, 124–25, *140*, *144*, 143, 145, *146*, 147, *148*, *149*, 150–51, *152*, 153–57, *158*, 159–65, 170, *175*, 182–84, 187, [Animation 5-3 larynx, voice quality], [Animation 5-4 larynx, pitch], [Animation 5-5 vocal fold cycle], [Animation 5-6 vocal fold cycle, continuous], [Video 5-1 normal larynx]; movements in wind playing, 129, 133–34, 202–3, 206; problems affecting, 172–80, *182*, 183, 187, 189
vocal fry. *See* pulse register
vocal ligament, *146*, 147, *148*, *149*, 150, 153, 157, *158*, 159, 177, [Animation 5-4 larynx, pitch], [Animation 5-7 vocal timbre], [Video 5-1 normal larynx]
vocal misuse, 176–77
vocal nodules, 176, [Video 5-3 edema nodules]
vocal polyps, 175
vocal tract, 113–14, 124–25, 143–73, 221; resonances in singing. *See* formants; resonances in wind playing, 202–3
vocal register, xiv, 144, 147, 153, 155, *156*, 157, *158*, 159–60, 179, [Animation 5-7 vocal timbre]
voice abuse, 176
voice: aging of, 177, *178*, 179–80, 187; breaking (*see* puberty, the voice and); pitch regulation of, 143, 150, 153–55, *158*, 159–60, [Animation 5-4 larynx, pitch]
vowel intelligibility, singing and, 167, *168*, 169, *170*, *171*

Wagner, Richard, 185
warm up, 75–76, 80, 86, 177
weight control, 342–44
Wernicke's area. *See* cortex, areas of
whispering, 155, 174, [Animation 5-3 larynx, voice quality]
white matter, 2, *9*, 10, 16, 219, *222*, 224, 249, 317
Williams, John, 37
windpipe. *See* trachea
Wolf, Virginia, 348
womb. *See* uterus

woodwind instruments, 7, 31, 73, 88, 92–93, 104, 128–29, 131, 133–35, 141, 196, 202, 207. Refer also to individual instruments

working memory, 311, 312, 315; failure of in stress, 334

wrist posture, problems arising from, 39, 59, 78, 82, 88, *89*, *90*, 93, *94*, 95, [Animation 2-3 piano posture], [Animation 3-4

retinacula of wrist], [Animation 3-5 wrist position]

writer's cramp. *See also* focal dystonia, 261–62, 265–66, 269

yoga, 40, 69, 73, 340, 342–43

zygomatic arch, 193, 197, 198

About the Author

Alan Watson is a senior lecturer in anatomy and neuroscience in the School of Biosciences at Cardiff University, and has had a lifelong interest in musical performance. He was born in Kirkcaldy in the kingdom of Fife, Scotland, and educated at Glenrothes High School. There he benefited from the excellent provision made for instrumental music by the local education authority, learning both the French horn and the flute. He took a B.Sc. in Zoology at the University of Edinburgh, and a Ph.D. in Neuroscience at St. Andrews University before postdoctoral studies at Cambridge University, where he held a Beit Memorial Fellowship for Medical Research. For the last twenty years he has taught gross anatomy and neuroscience to medical and science students at Cardiff University. He has published over sixty papers on neuroscience in professional journals and worked on an eclectic range of subjects that resembles the contents of the witches' cauldron in Shakespeare's *Macbeth* (eye of midge, gut of fish, leg of locust . . .). He has also dabbled in early keyboard and stringed instrument construction. In Cardiff he runs a course on the biological principles underlying musical performance for the Department of Lifelong Learning and also teaches on this subject at the Royal Welsh College of Music and Drama. There he works with staff and students on projects concerned with understanding breathing patterns in wind players and singers that are supported by the Wellcome Trust. He has also taught at the Royal College of Music in London and has given public lectures at venues such as the DANA Centre (London) and the British Association for Performing Arts Medicine, and at events ranging from science festivals to the Menuhin Violin Competition.